Optimization of Outcomes for Children After Solid Organ Transplantation

Guest Editors

VICKY LEE NG, MD, FRCPC
SANDY FENG, MD, PhD

PEDIATRIC CLINICS
OF NORTH AMERICA

www.pediatric.theclinics.com

T0372044

April 2010 • Volume 57 • Number 2

SAUNDERS an imprint of ELSEVIER, Inc.

W.B. SAUNDERS COMPANY

A Division of Elsevier Inc.

1600 John F. Kennedy Boulevard • Suite 1800 • Philadelphia, Pennsylvania 19103-2899

http://www.theclinics.com

THE PEDIATRIC CLINICS OF NORTH AMERICA Volume 57, Number 2
April 2010 ISSN 0031-3955, ISBN-13: 978-1-4377-1853-9

Editor: Carla Holloway
Developmental Editor: Theresa Collier

The Pediatric Clinics of North America (ISSN 0031-3955) is published bimonthly by Elsevier Inc., 360 Park Avenue South, New York, NY 10010-1710. Months of issue are February, April, June, August, October, and December. Periodicals postage paid at New York, NY and additional mailing offices. Subscription prices are $167.00 per year (US individuals), $378.00 per year (US institutions), $227.00 per year (Canadian individuals), $503.00 per year (Canadian institutions), $270.00 per year (international individuals), $503.00 per year (international institutions), $83.00 per year (US students and residents), and $142.00 per year (international and Canadian residents and students). To receive students/resident rare, orders must be accompanied by name of affiliated institution, date of term, and the signature of program/residency coordinator on institution letterhead. Orders will be billed at individual rate until proof of status is received. Foreign air speed delivery is included in all *Clinics* subscription prices. All prices are subject to change without notice. **POSTMASTER:** Send address changes to *The Pediatric Clinics of North America*, Elsevier Health Sciences Division, Subscription Customer Service, 3251 Riverport Lane, Maryland Heights, MO 63043. **Customer Service: 1-800-654-2452 (US and Canada). From outside of the US and Canada: 1-314-447-8871. Fax: 1-314-447-8029. For print support, E-mail: JournalsCustomerService-usa@elsevier.com. For online support, E-mail: JournalsOnlineSupport-usa@elsevier.com.**

Reprints. For copies of 100 or more, of articles in this publication, please contact the Commercial Reprints Department, Elsevier Inc., 360 Park Avenue South, New York, NY 10010-1710. Tel.: 212-633-3812; Fax: 212-462-1935; E-mail: reprints@elsevier.com.

The Pediatric Clinics of North America is also published in Spanish by McGraw-Hill Inter-americana Editores S.A., Mexico City, Mexico; in Portuguese by Riechmann and Affonso Editores, Rua Comandante Coelho 1085, CEP 21250, Rio de Janeiro, Brazil; and in Greek by Althayia SA, Athens, Greece.

The Pediatric Clinics of North America is covered in *MEDLINE/PubMed (Index Medicus)*, *Excerpta Medica*, *Current Contents*, *Current Contents/Clinical Medicine*, *Science Citation Index*, *ASCA*, *ISI/BIOMED*, and *BIOSIS*.

Printed and bound by CPI Group (UK) Ltd, Croydon, CR0 4YY

Transferred to Digital Print 2011

GOAL STATEMENT

The goal of the *Pediatric Clinics of North America* is to keep practicing physicians and residents up to date with current clinical practice in pediatrics by providing timely articles reviewing the state-of-the-art in patient care.

ACCREDITATION

The *Pediatric Clinics of North America* is planned and implemented in accordance with the Essential Areas and Policies of the Accreditation Council for Continuing Medical Education (ACCME) through the joint sponsorship of the University Of Virginia School Of Medicine and Elsevier.

The University Of Virginia School of Medicine is accredited by the ACCME to provide continuing medical education for physicians. The University of Virginia School of Medicine designates this educational activity for a maximum of 15 *AMA PRA Category 1 Credits*™ for each issue, 90 credits per year. Physicians should only claim credit commensurate with the extent of their participation in the activity.

The American Medical Association has determined that physicians not licensed in the US who participate in this CME activity are eligible for a maximum of 15 *AMA PRA Category 1 Credits*™ for each issue, 90 credits per year.

Credit can be earned by reading the text material, taking the CME examination online at http://www.theclinics.com/home/cme, and completing the evaluation. After taking the test, you will be required to review any and all incorrect answers. Following completion of the test and evaluation, your credit will be awarded and you may print your certificate.

FACULTY DISCLOSURE/CONFLICT OF INTEREST

The University of Virginia School of Medicine, as an ACCME accredited provider, endorses and strives to comply with the Accreditation Council for Continuing Medical Education (ACCME) Standards of Commercial Support, Commonwealth of Virginia statutes, University of Virginia policies and procedures, and associated federal and private regulations and guidelines on the need for disclosure and monitoring of proprietary and financial interests that may affect the scientific integrity and balance of content delivered in continuing medical education activities under our auspices.

The University of Virginia School of Medicine requires that all CME activities accredited through this institution be developed independently and be scientifically rigorous, balanced and objective in the presentation/discussion of its content, theories and practices.

All authors/editors participating in an accredited CME activity are expected to disclose to the readers relevant financial relationships with commercial entities occurring within the past 12 months (such as grants or research support, employee, consultant, stock holder, member of speakers bureau, etc.). The University of Virginia School of Medicine will employ appropriate mechanisms to resolve potential conflicts of interest to maintain the standards of fair and balanced education to the reader. Questions about specific strategies can be directed to the Office of Continuing Medical Education, University of Virginia School of Medicine, Charlottesville, Virginia.

The faculty and staff of the University of Virginia Office of Continuing Medical Education have no financial affiliations to disclose.

The authors/editors listed below have identified no financial or professional relationships for themselves or their spouse/partner:

Estella M. Alonso, MD; Luis A. Altamirano-Diaz, Medico-Cirujano, FRCP; Samantha J. Anthony, PhD(c), MSW; Lorraine E.Bell, MDCM, FRCPC; Tami Benton, MD; Kathleen M. Campbell, MD; Monique Choquette, MD; Jennifer Conway, MD; Maria DeAngelis, MScN, NP(Paediatrics); Anne I. Dipchand, MD; Jens W. Goebel, MD; Hartmut Grasemann, MD, PhD; Thomas G. Gross, MD, PhD; Carla Holloway (Acquisitions Editor); Binita M. Kamath, MBBChir, MRCP; Miriam Kaufman, MD; Shaf Keshavjee, MD, MSc, FRCSC, FACS; Beverly Kosmach-Park, MSN, CRNP; Kathy Martin, MN, NP(Paediatrics); Saeed Mohammad, MD; Vicky Lee Ng, MD, FRCPC (Guest Editor); Kim M. Olthoff, MD, FACS; Stacey Pollock BarZiv, PhD; Karen Rheuban, MD (Test Author); Minnie M. Sarwal, MD, PhD; Barbara Savoldo, MD, PhD; Susan M. Sawyer, MBBS, MD, FRACP; Vicki Seyfert-Margolis, PhD; Eyal Shemesh, MD; Simon Urschel, MD; and Angela Williams, MS, NP(PHNCP).

The authors/editors listed below identified the following professional or financial affiliations for themselves or their spouse/partner:

Upton Allen, MBBS, MSc, FRCPC is an industry funded research/investigator for Abbott Canada.

Yaron Avitzur, MD is a consultant for and is a shareholder in Lunguard.

Sandy Feng, MD, PhD (Guest Editor) has stock ownership/equity in Abbott, Amgen, Bristol Myers Squibb, Charles River Labs, Hospira, GSK, Johnson & Johnson, Medco, Merck, Pfizer, and Stryker; and is on the Governing Board, Editorial Board or other committee organizations for the American Journal of Transplant, American Association for the Study of Liver Disease, Organ Availability Committee, United Network for Organ Sharing, Scientific Advisory Committee, Roche Organ Transplant Fund, and ASTA: American Transplant Congress Planning Committee.

David Grant, MD is a consultant for Astellas.

Michael Green, MD, MPH is a consultant for Bristol Myers Squibb.

Angela Punnett, MD is on the Advisory Committee/Board for Genzyme.

Ron Shapiro, MD has received research grants from Astellas and Wyeth; is on the Data Monitoring Committee for Bristol-Myers Squibb and Stem Cells, Inc.; is the editor of eMedicine and an author for UpToDate; and is a key expert advisor for MedScape.

Melinda Solomon, MD, FRCPC is an industry funded research/investigator for Inspire Pharmaceutical Inc., Astellas Pharma, and Gilead Sciences.

Lori J. West, MD, DPhil is an industry funded research/investigator for Genzyme Canada, and is a consultant for Astellas Canada.

Disclosure of Discussion of Non-FDA Approved Uses for Pharmaceutical Products and/or Medical Devices

The University of Virginia School of Medicine, as an ACCME provider, requires that all faculty presenters identify and disclose any off-label uses for pharmaceutical and medical device products. The University of Virginia School of Medicine recommends that each physician fully review all the available data on new products or procedures prior to clinical use.

TO ENROLL

To enroll in the Pediatric Clinics of North America Continuing Medical Education program, call customer service at 1-800-654-2452 or visit us online at www.theclinics.com/home/cme. The CME program is available to subscribers for an additional fee of $195.00

Contributors

GUEST EDITORS

VICKY LEE NG, MD, FRCPC
Associate Professor, University of Toronto; Medical Director, Liver Transplant
Program; Staff Physician, Division of Pediatric Gastroenterology, Hepatology
and Nutrition, SickKids Transplant Center, The Hospital for Sick Children,
Toronto, Ontario, Canada

SANDY FENG, MD, PhD
Associate Professor, University of California San Francisco Division of Transplant Surgery,
Department of Surgery, San Francisco, California

AUTHORS

UPTON ALLEN, MBBS, MSC, FRCPC
Professor, Departments of Pediatrics and Health Policy Management & Evaluation,
University of Toronto; Division of Infectious Diseases, Hospital for Sick Children,
Toronto, Ontario, Canada

ESTELLA M. ALONSO, MD
Department of Pediatrics, Northwestern University Feinberg School of Medicine, Siragusa
Transplant Center, Children's Memorial Hospital, Chicago, Illinois

LUIS A. ALTAMIRANO-DIAZ, Medico-Cirujano, FRCP
Pediatric Heart Transplant Fellow, Department of Pediatrics, Division of Pediatric
Cardiology, University of Alberta, Edmonton, Alberta, Canada

SAMANTHA J. ANTHONY, PhD(C), MSW
Department of Social Work, SickKids Transplant Center, The Hospital for Sick Children,
Institute of Medical Science, University of Toronto, Toronto, Ontario, Canada

YARON AVITZUR, MD
Division of Gastroenterology, Hepatology and Nutrition; Transplant Centre, The Hospital
for Sick Children, Toronto, Ontario, Canada

LORRAINE E. BELL, MDCM, FRCPC
Associate Professor, Department of Pediatrics, McGill University; Director of Pediatric
Renal Transplantation, McGill University Health Centre - Montreal Children's Hospital,
Division of Nephrology, Montréal, Québec, Canada

TAMI BENTON, MD
Interim Psychiatrist-in-Chief, The Children's Hospital of Philadelphia, Behavioral Health
Center Assistant Professor of Psychiatry, Department of Psychiatry, University of
Pennsylvania School of Medicine, Philadelphia, Pennsylvania

KATHLEEN M. CAMPBELL, MD
Assistant Professor of Pediatrics and Medical Director of Pediatric Liver Transplant
Program, Division of Gastroenterology, Hepatology and Nutrition, Cincinnati
Children's Hospital Medical Center, Cincinnati, Ohio

MONIQUE CHOQUETTE, MD
Research Associate, Division of Gastroenterology, Hepatology and Nutrition,
Cincinnati Children's Hospital Research Foundation, Cincinnati, Ohio

JENNIFER CONWAY, MD
Labatt Family Heart Centre, Hospital for Sick Children, Toronto, Ontario, Canada

MARIA DEANGELIS, MScN, NP(Pediatrics)
Nurse Practitioner, Liver and Intestinal Transplant Program, Transplant Centre,
The Hospital for Sick Children, Toronto, Ontario, Canada

ANNE I. DIPCHAND, MD
Labatt Family Heart Centre, Hospital for Sick Children; Associate Professor of Pediatrics,
University of Toronto; Associate Director, SickKids Transplant Centre, Hospital for Sick
Children, University of Toronto, Toronto, Ontario, Canada

SANDY FENG, MD, PhD
Associate Professor, University of California San Francisco Division of Transplant
Surgery, Department of Surgery, San Francisco, California

JENS W. GOEBEL, MD
Associate Professor of Pediatrics and Medical Director of Kidney Transplantation,
Division of Nephrology and Hypertension, Cincinnati Children's Hospital Medical
Center, Cincinnati, Ohio

DAVID GRANT, MD
Transplant Centre; Division of General Surgery, The Hospital for Sick Children, Toronto,
Ontario, Canada

H. GRASEMANN, MD, PhD
Toronto Lung Transplant Program; Department of Pediatrics, Division of Respiratory
Medicine and Transplant Centre, The Hospital for Sick Children, University of Toronto,
Toronto, Ontario, Canada

MICHAEL GREEN, MD, MPH
Professor of Pediatrics, Surgery & Clinical and Translational Science, University
of Pittsburgh School of Medicine; Division of Infectious Diseases, Children's Hospital
of Pittsburgh, Pittsburgh, Pennsylvania

THOMAS G. GROSS, MD, PhD
Chief, Division of Hematology/Oncology/BMT, Nationwide Children's Hospital, Ohio
State University School of Medicine, Columbus, Ohio

BINITA M. KAMATH, MBBChir, MRCP
Assistant Professor, Department of Pediatrics, University of Toronto; Staff Physician,
Division of Gastroenterology, Hepatology and Nutrition, The Hospital for Sick Children,
Toronto, Ontario, Canada

MIRIAM KAUFMAN, MD
Adolescent Health Consultant, The Transplant Centre, The Hospital for Sick Children;
Professor of Pediatrics, Division of Adolescent Medicine, Department of Pediatrics,
The University of Toronto, Toronto, Ontario, Canada

S. KESHAVJEE, MD, MSc, FRCSC, FACS
Director, Toronto Lung Transplant Program; Chair, Division of Thoracic Surgery,
Toronto General Hospital, Toronto, Ontario, Canada

BEVERLY KOSMACH-PARK, MSN, CRNP
Clinical Nurse Specialist, Department of Transplant Surgery, Starzl Transplantation
Institute, Children's Hospital of Pittsburgh of UPMC, Pittsburgh, Pennsylvania

KATHY MARTIN, MN, NP(Pediatrics)
Nurse Practitioner, Heart Transplant Program, Transplant Centre, The Hospital for Sick
Children, Toronto, Ontario, Canada

SAEED MOHAMMAD, MD
Department of Pediatrics, Northwestern University Feinberg School of Medicine,
Siragusa Transplant Center, Children's Memorial Hospital, Chicago, Illinois

VICKY LEE NG, MD, FRCPC
Associate Professor, University of Toronto; Medical Director, Liver Transplant Program;
Staff Physician, Division of Pediatric Gastroenterology, Hepatology and Nutrition,
SickKids Transplant Center, The Hospital for Sick Children, Toronto, Ontario, Canada

KIM M. OLTHOFF, MD
Professor of Surgery, Department of Surgery, University of Pennsylvania; Director,
Transplant Center, The Children's Hospital of Philadelphia; Director, Liver Transplant
Program, Penn Transplant Institute, Philadelphia, Pennsylvania

STACEY POLLOCK BARZIV, PhD
Assistant Professor, Department of Pediatrics, SickKids Transplant Center, The Hospital
for Sick Children, University of Toronto, Toronto, Ontario, Canada

ANGELA PUNNETT, MD
Assistant Professor, Pediatrics; Education Program Director, Pediatric Hematology/
Oncology, Division of Hematology/Oncology, SickKids Hospital, University of Toronto,
Toronto, Ontario, Canada

MINNIE M. SARWAL, MD, PhD
Department of Pediatrics Nephrology, Stanford University Medical School, Stanford
University, Stanford, California

BARBARA SAVOLDO, MD, PhD
Associate Professor, Center for Cell and Gene Therapy, Baylor College of Medicine,
The Methodist Hospital and Texas Children's Hospital, Houston, Texas

SUSAN M. SAWYER, MBBS, MD, FRACP
Professor of Adolescent Health, Department of Pediatrics, The University of Melbourne,
Centre for Adolescent Health, Royal Children's Hospital; Murdoch Childrens Research
Institute, Melbourne, Australia

VICKI SEYFERT-MARGOLIS, PhD
Senior Advisor, Science Innovation and Policy, Office of the Chief Scientist, Office of the Commissioner, Food and Drug Administration, Silver Spring, Maryland

RON SHAPIRO, MD
Professor of Surgery, Robert J. Corry Chair in Transplantation Surgery, Director, Kidney, Pancreas, and Islet Transplantation, Thomas E. Starzl Transplantation Institute, University of Pittsburgh, Pittsburgh, Pennsylvania

EYAL SHEMESH, MD
Chief, Division of Behavioral Pediatrics, Department of Pediatrics; Associate Professor of Pediatrics and Psychiatry (Pending), Mount Sinai Medical Center; Mount Sinai School of Medicine, New York, New York

M. SOLOMON, MD, FRCPC
Toronto Lung Transplant Program; Department of Pediatrics, Division of Respiratory Medicine and Transplant Centre, The Hospital for Sick Children, University of Toronto, Toronto, Ontario, Canada

SIMON URSCHEL, MD
Pediatrician, Pediatric Cardiologist, Cardiac Transplant Research, Alberta Diabetes Institute, University of Alberta; Department of Pediatrics, Division of Pediatric Cardiology, University of Alberta, Edmonton, Alberta, Canada

LORI J. WEST, MD, DPhil
Professor of Pediatrics, Surgery and Immunology; Director, Cardiac Transplant Research; Department of Pediatrics, Division of Pediatric Cardiology, University of Alberta, Edmonton, Alberta, Canada

ANGELA WILLIAMS, MS, NP(PHNCP)
Nurse Practitioner, Renal Transplant Program, Transplant Centre, The Hospital for Sick Children, Toronto, Ontario, Canada

Contents

> In the last 40 years, orthotopic heart transplantation has been established as a realistic treatment strategy for infants and children with severe forms of congenital heart disease and cardiomyopathy. The evaluation, management, and outcomes of these patients have continued to improve. These achievements have advanced pediatric cardiac transplantation and allowed more attention to be focused on improving quality of life after transplantation and reducing the long-term complications.

> Lung transplantation is an accepted therapy for selected pediatric patients with severe end-stage vascular or parenchymal lung disease. Collaboration between the patients' primary care physicians, the lung transplant team, patients, and patients' families is essential. The challenges of this treatment include the limited availability of suitable donor organs, the toxicity of immunosuppressive medications needed to prevent rejection, the prevention and treatment of obliterative bronchiolitis, and maximizing growth, development, and quality of life of the recipients. This article describes the current status of pediatric lung transplantation, indications for listing, evaluation of recipient and donor, updates on the operative procedure, graft dysfunction, and the risk factors, outcomes, and future directions.

> Kidney transplantation in pediatric patients has become a routinely successful procedure, with 1- and 5-year patient survival rates of 98% and 94%, and 1- and 5-year graft survival rates of 93% to 95% and 77% to 85% (the range takes into account differences between living and deceased donors). These good outcomes represent the cumulative effect of improvements in pre- and posttransplant patient care, operative techniques, immunosuppression, and infection prophylaxis, diagnosis, and treatment. This article provides a brief historical overview, discusses the indications for transplantation, describes the evaluation process for the recipient and the potential donor, outlines the operative details, reviews the various causes of and risk factors for graft dysfunction, and analyzes outcomes.

> Pediatric liver transplant recipients represent an important target population for primary care health professionals as well as transplant practitioners. With improving patient and graft survival, new concerns now face health care professionals caring for the transplant community, namely the long-term complications of immunosuppressive therapy and the potential for withdrawal of immunosuppression, transplant recipients' quality of life, and the persistent shortage of donor organs leading to morbidity and mortality on the waiting list. These issues require constant collaboration between pediatricians, transplant hepatologists, transplant surgeons, nurses, dieticians, social workers, psychologists, and other supporting services.

> This article reviews the current status of pediatric intestinal transplantation, focusing on referral and listing criteria, surgical techniques, patient management, monitoring, complications after transplant, and short- and long-term patient outcome. Intestine transplantation has become the standard of care for children who develop life-threatening complications associated with intestinal failure. The results of intestinal failure treatment have significantly improved in the last decade following the establishment of gut rehabilitation programs and advances in transplant immunosuppressive protocols, surgical techniques, and posttransplant monitoring. The 1-year patient survival is now 80% and more than 80% of the children who survive the transplant are weaned off parenteral nutrition. Early referral for pretransplant assessment and careful follow-up after transplant with prompt recognition and treatment of transplant-related complications are key factors contributing to superior patient outcomes and survival. The best results are being obtained at high-volume centers with survival rates of up to 75% at 5 years.

> Effective immunosuppression is the key to successful organ transplantation, with success being defined as minimal rejection risk with concomitant minimal drug toxicities. Despite the general recognition of this fact, a paucity of appropriate clinical trials in children has contributed to lack of standardization of clinical management regimens, resulting in an extensive diversity of favored approaches. Nonetheless, although consensus has not been reached on the ideal approach to immunosuppression in pediatric transplantation, new drug therapies have contributed to a continuing improvement in graft and patient survival. Future clinical research must focus on diminishing the extensive burden of toxicities of these therapeutic agents in children.

> Effective prevention, diagnosis, and treatment of infectious diseases after transplantation are key factors contributing to the success of organ

transplantation. Most transplant patients experience different kinds of infections during the first year after transplantation. Children are at particular risk of developing some types of infections by virtue of lack of immunity although they may be at risk for other types due the effect of immunosuppressive regimens necessary to prevent rejection. Direct consequences of infections result in syndromes such as mononucleosis, pneumonia, gastroenteritis, hepatitis, among other entities. Indirect consequences are mediated through cytokines, chemokines, and growth factors elaborated by the transplant recipient in response to microbial replication and invasion, which contribute to the net state of immunosuppression among other effects. This review summarizes the major infections that occur after pediatric organ transplantation, highlighting the current treatment and prevention strategies, based on the available data and/or consensus.

The risk of developing cancer after solid organ transplantation (SOT) is about 5- to 10-fold greater than that of the general population. The cumulative risk of cancer rises to more than 50% at 20 years after transplant and increases with age, and so children receiving transplants are at high risk of developing a malignancy. Posttransplant lymphoproliferative disease (PTLD) is the most common cancer observed in children following SOT, accounting for half of all such malignancies. PTLD is a heterogeneous group of disorders with a wide spectrum of pathologic and clinical manifestations and is a major contributor to long-term morbidity and mortality in this population. Among children, most cases are associated with Epstein-Barr virus infection. This article reviews the pathology, immunobiology, epidemiology, and clinical aspects of PTLD, underscoring the need for ongoing systematic study of complex biologic and therapeutic questions.

As posttransplant longevity has increased, nonimmune complications related to the transplant and posttransplant course have emerged as important factors in defining long-term outcomes. The incidence of, and risk factors for these complications may vary by transplanted organ based on immunosuppressive protocols and preexisting risk factors. This article discusses the relevant nonimmune complications associated with posttransplant care, with a focus on risk factors and management strategies.

In the clinical arena of transplantation, tolerance remains, for the most part, a concept rather than a reality. Although modern immunosuppression regimens have effectively handled acute rejection, nearly all organs except the liver commonly suffer chronic immunologic damage that impairs organ function, threatening patient and allograft survival. In addition to the imperfect control of the donor-directed immune response, there are additional costs. First, there is the burden of mortality from infection and malignancy that can be directly attributed to a crippled immune system. Second, there are insidious effects on renal function, cardiovascular profile (hypertension, hyperglycemia, and dyslipidemia), bone health, growth, psychological and neurocognitive development, and overall quality of life. It is likely that the full consequences of lifelong immunosuppression on our pediatric transplant recipients will not be fully appreciated until survival routinely extends beyond 1 or 2 decades after transplantation. Therefore, it can be argued that the holy grail of transplantation tolerance is of the utmost importance to children who undergo solid organ transplantation.

One of the most critical differences between the posttransplant care of children and adults is the requirement in children to maintain a state of health that supports normal physical and psychological growth and development. Most children with organ failure have some degree of growth failure and developmental delay, which is not quickly reversed after successful transplantation. The challenge for clinicians caring for these children is to use strategies that minimize these deficits before transplantation and provide maximal opportunity for recovery of normal developmental processes during posttransplant rehabilitation. The effect of chronic organ failure, frequently complicated by malnutrition, on growth potential and cognitive development is poorly understood. This review presents a summary of what is known regarding risk factors for suboptimal growth and development following solid-organ transplant and describes possible strategies to improve these outcomes.

Long-term survival after pediatric solid organ transplantation is now the rule rather than the exception for increasing numbers of children with end-stage organ diseases. While transplantation restores organ function it does not necessarily return one to a normal life. Therefore, it is prudent to focus on assessment of not only traditional biologic outcomes but also the quality life for these children and their families. This article gives a brief overview of current definitions, conceptualizations, approaches to measurement of, and unique considerations in the evaluation of quality of life in children who have undergone solid organ transplant. Current understanding of quality of life in children who have undergone solid organ transplantation is reviewed, followed by limitations of current knowledge. Clinical implications are discussed and future research directions suggested.

Adolescents constitute a significant proportion of pediatric transplant patients, whether they have survived a transplant in early childhood (like most heart and liver recipients) or are transplanted in older childhood or adolescence, such as many renal transplant recipients. Their needs can be significantly different from either children or adults, as they are undergoing a major transformation that involves making educational and vocational decisions and commitments, establishing a new and more equal relationship with their parents, discovering their sexual identity, taking increasing responsibility for their health and creating the moral, philosophic, and ethical perspective that they will carry through their lives. This article discusses adolescent issues in transplantation.

Lorraine E. Bell and Susan M. Sawyer

The importance of transition to adult health care for young people with chronic conditions is increasingly recognized. Ensuring effective engagement with adult services for adolescents and young-adult solid-organ transplant recipients is as critical for immediate graft survival as it is for their future health and well-being. This article (1) examines the definitions of adolescence and emerging adulthood and some of the challenges of these phases of life, (2) discusses elements that may influence motivation and engagement and enhance communication and adherence for adolescents and young adults, (3) highlights important areas in education, vocational planning, and quality of life for transplant recipients, (4) reviews tasks and challenges during the transition, and (5) provides specific transition recommendations, for both transplant health care professionals and for primary care providers practicing outside transplant centers.

Maria DeAngelis, Kathy Martin, Angela Williams, and Beverly Kosmach-Park

Pediatric solid-organ transplant (SOT) recipients and their parents are often challenged to cope with new transplant regimens as well as common situations in the context of organ transplantation. Health care professionals will receive questions from parents and children regarding clinical transplant care as well as general pediatric concerns that seem unfamiliar to families now that their child has a transplant. The literature is limited in some areas of pediatric care after SOT, and there is little guidance for the health care practitioner. To help address gaps in the literature and provide guidance for health care professionals, this article reviews some of the most commonly asked questions regarding general care after SOT, parenting the child with a chronic illness, and growth and development. The answers provided stem from the literature in part but also the combined clinical experiences of transplant centers that over time have moved toward decreased limitations and full social integration.

RELATED INTEREST

Surgical Clinics of North America Volume 86, Issue 5 (October 2006)
Topics in Organ Transplatation for General Surgeons
Paul Morrissey, MD, *Guest Editor*
www.surgical.theclinics.com

THE CLINICS ARE NOW AVAILABLE ONLINE!

Access your subscription at:
www.theclinics.com

Preface:

Optimization of Outcomes for Children After Solid Organ Transplantation

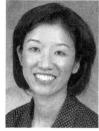 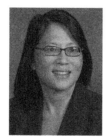

Vicky Lee Ng, MD, FRCPC   Sandy Feng, MD, PhD
Guest Editors

Solid organ transplantation is a life-saving treatment option for end-stage organ failure in children. With excellent graft and patient survival reported from all arenas of pediatric solid organ transplantation worldwide, it is not surprising, and entirely appropriate, that the success of pediatric solid organ transplantation in children is being defined by more than just survival rates. Conceptually, pediatric solid organ transplantation can be viewed as the replacement of a fatal disease with a chronic condition that poses its own risks of medical and psychosocial comorbidities—developing in spite of reinstated function of the previously failed native organ and recovery from the complications of end-stage organ disease. The commonly quoted mantra, "children are not simply little adults," is never more true than in the care of transplant recipients: pediatric transplant recipients, by nature of their young age, face a greater cumulative burden of lifelong immunosuppression and its ensuing complications. With the population of long-term survivors after pediatric transplantation ever increasing and greatly exceeding the numbers of newly transplanted recipients each year, *all* health care providers will undoubtedly find themselves encountering these special patients. A collaborative partnership and coordinated approach among primary care practitioners, pediatric health care providers, and allied health professionals both within and beyond the walls of the Pediatric Transplant program, as well as a commitment to self-management by patients and families, are essential ingredients to optimizing the long-term care and best outcomes for these children. This issue of *Pediatric Clinics of North America* is devoted to providing up-to-date, concise (and practical) reviews of the most common clinical issues confronting children who have undergone pediatric solid organ transplantation.

The first 5 articles provide an overview and status update of pediatric heart, liver, kidney, lung, and small bowel transplantation in 2010. The next 5 articles address

Pediatr Clin N Am 57 (2010) xv–xvi
doi:10.1016/j.pcl.2010.01.020
0031-3955/10/$ – see front matter © 2010 Elsevier Inc. All rights reserved.
pediatric.theclinics.com

the efficacy and toxicity conundrum of immunosuppression after pediatric solid organ transplantation, beginning with a review of the armamentarium and efficacy of immunosuppression agents available to the clinician in 2010 and culminating with an article addressing the advantages and potential of achieving the holy grail of transplantation. The following 4 articles address emerging trends and clinical challenges unique to children who have undergone transplantation, including the impact on growth and development, quality of life, adolescence and adherence, and transition to adult care. Last but certainly not least, the most commonly asked questions from parents and families of pediatric transplant patients are presented in a user-friendly Q and A format that can serve as a reference and resource for all physicians, nurse practitioners, trainees, and allied health professionals who care for these children.

In closing, we want to thank each author for their time and commitment to the preparation of this issue of *Pediatric Clinics of North America*. Highlighting the advances and future clinical challenges of pediatric transplantation in 2010, our goal remains to further optimize outcomes for these special children. We are also most grateful to Carla Holloway, Peg Ennis, and the editorial staff for the opportunity to share with the primary care practitioner and pediatricians some of the features that make pediatric solid organ transplantation unique, challenging, and always rewarding.

Vicky Lee Ng, MD, FRCPC
Division of Pediatric Gastroenterology
Hepatology and Nutrition
SickKids Transplant Center
The Hospital for Sick Children
Toronto, Canada

Sandy Feng, MD, PhD
UCSF Division of Transplant Surgery
Department of Surgery
San Francisco, CA, USA

E-mail addresses:
vicky.ng@sickkids.ca (V. Lee Ng)
sandy.feng@ucsfmedctr.org (S. Feng)

Heart Transplantation in Children

Jennifer Conway, MD[a], Anne I. Dipchand, MD[a,b],*

KEYWORDS

- Heart transplantation • Pediatrics • Assessment
- Outcomes

In the last 40 years, orthotopic heart transplantation has been established as a realistic treatment strategy for infants and children with severe forms of congenital heart disease and cardiomyopathy. The evaluation, management, and outcomes of these patients have continued to improve. These achievements have advanced pediatric cardiac transplantation and allowed more attention to be focused on improving quality of life after transplantation and reducing the long-term complications.

HISTORICAL NOTES

The first human pediatric heart transplant took place on December 6, 1967 in New York using an anencephalic donor with surface cooling and was performed off-pump (eg, without the use of a cardiopulmonary bypass machine).[1] The recipient died 6 hours later and it was another 16 years before the next heart transplant was carried out in the pediatric age range. Since then, there have been many advances in donor management, organ preservation, surgical techniques, postoperative care, and immunosuppressant agents, all contributing to what is now more than 7500 procedures performed worldwide. Pushing the boundaries has always been a hallmark of pediatric heart transplantation and in the last 25 years the field has also seen crossing of the blood group barrier[2] and transplanting across a positive crossmatch.[3] Both endeavors are part of the ongoing quest to maximize organ usage and steps toward achieving the ultimate goal in transplantation: tolerance.

INDICATIONS FOR LISTING

Pediatric heart transplantation is a treatment option for children with intractable heart failure or congenital heart disease not amenable to surgical palliation. The diversity in

[a] Labatt Family Heart Centre, Hospital for Sick Children, 555 University Avenue, Toronto, ON M5G 1X8, Canada
[b] SickKids Transplant Centre, Hospital for Sick Children, University of Toronto, 555 University Avenue, Toronto, ON M5G 1X8, Canada
* Corresponding author. Labatt Family Heart Centre, Hospital for Sick Children, 555 University Avenue, Toronto, ON M5G 1X8, Canada.
E-mail address: anne.dipchand@sickkids.ca

Pediatr Clin N Am 57 (2010) 353–373
doi:10.1016/j.pcl.2010.01.009
0031-3955/10/$ – see front matter © 2010 Elsevier Inc. All rights reserved.

pediatric.theclinics.com

underlying diagnosis and physiology, the broad age ranges, center-specific expertise and the small patient population have limited the development of universally accepted criteria for pediatric cardiac transplantation. Recent consensus guidelines and non-randomized trials continue to focus on the above 2 patient populations.[4,5] These guidelines are based primarily on expert opinion, as there is a lack of higher grades of evidence to guide transplant indications.[4,5] The clinical indications for transplantation can be classified into 2 main categories based on whether a transplantation is a life-saving or life-enhancing therapy. The life-saving indications include:

(1) Heart failure associated with symptomatic ventricular dysfunction secondary to myocardial disease or palliated congenital heart disease despite medical management. There are no specific quantitative values for ventricular function that guide listing for transplantation. Instead, importance is placed on the clinical consequences of decreased ventricular function, including growth failure or retardation and intractable cardiac symptoms despite optimal medical management. The need for ongoing ventilator, inotropic, or mechanical support to maximize cardiac output are also important markers of ventricular dysfunction
(2) Complex congenital heart disease with failed surgical correction or those lesions not amenable to surgical intervention because the risks of surgery and the survival outcomes are equal to or worse than transplantation
(3) Life-threatening arrhythmias resistant to medical or device management
(4) Unresectable cardiac tumors causing ventricular dysfunction or obstruction
(5) Unresectable ventricular diverticula
(6) Retransplantation for ventricular dysfunction or moderate graft vasculopathy.

Life-enhancing indications occur in the context of myocardial failure or palliated congenital heart disease associated with excessive disability, an unacceptable quality of life, or increased long-term morbidity. As pediatric and congenital heart disease patients are a diverse group, these categories encompass those patients who do not fit into the immediate life-saving categories. Examples include patients with[4,5]:

(1) Heart failure associated with progressive pulmonary hypertension that would preclude a transplant at a later time
(2) A restrictive cardiomyopathy due to the associated poor overall survival[6,7]
(3) A Fontan circulation and associated protein-losing enteropathy not reversible with medical therapy
(4) A failing Fontan circuit with a decline in exercise ability, quality of life, or ability to perform daily activities
(5) Congenital heart disease with atrioventricular valve regurgitation or aortic regurgitation not amenable to surgery
(6) Congenital heart disease and severe oxygen desaturations with no surgical options.

Current practice patterns reflect these indications as outlined in the data collected by the International Society of Heart and Lung Transplantation (ISHLT) and Pediatric Heart Transplant Study (PHTS). Both organizations collect data to characterize outcomes of pediatric transplantation from various centers around the world. The registry of the ISHLT is based on voluntary reporting from Canadian and European centers and mandatory reporting from all centers in the United States through the United Network for Organ Sharing (UNOS) data collection system.[8] The PHTS is a voluntary multicenter research registry designed to capture pre- and posttransplant outcomes data.[4]

The 2009 ISHLT report indicates that the number of reported pediatric heart transplants has remained stable during the last 3 years at 450/y.[8] In infants less than 1 year of age, congenital heart disease has remained the most common underlying diagnosis leading to heart transplantation (63%), followed by cardiomyopathies (31%). However, the proportion of infants receiving a transplant for cardiomyopathy has increased significantly, from 16% between 1988 and 1995 to 31% between 1996 and 2008.[8] This may reflect a shift in practice away from primary transplantation for hypoplastic left heart syndrome (HLHS) because of improved surgical outcomes.[9,10] Although the use of primary transplantation for congenital heart disease has decreased, it remains a viable treatment strategy for certain forms of congenital heart disease with poor long-term outcomes following surgical intervention. This category includes patients with single-ventricle anatomy associated with severe coronary artery stenosis, severe valvular stenosis or regurgitation, or ventricular dysfunction.[4,11,12]

Congenital heart disease is a less frequent indication for transplantation in the older population, with cardiomyopathies accounting for most of the transplantations in children aged from 1 to 10 years (55%) and adolescents (64%).[8]

EVALUATION OF THE RECIPIENT AND DONOR
Pretransplant Assessment

The pretransplant assessment is an essential part of the transplantation process as it helps identify patients with contraindications or potential complicating factors, those patients who may benefit from further medical or device management, and those who have an unrecognized reversible condition.[13,14] This assessment includes a thorough cardiac evaluation to delineate the cardiac anatomy and to define the hemodynamic profile (contraindications are discussed later in this article). Cardiac catheterization is often performed to assess the overall anatomy and pulmonary vasculature. Assessment of the other organ systems is included to ensure that there are no contraindications to transplantation or need for modification of standard treatments before or after transplantation. All noncardiac diseases should be evaluated and appropriate consultations should take place to help determine the associated long-term outcomes and morbidities. As part of the transplant assessment, the patient should undergo HLA typing, as the results may alter the intra- and postoperative management. Detailed psychosocial assessment of patients and their family members is essential to understand their support system, risk factors for noncompliance, and issues that would preclude transplantation, especially in the adolescent population. As these assessments are comprehensive, they are best performed within the context of a transplant-knowledgeable multidisciplinary team. Components of a typical assessment are outlined in **Table 1**.

Assessment of patients being considered for listing as fetuses differs somewhat because of the limitations in the diagnostic testing available. The workup includes a detailed maternal, prenatal, and family history. A detailed fetal echocardiogram and anatomic antenatal ultrasonography are required to define anatomy and to rule out associated anomalies. Additional testing includes amniocentesis for chromosomes, other genetic testing as indicated, and maternal screening for infectious diseases.[5,15] Indications for fetal listing are similar to those in the postnatal period and include single-ventricle anatomy with risk factors for surgical palliation (severe atrioventricular valve regurgitation, decreased function), HLHS in centers where transplantation is offered as primary therapy, unresectable cardiac tumors, right atrial isomerism syndromes, cardiomyopathies with poor ventricular function, and intractable arrhythmias. Ideally, candidates are listed once they are 35 weeks' gestational age

Table 1
Pretransplant assessment

Cardiology	Echocardiogram, electrocardiograph, chest radiograph, exercise test, cardiac catheterization, magnetic resonance imaging/magnetic resonance angiography, or computerized tomography angiography
Hematology/immunology	Blood group, HLA typing, PRA
Chemistry	Renal function, liver function, lipid profile, immunoglobulins
Infection	Serologies: Epstein-Barr virus, cytomegalovirus, varicella, herpes, human immunodeficiency virus, hepatitis titers
Multidisciplinary team	Social work, psychiatry, adolescent medicine, physiotherapy, occupational therapy, dietician
Additional consults	Genetics/metabolics, neurology, anesthesia, nephrology

or older, and have an estimated fetal weight greater than 2.5 kg to optimize pulmonary maturity. If a donor heart becomes available and there are no acceptable post-natal candidates, patients are delivered by cesarean section and undergo immediate transplantation.

Contraindications and Complicating Factors

The pretransplant assessment allows for the identification of factors that may complicate or completely exclude transplantation as a treatment option. The list of contraindications has been modified over the years, and several previous factors that would have excluded a transplant are now dealt with through a variety of strategies. In patients with complex congenital heart disease, the technical difficulties arising from unusual anatomy such as abnormal situs, systemic venous abnormalities, anomalous pulmonary venous drainage without stenosis, and some pulmonary artery anomalies no longer prohibit transplantation.[5,13] Previous sternotomy/thoracotomy, reversible pulmonary hypertension, noncardiac congenital abnormalities, kyphoscoliosis with restrictive pulmonary disease, nonprogressive or slowly progressive systemic diseases (genetic or isolated metabolic cardiomyopathies), and diabetes mellitus without end-organ damage no longer preclude cardiac transplantation.[5,13,14] Although the list of contraindications has decreased over the years, there are still several that must be ruled out before transplantation can occur[5,14,16]:

(1) Severe and irreversible end-organ damage or multisystem organ dysfunction
(2) Severe hypoplasia of the branch pulmonary arteries, because the distal branch pulmonary arteries are from the recipient and cannot be corrected with transplantation
(3) Severe pulmonary vein stenosis or atresia, because the recipient's pulmonary veins are connected to the donor's left atrium. Transplantation would not cure this anatomic problem and patients would be at high risk for pulmonary hypertension
(4) A severe or progressive noncardiac disease, such as a chromosomal, neurologic, or syndromic condition, that is associated with limited survival (eg, Duchenne muscular dystrophy, a systemic mitochondrial disorder, or an untreatable and multisystem metabolic disorder)
(5) Active infection
(6) Severe irreversible pulmonary hypertension
(7) Psychological issues: smoking, drug/alcohol abuse, unstable or chronic psychiatric conditions, life-threatening noncompliance

(8) Others: coexisting malignancy; morbid obesity; diabetes mellitus with end-organ damage; hypercoagulable states; retransplantation during an acute rejection episode.

Although discussion of all these contraindications is beyond the scope of this article, a better understanding of the role of pretransplant pulmonary hypertension is important. Pulmonary hypertension, specifically increased pulmonary vascular resistance (PVR), has been associated with significant right heart failure, graft loss, and increased mortality after transplantation.[17–21] PVR is best assessed during cardiac catheterization. If the PVR is found to be increased during a cardiac catheterization, the next step is to determine whether the pulmonary vascular bed is reactive to vasodilators. Patients who respond with a decrease in their PVR have reversible pulmonary hypertension, whereas those with no response are considered to have irreversible pulmonary hypertension. Cardiac transplantation is feasible in patients with a pulmonary vascular resistance indexed (PVRi) less than 6 Woods units/m^2 or a transpulmonary gradient (TPG) less than 15 mm Hg, or if inotropic support or pulmonary vasodilators are able to lower the PVRi to less than 6 Woods units/m^2 and TPG to less than 15 mm Hg.[4,19] The assessment of PVR may be difficult in certain forms of congenital heart disease as there are a variety of mechanisms that can lead to increased pulmonary artery pressures and resistance.[4] Therefore, in some conditions such as single ventricle lesions or those patients who have multiple sources of pulmonary blood flow, accurate assessment may not be possible.

Recently, the concept of irreversible pulmonary hypertension has been questioned because of improving drug therapy and the positive effects of mechanical support in patients believed to have irreversible pulmonary hypertension.[22–24] Therefore, the increasing use of mechanical support in the pediatric population may have the added benefit of increasing the number of patients eligible for isolated heart transplantation by lowering their PVR.

All of the above potential contraindications or complicating factors must be considered in the context of the risks of transplantation and the probability of short- (perioperative) and long-term survival given the ongoing shortage of donor organs that remains a limiting factor for solid-organ transplantation.

Sensitized Patients and Transplantation

As part of the routine testing all patients undergo a screening panel reactive antibody (PRA) test to look for the presence of anti-HLA antibodies. This is a test looking for pre-formed antibodies to a pool of potential donor antigens. A patient with a PRA higher than 10% is considered to be sensitized.[16] Increased PRA titers are seen in patients with a ventricular assist device (VAD), repaired congenital heart disease with homograft material, multiple blood transfusions, platelet transfusions, previous transplantation, or pregnancy.[25–27] Many of these risk factors, including the use of mechanical circulatory support, are important strategies for managing pediatric patients before and after listing for transplantation. Yang and colleagues[28] examined HLA sensitization rates in children supported with extracorporeal membrane oxygenation (ECMO) or a VAD. Their results suggest that younger patients supported on ECMO were unlikely to develop device-related HLA antibodies despite homograft use or blood transfusions. However, 66% of the patients supported with a VAD had new or additional HLA sensitization after 5 weeks of support. These patients tended to be older and supported for a longer period of time. The reason for this difference is unclear but has been postulated to be the result of impaired immune function secondary to the ECMO circuit, briefer exposure to the ECMO circuit, or possible age-related factors.[28] As the overall use of VADs increases in pretransplant management, and with the recent expansion of these devices to the neonatal and infant population, reevaluation of the risk factors and strategies to prophylaxically reduce sensitization will be needed.

Although the presence of HLA antibodies to a donor pool of antigens is not an absolute contraindication to transplantation, it continues to make these patients high-risk candidates. The presence of these antibodies increases the risk of antibody-mediated rejection, early graft failure, and decreased survival after transplantation.[25,26] Because of these risks, some centers list these patients with the requirement of a negative virtual or prospective crossmatch for donor-specific HLA antibodies at the time of transplantation or will not offer transplantation as a treatment strategy. Waiting for a negative crossmatch significantly increases the waiting-list time and identifying donor-specific antibodies before acceptance of a donor heart limits the donor pool to the local area because of time constraints.[29,30] Therefore, as an alternative several off-label treatment strategies intended to lower the pretransplant PRA levels or decrease the risk of antibody-mediated rejection after transplantation have been developed, including intraoperative plasma exchange, immune globulin, plasmapheresis, cyclophosphamide, rituximab, and antimetabolite treatment.[3,16,25,31,32] Implementation of treatment protocols using these strategies in both adult and pediatric studies have recently shown reasonable short and intermediate results after transplantation in those patients who were highly sensitized before transplantation.[3,30] As the pediatric outcomes are based on single centers studies, multicenter prospective studies are required to determine whether these results can be replicated and to decide on the optimal treatment regime. Listing a highly sensitized patient for heart transplantation should be performed in a center with experience and expertise in this high-risk population.

ABO Blood Group–Incompatible (ABO-I) Transplantation

Heart transplantation is usually contraindicated if a donor and recipient have incompatible blood groups because of the high risk of hyperacute rejection from preformed anti-A and anti-B antibodies (isohemagglutinins). Nevertheless, because of the limited number of organs available, attempts to transplant across blood groups have occurred. ABO blood group–incompatible (ABO-I) heart transplantation was pioneered in Toronto in the mid-1990s with a clear effect on waiting-list mortality[2,33] and excellent short- to intermediate-term outcomes.[34,35] Ten-year follow-up of the largest single-center cohort revealed no difference in survival, rejection, renal dysfunction, allograft vasculopathy, or posttransplant lymphoproliferative disorder.[34] ABO-I transplantations are increasingly being performed around the world and have been recognized as an important strategy to improve survival in infants following listing. It is still unclear which patients are best suited for this listing strategy and what is the upper age limit for tolerating an ABO-I transplant. Isohemagglutinins should routinely be checked as part of the pretransplant assessment in any patient less than 2 years of age, and in selected older patients at the discretion of an experienced transplant cardiologist.[34] Careful administration of appropriate blood products is paramount during and following ABO-I transplants to ensure the absence of isohemagglutinins against the donor or recipient.[2] **Table 2** lists the appropriate blood products to be used, based on the donor and recipient blood groups. As this is an essential part of the transplantation process, ABO-I heart transplantation should be performed in a center with the appropriate knowledge and infrastructure for management of the unique blood product needs.

Donor Evaluation

The suitability of the donor heart for transplantation and the management of the donor are vital parts of the transplantation process. Although most pediatric donors

Table 2
Blood products used during ABO-I transplants based on donor and recipient blood groups

Donor's Blood Group	Recipient's Blood Group	Antibodies to Avoid	Blood Products to be Used		
			Plasma	Red Cells	Platelets
AB	O	Anti-A vs graft Anti-B vs graft	AB	O	AB
B	O	Anti-B vs graft	AB or B	O	AB or B
A	O	Anti-A vs graft	AB or A	O	AB or A
AB	B	Anti-A vs graft Anti-B vs graft and recipient	AB	O or B	AB
A	B	Anti-A vs graft Anti-B vs recipient	AB	O or B	AB
AB	A	Anti-A vs graft and recipient Anti-B vs graft	AB	O or A	AB
B	A	Anti-A vs recipient Anti-B vs graft	AB	O or A	AB

Data from West LJ, Pollock-Barziv SM, Dipchand AI, et al. ABO-incompatible heart transplantation in infants. N Engl J Med 2001;344:793–800.

were previously healthy, the patient's history is essential to rule out any genetic, metabolic, or syndromic condition that may have cardiac involvement. The details of the mechanism of death are important to determine whether there has been any damage to the heart, such as a cardiac contusion after thoracic trauma or any risk of infection. Other pertinent information includes the donor's blood group, size and age, and the results of previous investigations including any electrocardiograms and echocardiograms.

To increase the donor pool for pediatric patients, strategies have been undertaken to accept oversized grafts. Recipients with oversized grafts, defined as a donor/recipient weight ratio greater than 2.5, were reported to have similar posttransplant outcomes to those with a ratio less than 2.5.[36,37] However, the one difference between these 2 groups was a higher incidence of delayed chest closure after transplantation when the weight ratio was greater than 2.5. Additional studies in patients with oversized grafts have also reported transient lobar collapse and greater left ventricle mass index.[38] Although oversized grafts have not been shown to affect outcomes, older donor age has been identified as a risk factor for poor outcomes. The donor age affects both the 1- and 5- year survival after transplantation with decreased 1-year survival in adolescents transplanted with hearts from donors more than 40 years of age.[39] In response to these findings, policies from the Canadian organ allocation system and the United Network for Organ Sharing in the United States specify that adolescent donor hearts are allocated to adolescent recipients preferentially.[5,16,40]

The suitability of the donor heart for transplantation can be altered by the brain death process and the subsequent management. Brain death has been shown to have a deleterious effect on ventricular function, with the right ventricle being particularly susceptible.[41] Therefore, the goals of treatment following brain death are to preserve ventricular function and prevent further myocardial damage. Intensive care management should focus on optimizing intravascular volume status, maintaining cardiac output with the lowest possible amount of inotropes, and preventing elevations in afterload.[42,43] An additional strategy that has been used successfully in donor management is hormonal resuscitation. This strategy has been shown to decrease the amount of inotropic support required and increase the suitability of the donor hearts for transplantation.[16,42]

During procurement, the donor heart is preserved using cardioplegia solution and cooled for transport. Carrying out this process efficiently serves to decrease the organ ischemic time. In adults, a donor ischemic time greater than 4 hours is a risk factor for decreased late survival.[44] This has not been the case in pediatric patients.[45,46] Ischemic times greater than 8 hours in children have not been shown to have an effect on long-term outcomes including survival, rejection, and allograft vasculopathy,[46] and recent analysis of the ISHLT registry revealed that ischemic time was not a risk factor for short term survival (1 year).[8]

TRANSPLANT SURGERY

The basic techniques for implantation of a cardiac donor allograft were initially described by Lower and Shumway[47] and have not changed greatly since this initial description. Patient size, heart location, situs, systemic venous, and pulmonary venous anatomy must all be taken into consideration. In some complex forms of congenital heart disease there may be a need to procure portions of branch pulmonary arteries, aorta, inferior vena cava, or the innominate vein to facilitate the anastamoses within the recipient, and this should be planned in the pretransplant assessment period.[48] There are objective differences in outcomes related to the type of surgical approach. The biatrial technique, anastomosis of the donor and recipient aortas, pulmonary arteries, and atrial cuffs, have been associated with conduction disturbances requiring pacemaker placement in 4% to 15%,[49] a higher thromboembolism risk, poor atrial synchrony, and more atrioventricular valvar regurgitation due to distortion of atrial anatomy.[50]

The bicaval approach, in which the right atrium is left intact because the donor and recipient's superior vena cava and inferior vena cava are anastomosed, has been reported to be associated with fewer tachyarrhythmias, slightly better hemodynamics, less tricuspid regurgitation, fewer pacemakers, and better exercise tolerance (**Figs. 1 and 2**).[51]

ALLOGRAFT DYSFUNCTION, REJECTION AND ALLOGRAFT VASCULOPATHY
Perioperative Allograft Dysfunction

Postoperative primary allograft failure is one of the most common causes of early mortality following transplantation. It can be characterized by the need for mechanical circulatory support or the use of multiple inotropes or vasopressors in the early post-transplant period.[17] Acute allograft dysfunction accounted for 6.5% of the total deaths and 31.4% of the deaths in the first 30 days after transplantation in 421 pediatric heart transplant recipients followed over a 20-year period.[52] Right ventricular (RV) dysfunction related to donor heart function, ischemic injury, and the recipient's PVR and reactivity are well-known perioperative factors leading to acute allograft dysfunction.[5,16,20] Other risk factors that have been identified for primary allograft failure include a diagnosis of congenital heart disease, need for mechanical support before transplantation, increased donor/recipient body-weight and body surface-area ratios, increased donor ischemic time, anoxia as the donor's cause of death, and increased cardiopulmonary resuscitation time.[17] Risk factors for death or graft loss associated with primary graft failure have not been clearly identified.

DIAGNOSIS IN PEDIATRIC HEART TRANSPLANT RECIPIENTS (Age: < 1 Year)

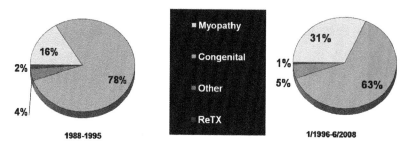

DIAGNOSIS IN PEDIATRIC HEART TRANSPLANT RECIPIENTS (Age: 1-10 Years)

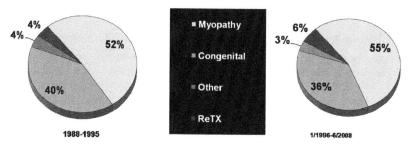

DIAGNOSIS IN PEDIATRIC HEART TRANSPLANT RECIPIENTS (Age: 11-17 Years)

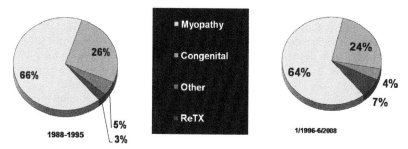

Fig. 1. Indications for cardiac transplantation, categorized by age, from the ISHLT database from 1998 to 2008. (*Data from* Kirk R, Edwards LB, Aurora P, et al. Registry of the international society for heart and lung transplantation: twelfth official pediatric heart transplantation report-2009. J Heart Lung Transplant 2009;28(10):993–1006.)

Postoperative management of these patients should focus on decreasing the PVR and RV afterload (pulmonary vasodilators and appropriate ventilation strategies), decreasing RV preload if the RV is known to be dilated and dysfunctional, maximizing coronary perfusion, maintaining systemic blood pressure, and optimizing oxygen delivery (inotropic support, ensuring adequate heart rate and atrioventricular synchrony, decreasing oxygen consumption).[5,16,20] Mechanical circulatory support may be necessary in some patients who have hemodynamic compromise from right or left ventricular dysfunction, and clinically significant stenosis contributing to

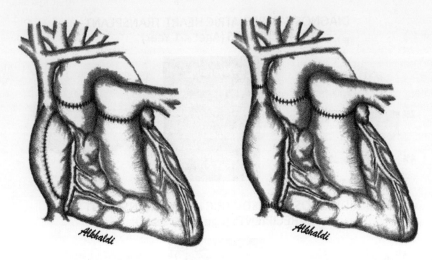

Biatrial Anastomosis   Bicaval Anastomosis

Fig. 2. Surgical techniques for heart transplantation. (*From* Alkhaldi A, Chin C, Bernstein D. Pediatric cardiac transplantation. Semin Pediatr Surg 2006;15:188–96; with permission.)

allograft dysfunction may be amenable to cardiac catheterization interventions or reoperation.[16,17,20]

Rejection

Rejection is the consequence of the recipient's immune response to foreign antigens. In transplantation, this reaction results in destruction of the graft tissue. There are 4 main forms of rejection: hyperacute, acute cellular rejection (ACR), antibody-mediated rejection, and chronic rejection.

Hyperacute rejection is due to preformed antibodies in the recipient, to donor antigens; predominantly blood group or anti-HLA antibodies.[14] This is a rare form of rejection in which tissue destruction manifests within minutes to hours of transplantation. It can be prevented by blood group matching, the use of a donor-specific crossmatch, and strategies to deal with preformed antibodies as discussed earlier.

Acute rejection continues to be a significant cause of morbidity and mortality after transplantation.[8] Acute rejection accounted for 17.8% of deaths overall in the PHTS data (Anne Dipchand, MD, Toronto, Canada, personal communication, PHTS annual report 2009). In the first 5 years after transplantation, rejection is the cause of death in 15% to 18% of patients, with this number decreasing to 6% by 10 years after transplantation.[6]

Rejection commonly occurs in the first year after transplantation with more than 50% to 60% of patients having experienced 1 episode,[8,53] and is associated with decreased late survival and allograft vasculopathy.[54,55] However, more recent data from the ISHLT registry suggests that rejection in the first year does not significantly change 3-year conditional survival (based on the ISHLT report, the term conditional survival is used to describe the survival statistics for those patients who are still alive 1 year after transplantation).[8]

Rejection with hemodynamic compromise is also more likely to occur in the first year and is associated with poor survival.[53,56] These significant episodes do not always correlate with the biopsy score and can be seen with antibody-mediated rejection (AMR).[54,56] Late rejection (defined as rejection occurring after the first year post transplant) is common and is seen in approximately 25% of patients.[57] Freedom from late rejection in the PHTS registry was reported as 73% at 3 years and 66% at 4 years after transplantation. Late rejection is associated with a high mortality, especially when hemodynamic compromise is present.[57] Risk factors for rejection, recurrent rejection, late rejection, and rejection with hemodynamic compromise include older age of recipients, nonwhite recipients, more than 1 episode of rejection in the first year, greater number of rejection episodes, and shorter time since last rejection episode.[53,56,57] Few studies have examined all of these events in the same patient population to determine whether there are any differentiating risk factors. Recently, Lammers and colleagues[58] reported on their single-center experience with acute rejection, including those with hemodynamic compromise. Multivariate analysis revealed that acute rejection was associated with the use of sirolimus, older age, male gender, and higher height and weight. For those with hemodynamic compromise, a univariate analysis identified sirolimus therapy, positive pretransplant cytomegalovirus (CMV) status, and non-Caucasian ethnicity as risk factors. A multivariate analysis was not reported.[58]

A less common form of rejection that is increasingly being recognized is B-cell mediated rejection or AMR. This type of rejection can be seen in patients with hemodynamic compromise and graft dysfunction with no histologic evidence of cellular rejection.[16] Typically, AMR is characterized by microvascular injury. AMR is probably the most common cause of biopsy-negative rejection, as screening for AMR has just recently been implemented in many centers. This type of rejection can be severe, difficult to treat, and has a worse prognosis than ACR. However, as noted earlier, there is increasing experience and success with diagnosing and managing AMR in the highly sensitized patient population.[25,26,30–32]

Many episodes of rejection occur without any detectable clinical symptoms, thus making endomyocardial biopsies the gold standard for screening and diagnosing rejection. The frequency of surveillance biopsies depends on the patient's age but, is also center-specific. Biopsies during episodes of rejection associated with cardiac symptoms, changes in cardiac function or wall thickness on echocardiogram, or hemodynamic compromise can aid in the immunologic management. Acute cellular rejection is characterized by varying degrees of lymphocytic infiltrate and myocyte necrosis on biopsy specimens. Biopsies are interpreted based on the revised ISHLT criteria that classify ACR into no rejection (0R), mild (1R), moderate (2R), and severe (3R). AMR is characterized by the presence of a positive immunofluoresence, vasculitis, or severe edema with no cellular infiltrates, and is classified into no acute AMR (AMR 0) and positive AMR (AMR 1).[16,59] As a cardiac biopsy is an invasive procedure with risks, there have been many efforts to identify a noninvasive screening tool for rejection, including echocardiography, tissue Doppler, gene profiling, and biochemical markers. Many of these tests have not shown the ability to consistently predict or diagnose rejection.[60,61] Recently, B-type natriuretic peptide levels have been shown to have a high sensitivity and negative predictive value for rejection in the pediatric population.[60] Further studies are required to confirm these findings.

Treatment of rejection depends on many factors including the type, grade, time after transplantation, clinical and hemodynamic effect, baseline immunosuppression and associated comorbidities.

Chronic Allograft Dysfunction

Chronic allograft dysfunction remains a common problem in all forms of solid-organ transplantation. This term is often used interchangeably with the terms chronic allograft vasculopathy or chronic rejection, especially in the heart transplant population. This problem contributes significantly to the limited long-term survival of the allograft and is one of the leading causes of death late after transplantation.[8,52] In the heart allograft, the coronary arteries develop uniform intimal proliferation and stenosis of the smaller branches, limiting blood supply to the allograft and resulting in chronic vascular injury.[62,63] This process is believed to be due to immune and nonimmune factors. Immune factors involved include cell-mediated and humoral injury to the vascular endothelium. This problem is potentially exacerbated or initiated by nonimmune factors such as ischemia-reperfusion injury, obesity, hyperlipidemia, smoking, and diabetes. Additional risk factors for the development of coronary allograft vasculopathy have been identified and include older age of the donor or recipient, early acute rejection, increased frequency of acute rejection, late rejection, CMV infection, and the absence of lipid-lowering agents.[8,14]

The true incidence of allograft vasculopathy in the pediatric population is unknown, with studies suggesting an incidence range between 3% and 43%.[64] However, a recent multi-institutional study using angiographic data reported an incidence of allograft vasculopathy of 17% at 5 years, with 6% of patients having moderate to severe disease.[63] Studies using intracoronary ultrasonography suggest that the incidence in pediatrics is even higher, with detection of intimal thickening in 75% of patients at 5 years with 37% having moderate to severe stenosis.[65] Within the ISHLT registry, 66% of patients are free of allograft vasculopathy at 10 years, but, once detected, the 3-year graft survival was only 45%.[8] Diagnosis of allograft vasculopathy is challenging and modalities include coronary angiography, exercise and pharmacologic stress testing or echocardiography, nuclear medicine scintigraphy, and intravascular ultrasonography. Once clinically significant disease is established, treatment is limited in the pediatric population with only 2 reports in the literature of coronary interventions in a small number of patients.[64,66]

Retransplantation

Retransplantation is a treatment option for patients with acute or chronic allograft failure on the basis of primary graft failure, rejection or significant allograft vasculopathy. Based on the 2009 ISHLT registry, retransplantation rates have been increasing and currently account for 5% of all pediatric transplants.[8] The interval between the primary transplant and retransplant, and the reason for retransplantation have significant effects on outcome. Early retransplantation for acute allograft failure or acute rejection is associated with a poor outcome. Retransplants occurring early (within 180 days) had a 1-year survival of 53% versus 86% for late retransplants.[67] Similar results were reported from the PHTS for early retransplantation with a 1-year survival of 56% compared with a 85% survival rate for patients with a primary transplant. However, there was no difference in outcomes in patients retransplanted more than 1 year after the initial transplantation compared with primary transplant recipients.[68]

RISK FACTORS AND OUTCOMES
Waiting-list Mortality

As with all forms of solid-organ transplantation, heart transplantation is limited by the availability of suitable donor organs. Those patients awaiting a heart transplant are at risk of dying if a donor organ does not become available. Pediatric cardiac transplant candidates, regardless of age, have the highest waiting-list mortality of all solid-organ recipients.[69] The mortality risk while on the waiting list can be attributed to several factors, including donor availability, status of the recipient, underlying diagnosis, age, and blood type.[9,15,70,71] There have been a variety of strategies to increase the donor pool and optimize treatment of patients, including the use of ABO-I hearts in infants, transplanting sensitized patients without a prospective negative crossmatch, and the use of mechanical circulatory support. In a recent analysis of 3098 pediatric patients between 1999 and 2006, risk factors for mortality while awaiting transplantation included ECMO support, ventilatory support, congenital heart disease, UNOS 1A status, dialysis use, and nonwhite ethnicity.[70] Status 1A patients were a heterogeneous group, with those requiring more invasive support such as ECMO having a higher mortality.[70,72] As not all status 1A patients are the same, these results may help to further modify the allocation system to improve survival in the higher-risk patients.

Infants have consistently been reported to have the highest waiting-list mortality (25%–30%) of all heart transplant candidates.[9,15,71] In this patient population, the infants with the highest risk of dying while on the waiting list are those requiring ECMO, ventilator support, or prostaglandins, those with congenital heart disease, infants less than 3 kg, and infants of nonwhite ethnicity.[71] The waiting-list mortality for infants has also been shown to vary based on organ allocation practices. The allocation system for pediatric donor hearts to an infant differs between Canada and the United States. In Canada the allocation of a donor heart is based on clinical status and not blood group compatibility.[33] This change in practice has significantly decreased the waiting-list mortality from 58% to 7% in infants less than 6 months of age.[33] These results have not been replicated in the United States as ABO-I transplantations are not uniformly performed across all centers, and the current allocation system prioritizes donor hearts to recipients of identical blood groups, followed by compatible blood groups, and then incompatible blood groups.[73] These recent studies highlight the need to reevaluate the current system of organ allocation to ensure that the highest-risk patients are prioritized.

Posttransplant Survival

Recent data from the ISHLT registry revealed that the overall 20-year survival for all pediatric heart transplant recipients is 40%, with 1-, 5- and 10-year survival reported as 80%, 68%, and 58% respectively.[8] Zuppan and colleagues[52] reported similar overall survivals of 85% at 1 year, 75% at 5 years, and 65% at 10 years.

The highest risk of dying is in the first 6 months after transplantation.[8] This is especially true for infant (<1 year) recipients. For those patients who survive to 1 year after transplantation, the conditional survival is 15 years for teenagers and 19 years for children transplanted between 1 and 10 years.[8] Conditional survival for infant recipients could not be calculated from the ISHLT data, with more than 70% still alive at 20 years after transplantation. Improvement in overall 5-year survival has also been reported in the current era (2000–2003), and has been attributed solely to the improved survival in the first 6 months after transplantation.[74] Improvements in the pre- and posttransplant management of pediatric cardiac transplant patients may account for these findings.

Survival is also related to underlying diagnosis.[52] A recent analysis from the PHTS revealed a better long-term survival (10 years) in patients transplanted for cardiomyopathy compared with noncardiomyopathy indications. Of those patients with a cardiomyopathy, dilated cardiomyopathy as an underlying diagnosis had the best outcomes.[72]

Risk factors for mortality at 1 year post transplantation include pretransplant support (ECMO, ventilation), diagnosis of congenital heart disease, higher pretransplant creatinine levels, retransplantation, PRA 10% or more, transplant center volume, and increased donor age.[8] Risk factors for mortality within 5 years of transplantation are similar, but female race was now identified as a risk factor and pretransplant creatinine was not.[8]

In the early postoperative period acute graft dysfunction and technical issues account for more than 50% of the deaths.[8,52] In a large single-center study, the

3 most common causes of death, independent of time after transplantation, were acute rejection (26%), infection (16%), and allograft vasculopathy (14%).[52] In those patients who survived beyond 1 year after transplantation, acute rejection (30%), allograft vasculopathy (23.5%), and infection (11.8%) accounted for most of the deaths. These findings differ slightly from the ISHLT registry in which mortality at 10 years after transplantation is secondary to allograft vasculopathy (28.5%) and graft failure (25.5%), with acute rejection being a less significant factor.[8]

Long-term Complications

Ongoing and close follow-up in pediatric transplant patients is essential for detecting transplant-related problems. Long-term follow-up is comprehensive and requires ongoing monitoring for rejection, infections, malignancies, complications of immunosuppression, growth, and development. A full discussion of all these issues is beyond the scope of this article, but a few key areas are discussed.

Posttransplant Surveillance

The hallmark of posttransplant surveillance is meticulous attention to the development of potential transplant-related complications and early intervention. In general, this involves routine annual follow-up of several systems, including renal, bones, blood pressure, and lipids. Most centers have routine bloodwork following hematologic parameters, renal and liver function tests, and therapeutic drug monitoring. Specific to heart transplantation is the cardiac follow-up that may consist of electrocardiogram, Holter monitor, echocardiography, cardiac catheterization and biopsy, graded exercise testing, and other tests at a frequency that is patient- and center-specific.

Infection

Infections are an important cause of early mortality after transplantation, and continue to pose risks for years afterwards.[8] Infection was the second leading cause of death reported within the PHTS (Anne Dipchand, MD, personal communication, 2009). Bacterial infections are the most common type of infection and primarily occur in the first month after transplantation.[75] They account for 60% of infections, with viral (30%), fungal (7%), and protozoan (2%) infections being less common. Routine serologic screening in the donor and recipient, routine posttransplant surveillance, and prophylactic or preemptive management strategies can help modulate the effect of infectious complications on posttransplant outcomes.

Renal Dysfunction and Hypertension

Renal insufficiency is important after solid-organ transplantation, with most patients experiencing some degree of dysfunction. Bharat and colleagues[76] reported that 84% of their pediatric heart transplant patients were free of at least mild dysfunction at 1 year, but this dropped to 33% by 5 years. Severe renal dysfunction, characterized by the need for dialysis, transplantation, or serum creatinine level greater than 221 μmol/L (2.5 mg/dL), is seen in 11% of recipients by 10 years.[8] The causes for renal dysfunction are multifactorial with predisposing factors often beginning in the pretransplant period, including low cardiac output state, the use of diuretic therapy, and mechanical support. Risk factors before and after transplantation for developing end-stage renal disease or chronic renal insufficiency include pretransplant dialysis, African American race, longer pretransplant stay in the intensive care unit, the use of ECMO, diagnosis of hypertrophic cardiomyopathy, longer duration on the waiting list, previous heart transplant, pretransplant diabetes, younger age at transplantation, and higher levels of calcineurin inhibitors.[77] Screening for renal dysfunction is an essential part of routine follow-up. Once renal dysfunction is recognized, efforts should be made to minimize the use of nephrotoxic drugs including the calcineurin inhibitors. Partial recovery can occur when calcineurin inhibitor exposure is decreased as there is potential for reversal.

Hypertension is also a common finding in the heart transplant population, with 69% of pediatric patients having hypertension at 8 years.[8] Treatment is essential to decrease the long-term risk for coronary artery vasculopathy and renal dysfunction, and includes diet modification, exercise, and antihypertensive therapy.

Malignancy

Malignancies continue to be an important cause of morbidity and mortality in the pediatric heart transplant population. Malignancy risk stems from the use of immunosuppression therapy after transplantation. Although in adults, skin and solid-organ malignancies contribute to this burden, posttransplant lymophoproliferative disease (PTLD) accounts for most malignancies in the pediatric population.[8] The development of PTLD is closely linked to the presence of an Epstein-Barr virus (EBV) infection, especially the acquisition of primary EBV after transplantation.[78] In the pediatric heart transplant population, freedom from malignancy is greater than 90% at 10 years.[8] Retrospective single-center studies and the PHTS registry have reported the overall incidence of PTLD to range from 3.5% to 8.4%.[78–80] Based on the PHTS data, survival with PTLD is 75% at 1 year, 68% at 3 years, and 67% at 5 years, with most deaths occurring in the first 2 years after diagnosis.[78] Death is usually secondary to progressive PTLD or graft loss from rejection.[78] The main goals of therapy depend on the histology and stage of the disease. The treatment strategies vary by the nature of the disease and the treating center, but include reducing immunosuppression, antivirals agents, surgical resection, radiation, chemotherapy, immune globulin, anti-CD 20 monoclonal antibodies (rituximab), and interferon-α.[78]

Growth and Development

Many patients experience poor growth before cardiac transplantation due to increased metabolic demands and decreased nutritional intake. There has been a discrepancy in the literature regarding the amount of catch-up growth that occurs after transplantation. Analysis of the PHTS database has shown that children have improved linear growth, although the overall z-score for height did not reach population norms by 6 years after transplantation.[81] Those patients with HLHS, or those transplanted at a younger age, had less capacity for catch-up growth. Other investigators have failed to identify any significant catch-up growth after transplantation.[82,83] These studies highlight the need for further research to better understand the potential for catch-up growth and what positively affects growth after transplantation.

Developmental assessments have shown mean physical and mental developmental scores in the low-normal range.[83–85] Most studies using cognitive testing have found that children receiving heart transplants have a 10 to 15 point IQ deficit compared with the control population.[86] Specific areas of deficit that have been identified include expressive language, short-term memory, visual-motor integration, and fine motor skills. Early identification of these issues is crucial in order to mobilize the appropriate resources to optimize developmental and neuropsychological outcomes.

Psychological Outcomes and Quality of Life

With improvement in survival after pediatric heart transplantation, focus has shifted to the importance of quality of life and functional status. Although the general perception is that pediatric patients following transplantation have a good quality of life, there are reports that suggest that these patients are at risk of behavioral and psychological sequelae.[86,87] School performance has been reported to be significantly lower than that of healthy children despite normal academic functioning, with a significant percentage having behavioral problems (8% at 6 months after transplantation, increasing to >26% by 3–5 years after transplantation).[88] Behavioral problems and less social competence have also been reported in other studies.[86] However, DeMaso and colleagues[89] found that 78.3% of their study population showed good psychological outcomes at a mean of 2.1 years after transplantation. This finding was reconfirmed in a longitudinal follow-up study (10 years) of the same patient cohort in which 73.3% were still assessed as having good psychological outcomes.[90] No correlation with posttransplant medical severity and psychological functioning was evident, but a correlation was found between psychological outcomes and family functioning. This finding highlights the importance of not only evaluating the patient but also evaluating the families, with reports in the literature of up to 40% of parents experiencing moderate to severe posttraumatic stress symptoms and 19% meeting criteria for posttraumatic stress disorder following transplantation.[91] Although most pediatric transplant recipients have the ability to adjust after transplantation there is ongoing need for psychological assessment and evaluation of family functioning to promote healthy psychological outcomes and reasonable quality of life.

SUMMARY

Overall survival after heart transplantation for pediatric recipients has greatly improved during the last 20 years. Despite this improvement, long-term complications continue to exist and ongoing surveillance by cardiac transplant teams and other health care professionals is essential. Although most transplant programs have their own institutional practices for surveillance, including frequency and nature of testing, continued vigilance is required when clinically assessing these patients to identify possible complications. As many patients with long-term complications are frequently asymptomatic routine surveillance coordinated by the transplant centers is essential. Therefore, an understanding of the regional transplant center's practices will assist in the overall care of the patient. Good communication with the transplant center will help the practitioner know when a referral is appropriate. However, there are some clues, although by no means an exhaustive list, that should prompt contact with the transplant center. These include patients presenting with cardiac symptoms or decreasing exercise tolerance, as these may be associated with rejection; an unusual course of a childhood illness, as most viral illness are well tolerated; and any unexplained symptoms that may be associated with posttransplant lymphoproliferative disease. Contact should also be made before starting any new medications to ensure that there is no interference with immunosuppression therapy. With all this being said, these patients are often complex and the regional transplant centers are an excellent resource for questions and assistance with management issues.

As pediatric heart transplantation continues to advance, further research is required in many areas including management of pediatric heart failure, development of less toxic immunosuppressive therapy, development of noninvasive techniques to diagnose rejection, and the assessment of preventative strategies for allograft vasculopathy. With these future directives in mind, the care of pediatric cardiac transplant recipients will continue to evolve to ensure the best quality of care for this unique patient population.

REFERENCES

1. Bailey LL. The evolution of infant heart transplant. J Heart Lung Transplant 2009; 28(12):1241–5.
2. West LJ, Pollock-Barziv SM, Dipchand AI, et al. ABO-incompatible heart transplantation in infants. N Engl J Med 2001;344:793–800.
3. Pollock-BarZiv SM, den Hollander N, Ngan B, et al. Pediatric heart transplantation in human leukocyte antigen sensitized patients: evolving management and assessment of intermediate-term outcomes in a high-risk population. Circulation 2007;116:172–8.
4. Canter CE, Shaddy RE, Bernstein D, et al. Indications for heart transplantation in pediatric heart disease. Circulation 2007;115(5):658–76.
5. Dipchand AI, Cecere R, Delgado D, et al. Canadian Consensus on Paediatric and Adult Congenital Heart Transplantation 2004. Can J Cardiol 2005;21(13):1145–8.
6. Weller RJ, Weintraub R, Addonizio LJ, et al. Outcome of restrictive cardiomyopathy in children. Am J Cardiol 2002;90:501–6.
7. Cetta F, O'Leary PW, Seward JB, et al. Idiopathic restrictive cardiomyopathy in childhood: diagnostic features and clinical course. Mayo Clin Proc 1995;70:634–40.
8. Kirk R, Edwards LB, Aurora P, et al. Registry of The International Society for Heart and Lung Transplantation: Twelfth Official Pediatric Heart Transplantation report-2009. J Heart Lung Transplant 2009;28:993–1006.
9. Chrisant MR, Naftel DC, Drummond-Webb J, et al. Fate of infants with hypoplastic left heart syndrome listed for cardiac transplantation: a multicenter study. J Heart Lung Transplant 2005;24:576–82.
10. Tweddell JS, Hoffman GM, Mussatto KA, et al. Improved survival of patients undergoing palliation of hypoplastic left heart syndrome: lessons learned from 115 consecutive patients. Circulation 2002;106:I82–9.
11. Mital S, Addonizio LJ, Lamour JM, et al. Outcome of children with end-stage congenital heart disease waiting for cardiac transplantation. J Heart Lung Transplant 2003;22:147–53.
12. Rosenthal DN, Dubin AM, Clifford Chin C, et al. Outcome while awaiting heart transplantation in children: a comparison of congenital heart disease and cardiomyopathy. J Heart Lung Transplant 2000;19:751–5.
13. Canter C. Preoperative assessment and management of pediatric heart transplantation. Prog Pediatr Cardiol 2000;11:91–7.
14. Canter CE, Kirklin JKIn: Pediatric heart transplantation. ISHLT Monograph Series, vol 2. Philadelphia (PA): Elsevier; 2007.
15. Pollock-Barziv SM, McCrindle BW, West LJ, et al. Waiting before birth: outcomes after fetal listing for heart transplantation. Am J Transplant 2008;8(2):412–8.
16. Haddad H, Issac D, Legare JF, et al. Canadian Cardiovascular Society Consensus: Conference update on cardiac transplantation 2008: executive summary. Can J Cardiol 2009;25(4):197–205.
17. Huang J, Trinkaus K, Huddleston CB, et al. Risk factors for primary graft failure after pediatric cardiac transplantation: importance of recipient and donor characteristics. J Heart Lung Transplant 2004;23:716–22.
18. Butler J, Stankewicz MA, Wu J, et al. Pre-transplant reversible pulmonary hypertension predicts higher risk for mortality after cardiac transplantation. J Heart Lung Transplant 2005;24:170–7.
19. Gajarski RJ, Towbin JA, Bricker JT, et al. Intermediate follow-up of pediatric heart transplant recipients with elevated pulmonary vascular resistance index. J Am Coll Cardiol 1994;23:1682–7.

20. Hoskote A, Carter C, Rees P, et al. Acute right ventricular failure after pediatric cardiac transplant: predictors and long-term outcome in current era of transplantation medicine. J Thorac Cardiovasc Surg 2010;139(1):146–53.
21. Gorlitzer M, Ankersmit J, Fiegl N, et al. Is the transpulmonary pressure gradient a predictor for mortality after orthotopic cardiac transplantation? Transpl Int 2005;18(4):390–5.
22. Liden H, Haraldsson A, Ricksten S-E, et al. Does pretransplant left ventricular assist device therapy improve results after heart transplantation in patients with elevated pulmonary vascular resistance? Eur J Cardiothorac Surg 2009;35: 1029–35.
23. Zimpfer D, Zrunek P, Sandner S, et al. Post-transplant survival after lowering fixed pulmonary hypertension using left ventricular assist devices. Eur J Cardiothorac Surg 2007;31:698–702.
24. Gandhi SK, Grady RM, Huddleston CB, et al. Beyond Berlin: heart transplantation in the "untransplantable". J Thorac Cardiovasc Surg 2008;136:529–31.
25. Jacobs JP, Quintessenza JA, Boucek RJ, et al. Pediatric cardiac transplantation in children with high panel reactive antibody. Ann Thorac Surg 2004;78: 1703–9.
26. Kobashigawa JA, Sabad A, Drinkwater D, et al. Pretransplant panel reactive-antibody screens. Are they truly a marker for poor outcome after cardiac transplantation? Circulation 1996;94:II294–7.
27. Shaddy RE, Hunter DD, Osborn KA, et al. Prospective analysis of HLA immunogenicity of cryopreserved valved allografts used in pediatric heart surgery. Circulation 1996;94:1063–7.
28. Yang J, Schall C, Smith D, et al. HLA sensitization in pediatric pre-transplant cardiac patients supported by mechanical assist devices: the utility of Luminex. J Heart Lung Transplant 2009;28:123–9.
29. Holt DB, Lublin DM, Phelan DL, et al. Mortality and morbidity in pre-sensitized pediatric heart transplant recipients with a positive donor crossmatch utilizing peri-operative plasmapheresis and cytolytic therapy. J Heart Lung Transplant 2007;26:876–82.
30. Wright EJ, Fiser WP, Edens E, et al. Cardiac transplant outcomes in pediatric patients with pre-formed anti-human leukocyte antigen antibodies and/or positive retrospective crossmatch. J Heart Lung Transplant 2007;26:1163–9.
31. Pisani BA, Mullen GM, Malinowska K. Plasmapheresis with intravenous immunoglobulin G is effective in patients with elevated panel reactive antibody prior to cardiac transplantation. J Heart Lung Transplant 1996;18:701–6.
32. Larson DF, Elkund DK, Arabia F, et al. Plasmapheresis during cardiopulmonary bypass: a proposed treatment for presensitized cardiac transplantation patients. J Extra Corpor Technol 1999;31:177–83.
33. West L, Karamlou T, Dipchand AI, et al. Impact on outcomes after listing and after transplantation of a strategy to accept ABO blood group incompatible donor hearts for neonates and infants. J Thorac Cardiovasc Surg 2006;131(2): 455–61.
34. Dipchand AI, Pollock BarZiv S, West L, et al. ABO-incompatible heart transplantation: the first 10 years. Am J Transplant 2009;10(2):389–97.
35. Roche SL, Burch M, O'Sullivan J, et al. Multicenter experience of ABO-incompatible pediatric cardiac transplantation. Am J Transplant 2008;8(1):208–15.
36. Razzouk AJ, Johnston JK, Larsen RL, et al. Effect of oversizing cardiac allografts on survival in pediatric patients with congenital heart disease. J Heart Lung Transplant 2005;24(2):195–9.

37. Fullerton DA, Gundry SR, de Begona AJ, et al. The effects of donor-recipient size discrepancy in infant and paediatric heart transplantation. J Thorac Cardiovasc Surg 1992;104(5):1314–9.
38. Kertesz NJ, Gajarski RJ, Towbin JA, et al. Effect of donor-recipient size mismatch on left ventricular remodelling after pediatric orthotopic heart transplantation. Am J Cardiol 1995;76(16):1167–72.
39. Chin C, Miller J, Robbins R, et al. The use of advanced-age donor hearts adversely affects survival in pediatric heart transplantation. Pediatr Transplant 1999;3(4):309–14.
40. United Network for Organ Sharing. Allocation of pediatric donor hearts to pediatric heart candidates. United Network for Organ Sharing Policy 3.7: organ distribution: the distribution of thoracic organs. Available at: http://www.unos.org/PoliciesandBylaws2/policies/pdfs/policy_9.pdf. Last Revised Nov 17, 2009. Accessed January, 2010.
41. Novitzky D. Detrimental effects of brain death on the potential organ donor. Transplant Proc 1997;29:3770–2.
42. Shemie SD, Ross H, Pagliarello J, et al. Organ management in Canada: recommendations of the Forum on Medical Management to Optimize Donor Organ Potential. CMAJ 2006;174(6):S13–30.
43. Berman M, Barker A, Betts G. Transforming the "unacceptable" donor: fifteen years later. J Heart Lung Transplant 2008;27(2):S225.
44. Del Rizzo DF, Menkis AH, Pflugfelder PW, et al. The role of donor age and ischemic time on survival following orthotopic heart transplantation. J Heart Lung Transplant 1999;18:310–9.
45. Kawauchi M, Gundry SR, de Begona JA, et al. Prolonged preservation of human pediatric hearts for transplantation: correlation of ischemic time and subsequent function. J Heart Lung Transplant 1993;12(Pt 1):55–8.
46. Scheule A, Zimmerman G, Johnston J, et al. Duration of graft cold ischemia does not affect outcomes in pediatric heart transplant recipients. Circulation 2002;106:1163–7.
47. Trento A, Czer LS, Blanche C. Surgical techniques for cardiac transplantation. Semin Thorac Cardiovasc Surg 1996;8:126–32.
48. Del Nido PJ, Bailey L, Kirklin JK. Surgical techniques in pediatric heart transplantation. Chapter 6. In: Canter CE, Kirklin JK, editors. Pediatric heart transplantation, ISHLT Monograph Series, vol. 2. Philadelphia (PA): Elsevier; 2007. p. 83–102.
49. Blanche C, Czer LS, Trento A, et al. Bradyarrhythmias requiring pacemaker implantation after orthotopic heart transplantation: association with rejection. J Heart Lung Transplant 1992;11:446–52.
50. Angermann CE, Spes CH, Tammen A, et al. Anatomic characteristics and valvular function of the transplanted heart: transthoracic versus transesophageal echocardiographic findings. J Heart Transplant 1990;9:331–8.
51. Milano CA, Shah AS, Van Trigt P, et al. Evaluation of early postoperative results after bicaval versus standard cardiac transplantation and review of the literature. Am Heart J 2000;140:717–21.
52. Zuppan CW, Wells LM, Kerstetter JC, et al. Cause of death in pediatric and infant heart transplant recipients: review of a 20-year, single-institution cohort. J Heart Lung Transplant 2009;28(6):579–84.
53. Chin C, Naftel DC, Singh TP. Risk factors for recurrent rejection in pediatric heart transplantation: a multicenter experience. J Heart Lung Transplant 2004;23:178–85.
54. Wu GW, Kobashigawa JA, Fishbein MC, et al. Asymptomatic antibody-mediated rejection after heart transplantation predicts poor outcomes. J Heart Lung Transplant 2009;28:417–22.

55. Boucek MM, Aurora P, Edwards LB, et al. Registry of the International Society for Heart and Lung Transplantation: tenth official pediatric heart transplantation report–2007. J Heart Lung Transplant 2007;26(8):796–807.

56. Pahl E, Naftel D, Canter C, et al. Death after rejection with severe hemodynamic compromise in pediatric heart transplant patients: a multi-institutional study. J Heart Lung Transplant 2001;20:279–87.

57. Webber SA, Naftel DC, Parker J, et al. Late rejection episodes more than 1 year after pediatric heart transplantation: risk factors and outcomes. J Heart Lung Transplant 2003;22:869–75.

58. Lammers AE, Roberts P, Brown K, et al. Acute rejection after pediatric heart transplantation: far less common and less severe. Transpl Int 2010;23:38–46.

59. Reed EF, Demetris AJ, Hammond E, et al. Acute antibody-mediated rejection of cardiac transplants. J Heart Lung Transplant 2006;25(2):153–9.

60. Rossano JW, Denfield SW, Kim JJ, et al. B-type natriuretic peptide is a sensitive screening test for acute rejection in pediatric heart transplant patients. J Heart Lung Transplant 2008;27:649–54.

61. Dodd DA, Cabo J, Dipchand AI. Acute rejection: natural history, risk factors, surveillance, and treatment. Chapter 9. In: Canter CE, Kirklin JK, editors. Pediatric heart transplantation, ISHLT Monograph Series, vol. 2. Philadelphia (PA): Elsevier; 2007. p. 139–56.

62. Valantine H. Cardiac allograft vasculopathy after heart transplantation: risk factors and management. J Heart Lung Transplant 2004;23:S187–93.

63. Pahl E, Naftel D, Kuhn M, et al. The incidence and impact of transplant coronary artery disease in pediatric recipients: a 9 year multi-institutional study. J Heart Lung Transplant 2005;24(6):645–51.

64. Shaddy RE, Revenaugh JA, Orsmond GS, et al. Coronary artery interventional procedures in pediatric heart transplant recipients with cardiac allograft vasculopathy. Am J Cardiol 2000;85:1370–2.

65. Dent C, Canter C, Hirsch R, et al. Transplant coronary artery disease in pediatric heart transplant recipients. J Heart Lung Transplant 2000;19(3):240–8.

66. Tham EB, Yeung AC, Cheng CW, et al. Experience of percutaneous coronary interventions in the management of pediatric cardiac allograft vasculopathy. J Heart Lung Transplant 2005;24(6):769–73.

67. Mahle WT, Vincent RN, Kanter KR. Cardiac retransplantation in childhood: analysis of data from the United Network for Organ Sharing. J Thorac Cardiovasc Surg 2005;130:542–6.

68. Chin C, Naftel D, Pahl E, et al. Cardiac re-transplantation in pediatrics: a multi-institutional study. J Heart Lung Transplant 2006;25:1420–4.

69. McDiarmid S. Death on the pediatric waiting list: scope of the problem. Paper presented at Summit on Organ Donation and Transplantation. San Antonio (TX), March 28–29, 2007.

70. Almond CS, Thiagarajan RR, Piercey GE, et al. Waiting list mortality among children listed for heart transplantation in the United States. Circulation 2009;119: 717–27.

71. Mah D, Singh TP, Thiagarajan RR, et al. Incidence and risk factors for mortality in infants awaiting heart transplantation in the USA. J Heart Lung Transplant 2009; 28:1292–8.

72. Dipchand AI, Naftel DC, Feingold B, et al. Outcomes of children with cardiomyopathy listed for transplant: a multi-institutional study. J Heart Lung Transplant 2009;28(12):1312–21.

73. Everitt MD, Donaldson AE, Casper C, et al. Effect of ABO-Incompatible listing on infant heart transplant waitlist outcomes: analysis of the United Network for Organ Sharing (UNOS) database. J Heart Lung Transplant 2009;28:1254–60.

74. Singh TP, Edwards LB, Kirk R, et al. Era effect on post-transplant survival adjusted for baseline risk factors in pediatric heart transplant recipients. J Heart Lung Transplant 2009;28:1285–91.

75. Schowengerdt KO, Naftel DC, Seib PM, et al. Infection after pediatric heart transplantation: results of a multiinstitutional study. J Heart Lung Transplant 1997;16:1207–16.

76. Bharat W, Manlhiot C, McCrindle BW, et al. The profile of renal function over time in a cohort of pediatric heart transplant recipients. Pediatr Transplant 2009;13(1):111–8.

77. Sachdeva R, Blaszak RT, Ainley KA. Determinants of renal function in pediatric heart transplant recipients: long-term follow-up study. J Heart Lung Transplant 2007;26:108–13.

78. Webber SA, Naftel DC, Fricker FJ, et al. Lymphoproliferative disorders after paediatric heart transplantation: a multi-institutional study. Lancet 2006;367:233–9.

79. Kulikowsa A, Boslaugh SE, Huddleston CB, et al. Infectious, malignant, and auto-immune complications in pediatric heart transplant recipients. J Pediatr 2008;152:671–7.

80. Mendonza F, Kunitake H, Laks H, et al. Post-transplant lymphoproliferative disorder following pediatric heart transplant. Pediatr Transplant 2006;10(1):60–6.

81. Ibrahim J, Canter C, Chinnock R, et al. Linear and somatic growth following pediatric heart transplantation. J Heart Lung Transplant 2002;21:63.

82. Peterson RE, Perens GS, Alejos JC, et al. Growth and weight gain of prepubertal children after cardiac transplantation. Pediatr Transplant 2008;12(4):436–41.

83. Trimm RF. Session VII: physiological and psychological growth and development in pediatric heart transplant recipients. J Heart Lung Transplant 1991;10:848–55.

84. Freier M, Babikian T, Pivonka J, et al. A longitudinal perspective on neurodevelop-mental outcome after infant cardiac transplantation. J Heart Lung Transplant 2004;23(7):857–64.

85. Ikle L, Hale K, Fashaw L, et al. Developmental outcome of patients with hypo-plastic left heart syndrome treated with heart transplantation. J Pediatr 2003;142(1):20–5.

86. Uzark K, Spicer R, Beebe DW. Neurodevelopmental outcomes in pediatric heart transplant recipients. J Heart Lung Transplant 2009;28:1306–11.

87. Uzark KC, Sauer SN, Lawrence KS, et al. The psychosocial impact of pediatric heart transplantation. J Heart Lung Transplant 1992;11:1160–7.

88. Wray J, Long T, Radley-Smith R, et al. Returning to school after heart or heart-lung transplantation: how well do children adjust? Transplantation 2001;72:100–6.

89. DeMaso DR, Twente AW, Spratt EG, et al. The impact of psychological func-tioning, medical severity, and family functioning in pediatric heart transplantation. J Heart Lung Transplant 1995;14:1102–8.

90. DeMaso DR, Kelley SD, Bastardi H, et al. The longitudinal impact of psycholog-ical functioning, medical severity, and family functioning in pediatric heart trans-plantation. J Heart Lung Transplant 2004;23(4):473–80.

91. Farley LM, DeMaso DR, D'Angelo E, et al. Parenting stress and parental post-traumatic stress disorder in families after pediatric heart transplantation. J Heart Lung Transplant 2007;26(2):120–6.

Pediatric Lung Transplantation

M. Solomon, MD, FRCPC[a,b],*, H. Grasemann, MD, PhD[a,b],
S. Keshavjee, MD, MSc, FRCSC[a,c]

KEYWORDS

- Lung transplantation • Pediatrics • Bronchiolitis obliterans
- Cystic fibrosis • Pulmonary hypertension

HISTORICAL NOTES

Compared with transplantation of other organs, lung transplantation is a young field that continues to grow. Lung transplantation is an important treatment option in children with acquired or congenital lung diseases. The first human lung transplantation was attempted in 1963 by Hardy, as reported in the *New England Journal of Medicine*,[1] but the world's first long-term successful lung transplantation was achieved in Toronto in 1983. Successful heart-lung transplantation and lung transplantation in adults during the early 1980s were followed by the application of lung transplantation in the pediatric population. The first reported pediatric lung transplant occurred in Toronto in 1987 in a 16-year-old boy with familial pulmonary fibrosis,[2] which, along with other early reports of success in children, led to an increased use of this procedure in children.

From 1986 to June 2008, 1278 pediatric lung transplant and 549 heart-lung transplant procedures were reported to the registry of the International Society of Heart & Lung Transplant (ISHLT).[3] The number of lung transplantations performed annually has varied between 20 and 87. In 2007, 93 pediatric lung transplant and 8 heart-lung transplant procedures were reported. To date, this is the highest number of pediatric lung transplants reported in a single year to this registry. According to the 2009 ISHLT Registry report, there are 36 centers worldwide that perform lung transplants in children. These numbers suggest that each center performs 2 to 3 transplants per year on average. In fact, 1 center reported 10 to 19 transplants per year, 3 centers reported 5 to 9 transplants per year, and the remainder performed 4 or fewer procedures annually.

[a] Toronto Lung Transplant Program
[b] Department of Pediatrics, Division of Respiratory Medicine and Transplant Centre, The Hospital for Sick Children, University of Toronto, 555 University Avenue, Toronto, ON M5G 1X8, Canada
[c] Division of Thoracic Surgery, Toronto General Hospital, 200 Elizabeth Street, 9N-946, Toronto, ON M5G 2C4, Canada
* Corresponding author. Department of Pediatrics, Division of Respiratory Medicine and Transplant Centre, The Hospital for Sick Children, University of Toronto, 555 University Avenue, Toronto, ON M5G 1X8, Canada.
E-mail address: melinda.solomon@sickkids.ca

Pediatr Clin N Am 57 (2010) 375–391
doi:10.1016/j.pcl.2010.01.017
0031-3955/10/$ – see front matter Crown Copyright © 2010 Published by Elsevier Inc. All rights reserved.

The overall number of heart-lung transplant procedures has decreased in recent years because of the recognition that isolated lung transplantation or isolated heart transplantation can be used in many conditions once believed to require combined heart-lung transplantation, such as primary pulmonary hypertension (PPH). Even severe right-sided ventricular dysfunction will generally recover when the right ventricle is unloaded after lung transplant. Presently heart-lung transplantation is indicated only in patients with end-stage heart and lung failure or for complex congenital heart and lung disease. Heart-lung transplants are uncommonly performed in North America and are now concentrated in only a few centers. The number of infant lung transplants remains low at less than 10 procedures per year since 1997, with most being performed in the United States. In addition, the number of living donor procedures in pediatric recipients has markedly decreased, with only 3 procedures reported from 2005 to 2007. The numbers of this procedure were highest in 1998 and 1999 when 14 cases were reported per year.[3]

This article describes the current status of pediatric lung transplantation, indications for listing, evaluation of recipient and donor, updates on the operative procedure and graft dysfunction, and the risk factors, outcomes, and future directions.

INDICATIONS FOR LISTING

Lung transplantation in children should be considered in carefully selected patients only. Progressive lung disease or life-threatening pulmonary vascular disease for which there is no further medical therapy are indications for lung transplantation. The indications for transplantation in childhood differ by age group.[4]

A summary of the underlying diagnoses for which lung transplantation may be indicated in children is presented in **Fig. 1**. Most pediatric patients (~60%) receiving a

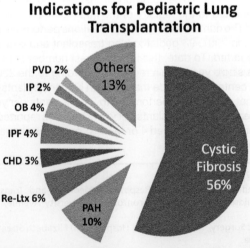

Indications for Pediatric Lung Transplantation

PVD 2%
IP 2%
OB 4%
IPF 4%
CHD 3%
Re-Ltx 6%
PAH 10%
Others 13%
Cystic Fibrosis 56%

Fig. 1. Indications for pediatric lung transplantation according to the ISHLT Registry data. CHD, congenital heart diseases; IP, interstitial pneumonitis; IPF, idiopathic pulmonary fibrosis; OB, obliterative bronchiolitis (not re-transplant); PAH, pulmonary arterial hypertension; PVD, pulmonary vascular disease; Re-Ltx, repeat lung transplant. (*Data from* Aurora P, Edwards LB, Christie JD, et al. Registry of the international society for heart and lung transplantation: twelfth official pediatric lung and heart/lung transplantation report-2009. J Heart Lung Transplant 2009;28(10):1023–30.)

lung transplant are patients with severe advanced cystic fibrosis (CF) lung disease, although the number of transplants for this indication is decreasing. Other indications within the pediatric age range include pulmonary hypertension, obliterative bronchiolitis (OB; retransplant or nontransplant related), interstitial lung disease, and congenital heart disease. Less common indications in children include Eisenmenger syndrome, pulmonary fibrosis, and bronchiectasis.[3]

Indications for lung transplantation in infants include primary and secondary pulmonary hypertension, congenital heart disease (such as tetralogy of Fallot with absent pulmonary valves), primary pulmonary vascular conditions (pulmonary vein stenosis or alveolar capillary dysplasia), bronchopulmonary dysplasia, and surfactant B deficiency.[5] Infants with other surfactant disorders, such as surfactant protein C deficiency[6] and disorders of the ABCA3 transporter,[7] can also potentially benefit from lung transplantation.

In contrast, most adults are transplanted for chronic obstructive pulmonary disease (COPD) (36%) and idiopathic pulmonary fibrosis (21%), and approximately 16% for CF.[8] According to the American Society of Transplantation consensus statement,[4] regardless of diagnosis, all lung transplant candidates should possess:

1. A clear diagnosis or adequately delineated trajectory of illness despite optimal medical therapy that puts the individual child at risk of dying without a lung transplant
2. An adequate array of family support personnel
3. Adequate access to transplant services and medications after transplantation
4. Adequate evidence of willingness and ability on the part of patient and parent to adhere to the rigorous therapy, daily monitoring, and re-evaluation schedule after transplant.

Contraindications for lung transplantation are similar for adults and children. They include active malignancy, active sepsis, active tuberculosis, severe neuromuscular disease, refractory nonadherence, multiple organ dysfunction, human immunodeficiency virus (HIV), and hepatitis C infection with histologic liver disease. There is also a list of relative contraindications including issues such as chronic airway infection with multiply resistant organisms, mechanical ventilation, and renal insufficiency.[4] This list varies from center to center and will change over time.

In most centers airway colonization with *Burkholderia cepacia* is considered an absolute contraindication, specifically with *Burkholderia cenocepacia* (genomovar III). However, a few centers, such as Toronto, are successfully transplanting CF patients infected with this organism. Several centers reported increased early posttransplant morbidity and mortality due to *B cepacia* in the 1990s[9,10] with genomovar III–positive recipients being at the highest risk.[11,12] However, more recent data show that the risk for poor transplant outcome varies between *Burkholderia* species and this should be taken into account during the assessment of candidates. A recent study in the United States using multivariate Cox survival models to assess hazard ratios of infection with *Burkholderia* species found no significant difference in survival based on *Burkholderia* infection status in CF patients on the waiting list for lung transplantation. However, infection with the nonepidemic strain of *B cenocepacia* resulted in a significantly increased risk of posttransplant mortality compared with uninfected control subjects.[13] It has also been shown that *B cenocepacia* strain E12, which is more common in Canada and the United Kingdom, results in increased mortality in CF patients, with and without lung transplantation.[12,14,15] Patients with *Burkholderia gladioli* were also found to have an increased posttransplant mortality risk, whereas there was no increased risk for CF patients infected with *Burkholderia multivorans*.[13] This is not to say that poor outcomes have not been reported in patients with *B multivorans*.

The Toronto Group continues to be the center with the largest *B cepacia complex* experience in CF patients in the world and, with the use of a strategy of multiple antibiotic synergy testing, triple antibiotics, and regimens including reduced immunosuppressive drug level targets after transplantation, hopefully it will continue to decrease the post-transplant morbidity and mortality in this high-risk group of lung transplant recipients.

EVALUATION OF RECIPIENT AND DONOR
Evaluation of the Lung Donor

Donors are selected on the basis of medical history, chest radiographs, oxygenation, bronchoscopy findings, and intraoperative evaluation. The ISHLT criteria for ideal lung donors are: age less than 55 years; smoking history of less than 20 pack-years; no chest trauma; duration of mechanical ventilation less than 48 hours; no history of asthma; no history of cancer; negative Gram stain on bronchoalveolar lavage (BAL); arterial partial pressure of oxygen greater than 300 mm Hg on positive end-expiratory pressure of 5 cm H_2O and inspired oxygen 100%; clear chest radiograph; and clear bronchoscopy. It is recognized that few donors meet all these criteria to be defined as ideal and, when these criteria are not met, potential donors are then classified as extended donors.

Several factors may lead to the unsuitability of lungs for transplantation. These include significant pulmonary contusion, pneumonia, pulmonary aspiration, and pulmonary edema.[16] Because many donors sustain severe brain injuries via blunt trauma, chest trauma can lead to pulmonary contusions. Obviously the term "significant pulmonary contusion" allows judgment by the transplant surgeon. Fat embolisms can be a complicating factor as reperfusion of the embolized lung may lead to activation of a cascade of inflammation, which can lead to major graft dysfunction early after transplant. A retrograde flush with preservation solution via the pulmonary veins following the initial instillation of preservation solution into the main pulmonary artery can potentially be performed to flush out pulmonary emboli. Protective ventilation strategies are used to recruit collapsed alveoli. Pulmonary edema (neurogenic and other types), often a significant problem in brain-dead donors, can be improved by active fluid management of the multiorgan donor to maintain euvolemia.[16]

The evaluation of donor lungs is standardized. A complete general clinical evaluation of the donor is performed that includes an assessment for blunt trauma, a chest radiograph, and review of the ventilator settings. Flexible bronchoscopy is performed to assess for aspiration and pneumonia, and to acquire a bronchial wash to be sent for microbiology cultures and to evaluate for anatomic abnormalities of the airways. As stated earlier, the ideal donor has a Pao_2/Fio_2 ratio greater than 300 mm Hg and has minimal, if any, lung infiltrates. The lungs, once harvested, are preserved using a standardized protocol using Perfadex cold flush preservation before implantation.

Evaluation of Recipients

The assessment is performed to determine a patient's suitability for lung transplantation and therefore is an in-depth review. There is a standard list of investigations and consultations that needs to be completed.[17] Additional investigations may be added for specific underlying diagnoses or on an individualized basis. For instance, an abdominal ultrasound or a computerized tomography (CT) scan of the sinuses may be added to assess a patient with CF. The assessment includes laboratory tests:

ABO group, hematology and biochemistry, viral serology (HIV, hepatitis B surface antigen/antibody/core antibody, hepatitis C antibody, cytomegalovirus [CMV], Epstein-Barr virus [EBV], varicella, toxoplasma, antibodies to childhood immunizations), urinalysis, sputum cultures including sensitivities/mycobacteria/fungus, tuberculin skin test, measurement of bone mineral density, a chest radiograph, CT scan of chest and neck, quantitative ventilation-perfusion scan, complete pulmonary function tests, 6-minute walk test, electrocardiogram, and cardiac echo. In addition, the assessment should include consultations from the transplant respirologist, transplant surgeon, nurse transplant coordinator, dietician, social worker, pharmacist, anesthetist, psychiatrist, and possibly infectious disease and cardiology consultants.

TRANSPLANT SURGERY

Technically, lung and heart-lung transplant procedures in children are essentially the same as in adults.[18,19] However, there is significantly more frequent use of cardiopulmonary bypass (CPB) in children. Although most adult bilateral lung transplant procedures can be performed as sequential single lung transplants using isolated lung ventilation through a double-lumen endotracheal tube, these tubes are often not available for smaller pediatric sizes, thus most pediatric transplants in younger or smaller children are performed on CPB. In addition, all patients with pulmonary hypertension are usually done on CPB. In the Toronto Program only 44% of transplants are done on CPB, but in the pediatric age group (<18 years), most are done on CPB. The use of CPB is essential in some cases, particularly in pulmonary hypertension and in hemodynamically unstable patients. Disadvantages of using CPB include heparinization with increased risk of bleeding and increased blood product use, coagulopathy, red blood cell trauma, activation of complement, neutrophil activation, and a systemic inflammatory response that may contribute to allograft injury at reperfusion. The use of CPB has been associated with increased risks of bleeding and early graft dysfunction.

Bilateral Lung Transplant

The most common pediatric lung transplant procedure currently performed is the bilateral sequential lung transplant. In this procedure each lung is sequentially implanted separately. The pulmonary artery and veins to that lung are divided. The native lung with the least perfusion is excised first. The bronchial anastomosis is performed first. Usually an end-to-end anastomosis is performed using an absorbable running suture for the membranous wall and interrupted absorbable sutures for the cartilaginous wall (polydioxone suture). Telescoping is done only if the discrepancy is severe. Next, the anastomosis of the main pulmonary artery is completed followed by the atrial anastomosis, which approximates a cuff of donor left atrium surrounding the 2 pulmonary veins to the recipient left atrium. The transplanted lung is then gently reinflated and ventilated. Reperfusion occurs slowly as the pulmonary artery clamp is released gradually over 10-minute period. The procedure is then repeated on the contralateral side. If the donor lungs are larger than required, options include performing lobar transplants (ie, right lower lobe and left lower lobe) or performing a wedge resection using a linear staple. In the Toronto center, 15% of the pediatric transplant patients have received lobar transplants.

Single Lung Transplant

This procedure is most commonly used in the adult population. Single lung transplants are rarely performed in children because most underlying diagnoses indicate bilateral lung transplantation, such as CF or pulmonary hypertension. Single lung transplantation may occasionally be a consideration in unique situations such as when the patient has had a previous pneumonectomy.

Living Related Donor Lung Transplant

This procedure was initiated in 1993 due to the higher demand than supply for patients waiting for a lung transplant, along with a scarcity of deceased donor organs. A living related donor lung transplant (LDLT) requires 2 living donors to each undergo 1 lower lobectomy. A right lower lobe is removed from 1 donor and a left lower lobe from the other. These lobes are then implanted into the recipient in place of the whole right and left lung, respectively. The most common indication for LDLT in North America is CF, with retransplantation being second.[20] It is well suited for children because the donors must be bigger than the recipients. However, the procedure is limited in younger/smaller children because of the size mismatch between adult donor lobes and the pediatric thorax. The most important surgical difference between LDLT and deceased donor lung transplant (DDLT) is that a single pulmonary vein drains the donor lobe, as a cuff of donor left atrium is not harvested from the living donor (as described earlier), thus there is an end-to-end anastomosis of 1 living donor's pulmonary vein and 1 recipient pulmonary vein for each side.[21]

Donor evaluations and care are provided by physicians who are independent of the pediatric lung transplant team. The advantages of this procedure include a planned operating room time, a shorter ischemic time, and an increase in the pool of donor organs. There is also an increased risk of the donor lung being undersized for the chest cavity.

Published results after 10 years of experience that included 39 pediatric lung transplant recipients found no difference in the actuarial survival between adults and pediatric recipients of LDLT, despite this being a sicker cohort with greater than 50% of the recipients being hospital bound and 18% being ventilator-dependent at the time of the procedure. Infection was the predominant cause of death in this patient group.[22]

Donor outcomes have been published with no reported deaths. However, major complications have included pleural effusion, bronchial stump fistula, bilobectomy, hemorrhage phrenic nerve injury, pulmonary artery thrombosis, bronchial stricture, and persistent air leak. Minor complications include persistent air leak, arrhythmia, and pneumonia.[23,24]

Clearly, deceased donor lung transplantation is the preferred option wherever possible to avoid the risk to 2 healthy donors. However, LDLT is an acceptable alternative when the recipient is not likely to survive long enough to receive deceased donor organs. With the improved lung allocation system (LAS) in the United States, sicker patients are now being appropriately allocated donor organs and the number of LDLTs performed has dropped drastically.

COMPLICATIONS

Posttransplant complications can be categorized into 3 phases: immediate phase, which includes the first few days after transplant; the early phase, which includes the first 3 months; and the late phase, which includes the period after the first 3 months.

Immediate Phase Complications

These include hyperacute rejection, primary graft dysfunction (PGD), ischemia-reperfusion injury, surgical complications, and infections.

Hyperacute rejection

This complication is as a result of circulating preformed recipient serum antibodies that bind to donor tissue antigens and cause complement-mediated graft injury. Endothelial cells lining the blood vessels of the new organ are the principal targets. Preformed antibodies that are generally attributed to prior blood transfusions, a previous transplant, or pregnancy, may be directed at HLA or endothelial antigens. True hyperacute rejection is rare, but when severe, can result in early graft failure. To evaluate the risk for this complication, testing for panel reactive antibodies (PRA) is performed during the assessment process. PRAs include a mix of 60 to 100 different samples that express a wide range of antigens tested with the recipient serum. The percentage of the cell samples to which the serum binds in the panel is reported. Other more sensitive methodologies include flow cytometer and beads coated with purified major histocompatibility complex (MHC) antigens rather than cells. For patients with positive PRAs, a virtual crossmatch can be done before transplant, followed by an actual crossmatch at the time of the transplant using donor leukocytes. If there is a positive actual crossmatch, the recipient is treated with intraoperative and postoperative plasmapheresis and thymoglobulin followed by intravenous immunoglobulins.

Primary graft dysfunction

PGD represents a severe form of acute injury to the allograft with clinical, radiographic, and histologic features similar to those of acute respiratory distress syndrome. PGD is characterized by patchy pulmonary infiltrates, a low ratio of arterial oxygen to the fraction of inspired oxygen, diminished lung compliance, and pathologic findings of diffuse alveolar damage.[25]

PGD is the end result of a series of hits occurring from the time of brain death to lung reperfusion after transplant. Although it is recognized that ischemic reperfusion injury is a major contributor to PGD, it is clearly part of a multifactorial/multihit injury process. Other injuries occurring in the donor before the retrieval process and during lung preservation can contribute to and amplify the manifestations of PGD. Thus it is important that attention be paid to the assessment of donor lungs, effective technique of lung preservation, and careful management of transplanted lungs after reperfusion, to reduce the severity of ischemic reperfusion injury and the incidence of PGD.[26]

Several studies have found that PPH is a recipient risk factor independently associated with the development of PGD.[27–29] This may be because patients with PPH, compared with other causes of pulmonary hypertension, are different in chronicity and degree of right ventricular morphologic changes and have more severe cardiac dysfunction. Secondary pulmonary hypertension has also been implicated as a potential risk factor for PGD, but the strongest and most clearly established recipient risk factor remains the diagnosis of PPH. Other reports showed a link between early PGD and subsequent development of bronchiolitis obliterans syndrome (BOS).[30] It was further suggested that PGD may contribute to nearly half of the short-term mortality after lung transplantation.[31] Survivors of PGD even have increased risk of death extending beyond the first posttransplant year. Christie and colleagues[31] found that the relationship of PGD with mortality among 1-year survivors was remarkable, with a relative increase in the risk of mortality in the next 4 years. Suggested reasons for these finding were a lingering effect after prolonged critical illness or the potential for increased immunogenicity of the allograft as a sequel of earlier severe lung injury.[31]

It is important to continue the search for a better understanding of risk factors and of ways to prevent PGD as it remains not only a major cause of early death after lung transplant but also increases risk of mortality among patients who survive at least 1 year after PGD. Treatment includes supportive care, such as mechanical ventilation, and pharmacologic interventions, such as PGE$_1$[32] or nitric oxide,[33] and, in severe cases, extracorporeal membrane oxygenation (ECMO) has been used with success.

Ischemia reperfusion injury

Ischemia-reperfusion induced lung injury continues to be a frequent complication of lung transplantation within the first few days after the procedure. As mentioned earlier, it is a significant contributor to the PGD, which is characterized by nonspecific alveolar damage, lung edema, and hypoxemia occurring within 72 hours after transplant.[26] The clinical spectrum can range from mild hypoxemia associated with a few infiltrates on chest radiograph to a clinical scenario similar to severe respiratory distress syndrome requiring positive-pressure ventilation, pharmacologic therapy, and occasionally even ECMO.[27] Furthermore, it has been recognized that, if this injury is severe, it can lead to an increased risk of acute rejection that could ultimately result in significant graft dysfunction in the long-term.[34] Whether severe ischemia-reperfusion injury increases the risk of chronic rejection remains controversial because some studies have found that there is a relationship[34] and others have not.[35]

Many strategies to prevent lung dysfunction have been studied and used, including optimization of the lung preservation solution,[36,37] and optimizing of volume, pressure, and temperature of the flush solution. In addition, a retrograde flush has been found to have added benefit. Low reperfusion pressure and a protective ventilation strategy during the early reperfusion phase may also decrease lung dysfunction. In established ischemic reperfusion injury, inhaled nitric oxide has been used as it can improve ventilation-perfusion mismatch and decrease pulmonary artery pressures without affecting systemic pressures. Further treatments include supportive care, such as mechanical ventilation, and ECMO in severe cases.[26] Overall, this injury continues to be a significant cause of morbidity and mortality after lung transplantation and further work on its prevention and treatment will decrease its effect on survival and graft function.

Surgical Complications

Surgical complications include postoperative bleeding or airway anastomotic complications, phrenic nerve injury, chylothorax, and wound infection.

Airway complications

Airway complications include dehiscence or stenosis of the airway anastomosis. Pediatric airways are different from adult airways in that they are smaller and have bronchial cartilage that has a higher compliance. However, reports from the mid-1990s in adults showed the rates of airway complications to be between 9% and 15% of the anastomoses at risk, with a related mortality of 2% to 3%,[38,39] and similar rates have been reported in pediatrics.[40] More recently, Meyers and colleagues[41] reported that the frequency of treated airway complications did not differ between adults and children (9% vs 11%). Narrowing at the level of the suture line continues to be seen in a small number of patients. The clinical presentation includes wheezing, along with an obstructive pattern on spirometry and occasionally a biphasic flow volume loop.[4] Airway anastomotic narrowing can be treated with rigid bronchoscopic or balloon dilatation of the affected region. Balloon dilatation can be less traumatic and provide more accurate dilatation of the stenotic segment than rigid bronchoscopy dilatations. Stents are generally avoided in children with potential for airway growth, are difficult to remove, and can cause problems with exuberant granulation tissue growing through the wire mesh. In infants, significant airway malacia can occur, and one option is early tracheostomy to allow weaning from mechanical ventilation over weeks. In one study, independent predictors for airway complications in children included preoperative *B cepacia*, postoperative fungal lung infection as well as days on mechanical ventilation.[40] Although airway complications can be a significant cause of morbidity, most are successfully treated and patient outcomes are generally not adversely affected.

Infection

The risk of infection continues throughout all posttransplant phases but, because of the higher level of immunosuppression used in the first month after transplant and the use of induction agents in some centers, it is higher early after transplant. Prophylactic antibiotics are generally given in the perioperative period. The choice of antibiotics is initially based on known recipient organisms and can be adjusted once donor bronchial lavage culture results are available. In the absence of known recipient lower respiratory tract organisms, prophylaxis is given according to center-specific lung transplant antibiotic prophylaxis protocols that may include cefuroxime or piperacillin-tazocin.

Early Complications

Complications that occur during the early phase (first 3 months) after transplant include acute rejection, infection, airway complications, and medication side effects.

Acute rejection

Acute cellular rejection, which is T cell mediated, is common in the first year after lung transplantation, especially during the first 3 months. Diagnosing acute rejection in the lung allograft is more difficult than in other solid-organ transplants. The problem is that the presentation of rejection can be similar to that of infection. The histopathologic diagnosis is also not always accurate in the acute rejection of the lung. Often the diagnosis is made on clinical suspicion based on a constellation of symptoms and signs, and confirmed by the response to therapy. Early acute rejection episodes can present with fever, chills, malaise, increased chest tightness, cough, and dyspnea. Physical examination may reveal crackles on auscultation and/or evidence of pleural effusion, with radiograph illustrating interstitial infiltrates with or without a pleural effusion. With later rejection episodes the patient may be asymptomatic, or present with deterioration in pulmonary function tests with a decrease in FEV_1 (forced expiratory volume in the first second of expiration) revealing airflow limitation. In principle, a 10% drop from baseline FEV_1 is considered significant. If the rejection episode is more severe, the patient can present with dyspnea and hypoxia and infiltrates on chest radiograph.

In our and other centers, routine monitoring for acute rejection episodes is performed through daily home spirometry, regular pulmonary function testing, chest radiographs, and routine surveillance transbronchial lung biopsies at 2 and 6 weeks, and 3, 6, 9 and 12 months after transplant. Transbronchial lung biopsies have been the mainstay of lung allograft evaluation. The ISHLT consensus paper[42] continues to advocate for at least 5 biopsy pieces of well-expanded lung parenchyma required for an assessment of acute rejection. The bronchoscopist may need to obtain more than 5 biopsy samples to provide the minimum of adequate tissue for evaluation. Generally, transbronchial biopsies are taken from 2 lobes of 1 lung because rejection may be patchy and multiple biopsies from different lobes increases the chance of picking up rejection. It has been shown that infants and toddlers have a lower incidence of acute rejection compared with older children.[43]

A pathologic diagnosis of acute cellular rejection is based on the presence of perivascular and interstitial mononuclear cell infiltrates in the lung biopsy samples. The distribution of the mononuclear cells, including extension beyond the vascular adventitia into adjacent alveolar septa, forms the basis of the histologic grade.[42] Acute rejection may be accompanied by subendothelial infiltration and also by lymphocytic bronchitis and bronchiolitis. Grading for acute pulmonary allograft rejection according to the ISHLT classification includes grade 0 to 4, with A0 being no acute rejection, A1 minimal, A2 mild, A3 moderate, and A4 severe acute rejection. The categories of small airways involvement (ie, lymphocytic bronchiolitis) are problematic as these B grades were shown to have significant problems with inter- and intraobserver variability. New recommendations are needed to improve reproducibility. It is unclear to what extent humoral rejection, which is antibody mediated, occurs among lung transplant recipients.

Methylprednisolone pulse at 10 mg/kg/dose daily for 3 days followed by augmented oral prednisone is the treatment of acute cellular rejection. Overall, the response to this treatment, if the diagnosis is correct, is quick, with improvement of symptoms and pulmonary function test results over several days. Treatment options for humoral rejection include plasmapheresis for antibody removal and immunoglobulin infusion.

Infection
With the high-dose triple immunosuppression used, the risk of infection is high. Infections occur in 60% to 90% of recipients. Similar to other ventilated patients, lung transplant recipients are at risk for ventilator-associated infections but also for other lower respiratory tract infections. The clinical dilemma is often whether a presentation with hypoxia, increased white blood cell count, and infiltrates on chest radiograph with or without fever is related to infection or acute allograft rejection. For a definitive diagnosis, a bronchoscopy and BAL, with or without transbronchial biopsies, is performed. If bacterial infection is found, antibiotic treatment is based on the organisms and their sensitivities. Inhaled antibiotics are an alternative or adjunctive strategy to systemic antibiotic treatment, for instance in *Pseudomonas* lung infection. Cotrimoxazole prophylaxis is used to prevent *Pneumocystis jiroveci* pneumonia.

Viral infections
Early-phase respiratory viral infections can have a significant effect on morbidity and mortality. A study evaluating respiratory viral infections within 1 year after lung transplantation in children found that the most frequently documented viral pathogens were adenovirus, rhinovirus, respiratory syncytial virus, and parainfluenza virus, and that respiratory viral infections occurred in 14% of subjects in their cohort with seasonal variation.[44] Subjects with respiratory viral infections during the first hospitalization for transplantation had an increased risk of death or retransplantation within 1 year compared with all subjects and with those who had infections after their initial hospitalization.

Cytomegalovirus
CMV after lung transplantation remains a serious infectious complication, especially in CMV-negative recipients receiving CMV-positive donor lungs (ie, mismatch). Pediatric patients are at increased risk for mismatch because they are more likely to be CMV negative. The incidence of CMV episodes in a recent multicenter retrospective study of pediatric lung transplant recipients was 30%,[45] which is similar to a previous study.[46] CMV infection/disease was found to be associated with increased mortality after pediatric lung transplantation. CMV disease most commonly includes pneumonitis, but can also involve the liver, small bowel, and retina. The use of prophylactic treatment with antiviral drugs such as ganciclovir/valganciclovir has a significant effect on CMV infection and disease.[47] The approach to prophylaxis/treatment varies between centers, as do the means of diagnosis and surveillance. The optimal duration

of prophylaxis is uncertain. Surveillance using quantitative polymerase chain reaction to measure viral load in the blood is most common, and increased risk for CMV infection clearly exists after prophylaxis is stopped, so diligent, regular surveillance for early CMV detection is essential. Preemptive therapy with ganciclovir/valganciclovir may be warranted if significant increases in serum EBV titers occur.

Fungal infections
Antifungal prophylaxis after lung transplantation is used in most pediatric centers. Itraconazole or voriconazole are most commonly used, and nebulized amphotericin B is another option. Fungal infections are common in pediatric lung recipients and a recent retrospective, multicenter study revealed a prevalence of 10.5%[48] and found that pulmonary fungal infections were independently associated with a decreased 12-month posttransplant survival.

Medication side effects
Most pediatric lung transplant recipients remain on triple immunosuppression that typically includes a calcineurin inhibitor (cyclosporine or tacrolimus), an antimetabolite (azathioprine or mycophenolate mofetil) and systemic steroids as maintenance therapy. Complications associated with these medications include hypertension, diabetes (most commonly in recipients with CF), renal dysfunction, and neurologic complications such as seizures, which are typically related to calcineurin inhibitor use. The seizures are believed to be due to cerebral vasoconstriction and the resultant cerebral ischemia. According to the 2009 ISHLT Registry report on lung transplantation, the prevalence of hypertension is 43%, renal dysfunction 10.5%, and diabetes 27% at 1 year, and within 5 years these numbers increase to 69%, 22%, and 33%, respectively.[3]

Late Complications

Complications that occur during the late posttransplant phase include BOS, renal dysfunction, and malignancy.

BOS
Despite the improvements in outcome that have been made in lung transplantation in recent years, progressive airways obstruction and graft dysfunction still develop frequently. Chronic allograft dysfunction is clinically known as BOS, and is defined as a progressive decline in FEV_1 in the absence of other acute events such as rejection or infection. OB is a chronic graft dysfunction process that is histologically characterized by fibroproliferative tissue remodeling with excessive amounts of extracellular matrix deposition resulting in small airway occlusion with sparing of the alveoli and interstitium.[49] The cause of this process remains elusive.

The prevalence of BOS increases with time after transplant. The ISHLT Registry reports a prevalence of 14% within 1 year and approximately 50% within 5 years.[3] The prevalence of BOS in adult lung transplant recipients was 28% by 2.5 years, 51% by 5 years, and 74% by 10 years.[8] There is evidence that infants/toddlers may have a lower risk for the development of OB.[43]

The onset of BOS is insidious, with gradual progressive exertional dyspnea. Patients can also present with a viral-like illness with an acute or subacute cough associated with a wheeze. Treatment with bronchodilators produces no significant response. Auscultation of the lung can be normal or reveal fine crackles with or without a wheeze. The pattern of BOS progression varies. Generally, once established OB/BOS is progressive and results in severe airway obstruction and gradual respiratory failure, but progression may also plateau. Chest radiographs can be normal except for mild hyperinflation. However, high-resolution CT scans often show a mosaic pattern that is most prominent on expiratory views. This pattern is consistent with variable air trapping in various lung zones/areas. Pulmonary function test results are particularly characterized by an irreversible decrease in FEV_1 and FEF_{25-75} (forced expiratory flow between 25% and 75% of forced vital capacity) due to airway obstruction.

The diagnosis of OB may be made by transbronchial lung biopsies, but, because OB is often patchy in distribution, it can be difficult to diagnose simply by pathology. Because of the low sensitivity and specificity of transbronchial biopsies,[50,51] the BOS clinical criteria were created (**Table 1**).[52] The measurement of exhaled nitric oxide may also be useful for the evaluation of BOS, but currently no published data are available for pediatric lung transplant recipients.

The cause of chronic allograft dysfunction remains unclear, but several risk factors have been noted, including immunologic and nonimmunologic factors. Late or recurrent refractory acute rejection and lymphocytic bronchiolitis seem to be the most convincing factors.[53] Glanville and colleagues[54] found in a large cohort that severity of lymphocytic bronchiolitis detected on transbronchial biopsies was the most significant risk factor for the development of BOS. There is also evidence that CMV may be associated with BOS pathogenesis, and perhaps prolonged antiviral prophylaxis could decrease CMV infection rate and the occurrence of BOS.[55] Other risk factors include the ages of donor and recipient, ischemia reperfusion injury, HLA mismatches, infection, and gastroesophageal reflux with aspiration.

Effective treatment of BOS is extremely limited. Stabilization can sometimes be achieved by changes in immunosuppression, such as switching cyclosporine to tacrolimus.[56] This change has arrested the FEV_1 decline in 50% to 90% of patients with better results if the change was done early. Similar findings were noted with the switch from azathioprine to mycophenolate mofetil. Other medications that have been attempted include pulse steroids, methotrexate,[57] cyclophosphamide,[58] cytolytic therapy,[59] inhaled cyclosporine,[60] total lymphoid irradiation,[61] and photophoresis.[62,63] However, despite this extensive list of potential strategies, treatment success has been fairly limited and improvement of lung function is uncommon, probably because the fibroproliferative process is not reversible. Azithromycin and other macrolides seem to have some role in treatment. In one study, 3 months of treatment with azithromycin were associated with protection from disease progression (as measured by an increase in FEV_1 of 10% or more after 3 months of treatment) and death.[64]

Because children less than 5 years of age are often unable to perform pulmonary function tests (PFTs), making the diagnosis based on the FEV_1 criteria alone can be difficult in this age range. Infant PFT machines exist, but as these measure $FEV_{0.5}$ the classic BOS criteria cannot be used. However, it is recommended that declines

Table 1 Classification of BOS	
Stage	**Spirometry Result**
BOS 0	$FEV_1 > 90\%$ of baseline and $FEF_{25-75} > 75\%$ of baseline
BOS 0-p	FEV_1 81%–90% of baseline or $FEF_{25-75} \leq$ of baseline
BOS 1	FEV_1 66%–80% of baseline
BOS 2	FEV_1 51%–65% of baseline
BOS 3	FEV_1 50% or less of baseline

Abbreviations: FEF_{25-75}, mid-expiratory flow rates; FEV_1, forced expiratory volume in 1 second; p, potential.

in lung function be expressed as percent of predicted volumes instead of absolute volumes for BOS scores, because of lung and airway growth.[5,52]

Renal dysfunction

Chronic renal insufficiency is common in pediatric lung transplant recipients, with a prevalence of 10% at 1 year, 23% at 5 years, and 35% at 7 years after transplant.[3] Glomerular filtration rate (GFR) is often used to measure renal function. A single-center study revealed that renal function declined by 33% within 3 months after transplant, and advanced chronic kidney disease occurred in almost half of the patients studied after a median of 23 months.[65] It is clear that many children have a decline in renal function due to the effects of calcineurin inhibitor and other nephrotoxic drugs.

Malignancy

The incidence of malignancies increases with time after transplant with EBV-related posttransplant lymphoproliferative disease (PTLD) being the most common. Among other factors, this is presumably because children are more likely than adults to be naïve to EBV infection before transplant. Therapy for PTLD includes empiric reduction in immunosuppression antiviral drugs, monoclonal antibodies specifically targeting the B-lymphocyte antigen CD20 (eg, rituximab), or chemotherapy, when appropriate.[66,67]

OUTCOME

Survival after lung transplantation is similar in children and adult recipients, and has improved in recent years. Children transplanted between 2002 and 2007 had a 1-year survival of 83% and a 4-year survival of 50%.[3] Outcome seems better in children aged less than 12 years at transplant than in adolescents, but, nevertheless, survival after lung transplantation in general is worse than with other pediatric solid organ transplantation. However, it is evident that equivalent or better outcomes can be achieved in select high-volume experienced centers.

BOS accounts for more than 40% of deaths by 5 years after transplant, whereas early deaths are caused by infectious complications and graft failure.[3] The functional status of most long-term survivors is good, with 84% of 5-year survivors reporting no limitations in activity.

SUMMARY

Lung transplantation remains an accepted therapy for selected pediatric patients with severe end-stage vascular or parenchymal lung disease. Once discharged from the hospital, collaboration between the patients' primary care physicians and the lung transplant team is essential for long-term follow-up. The roles of the primary care physicians include general aspects of pediatric care, from completing immunizations to assessment and management of acute illnesses, such as respiratory infections or fevers. Awareness of complications specific to the immunocompromised organ recipient include consideration of CMV, EBV, or opportunistic infections, the presence of PTLD, or other complications. Live vaccines are contraindicated after transplant, and some antibiotics can significantly alter the blood levels of the immunosuppressive medications. Primary care physicians and the lung transplant team need to work in a partnership with these patients and their families. The transplant team and specialized center continue to follow these patients for posttransplant-specific surveillance of the allograft function and other organ systems.

Lung transplantation in children with otherwise untreatable respiratory failure can result in improved survival and significantly increased quality of life. The challenges of this treatment include the limited availability of suitable donor organs, the toxicity of immunosuppressive medications needed to prevent rejection, the prevention and treatment of OB, as well as maximizing growth, development, and quality of life of the recipients.

REFERENCES

1. Hardy JD, Webb WR, Dalton ML Jr, et al. Lung homotransplantations in man. JAMA 1963;186:1065–74.
2. Mendeloff EN. The history of pediatric heart and lung transplantation. Pediatr Transplant 2002;6(4):270–9.
3. Aurora P, Edwards LB, Christie JD, et al. Registry of the International Society for Heart and Lung Transplantation: twelfth official pediatric lung and heart/lung transplantation report-2009. J Heart Lung Transplant 2009;28(10):1023–30.
4. Faro A, Mallory GB, Visner GA, et al. American Society of Transplantation executive summary on pediatric lung transplantation. Am J Transplant 2007;7(2):285–92.
5. Sweet SC. Pediatric lung transplantation. Proc Am Thorac Soc 2009;6(1):122–7.
6. Nogee LM, Dunbar AE 3rd, Wert SE, et al. A mutation in the surfactant protein C gene associated with familial interstitial lung disease. N Engl J Med 2001;344(8):573–9.
7. Shulenin S, Nogee LM, Annilo T, et al. ABCA3 gene mutations in newborns with fatal surfactant deficiency. N Engl J Med 2004;350(13):1296–303.
8. Christie JD, Edwards LB, Aurora P, et al. The Registry of the International Society for Heart and Lung Transplantation: twenty-sixth official adult lung and heart-lung transplantation report-2009. J Heart Lung Transplant 2009;28(10):1031–49.
9. Snell GI, de Hoyos A, Krajden M, et al. Pseudomonas cepacia in lung transplant recipients with cystic fibrosis. Chest 1993;103(2):466–71.
10. Chaparro C, Maurer J, Gutierrez C, et al. Infection with Burkholderia cepacia in cystic fibrosis: outcome following lung transplantation. Am J Respir Crit Care Med 2001;163(1):43–8.
11. Aris RM, Routh JC, LiPuma JJ, et al. Lung transplantation for cystic fibrosis patients with Burkholderia cepacia complex. Survival linked to genomovar type. Am J Respir Crit Care Med 2001;164(11):2102–6.
12. De Soyza A, McDowell A, Archer L, et al. Burkholderia cepacia complex genomovars and pulmonary transplantation outcomes in patients with cystic fibrosis. Lancet 2001;358(9295):1780–1.
13. Murray S, Charbeneau J, Marshall BC, et al. Impact of Burkholderia infection on lung transplantation in cystic fibrosis. Am J Respir Crit Care Med 2008;178(4):363–71.
14. Jones AM, Dodd ME, Govan JR, et al. Burkholderia cenocepacia and Burkholderia multivorans: influence on survival in cystic fibrosis. Thorax 2004;59(11):948–51.
15. Ledson MJ, Gallagher MJ, Jackson M, et al. Outcome of Burkholderia cepacia colonisation in an adult cystic fibrosis centre. Thorax 2002;57(2):142–5.
16. Mallory GB Jr, Schecter MG, Elidemir O. Management of the pediatric organ donor to optimize lung donation. Pediatr Pulmonol 2009;44(6):536–46.
17. Maurer JR, Frost AE, Estenne M, et al. International guidelines for the selection of lung transplant candidates. The International Society for Heart and Lung Transplantation, the American Thoracic Society, the American Society of Transplant Physicians, the European Respiratory Society. J Heart Lung Transplant 1998;17(7):703–9.

18. Spray TL, Mallory GB, Canter CB, et al. Pediatric lung transplantation. Indications, techniques, and early results. J Thorac Cardiovasc Surg 1994;107(4):990–9.
19. Boasquevisque CH, Yildirim E, Waddel TK, et al. Surgical techniques: lung transplant and lung volume reduction. Proc Am Thorac Soc 2009;6(1):66–78.
20. Sweet SC. Pediatric living donor lobar lung transplantation. Pediatr Transplant 2006;10(7):861–8.
21. Starnes VA, Barr ML, Cohen RG. Lobar transplantation. Indications, technique, and outcome. J Thorac Cardiovasc Surg 1994;108(3):403–10.
22. Starnes VA, Bowdish ME, Woo MS, et al. A decade of living lobar lung transplantation: recipient outcomes. J Thorac Cardiovasc Surg 2004;127(1):114–22.
23. Bowdish ME, Barr ML, Schenkel FA, et al. A decade of living lobar lung transplantation: perioperative complications after 253 donor lobectomies. Am J Transplant 2004;4(8):1283–8.
24. Battafarano RJ, Anderson RC, Meyers BF, et al. Perioperative complications after living donor lobectomy. J Thorac Cardiovasc Surg 2000;120(5):909–15.
25. Christie JD, Kotloff RM, Pochettino A, et al. Clinical risk factors for primary graft failure following lung transplantation. Chest 2003;124(4):1232–41.
26. de Perrot M, Liu M, Waddell TK, et al. Ischemia-reperfusion-induced lung injury. Am J Respir Crit Care Med 2003;167(4):490–511.
27. King RC, Binns OA, Rodriguez F, et al. Reperfusion injury significantly impacts clinical outcome after pulmonary transplantation. Ann Thorac Surg 2000;69(6):1681–5.
28. Khan SU, Salloum J, O'Donovan PB, et al. Acute pulmonary edema after lung transplantation: the pulmonary reimplantation response. Chest 1999;116(1):187–94.
29. Boujoukos AJ, Martich GD, Vega JD, et al. Reperfusion injury in single-lung transplant recipients with pulmonary hypertension and emphysema. J Heart Lung Transplant 1997;16(4):439–48.
30. Daud SA, Yusen RD, Meyers BF, et al. Impact of immediate primary lung allograft dysfunction on bronchiolitis obliterans syndrome. Am J Respir Crit Care Med 2007;175(5):507–13.
31. Christie JD, Kotloff RM, Ahya VN, et al. The effect of primary graft dysfunction on survival after lung transplantation. Am J Respir Crit Care Med 2005;171(11):1312–6.
32. de Perrot M, Fischer S, Liu M, et al. Prostaglandin E1 protects lungs from ischemia-reperfusion injury: a shift from pro- to anti-inflammatory cytokines. Transplantation 2001;72(9):1505–12.
33. Shargall Y, Guenther G, Ahya VN, et al. Report of the ISHLT Working Group on primary lung graft dysfunction part VI: treatment. J Heart Lung Transplant 2005;24(10):1489–500.
34. Fiser SM, Tribble CG, Long SM, et al. Ischemia-reperfusion injury after lung transplantation increases risk of late bronchiolitis obliterans syndrome. Ann Thorac Surg 2002;73(4):1041–7 [discussion: 1047–8].
35. Fisher AJ, Wardle J, Dark JH, et al. Non-immune acute graft injury after lung transplantation and the risk of subsequent bronchiolitis obliterans syndrome (BOS). J Heart Lung Transplant 2002;21(11):1206–12.
36. Keshavjee SH, Yamazaki F, Cardoso P, et al. A method for safe 12 hour pulmonary preservation. J Thorac Cardiovasc Surg 1989;98:529–34.
37. Fischer S, Matte-Martyn A, dePerrot M, et al. Low potassium dextran preservation solution improves lung function after human lung transplantation. J Thorac Cardiovasc Surg 2001;121(3):594–6.

38. Date H, Trulock EP, Arcidi JM, et al. Improved airway healing after lung transplantation. An analysis of 348 bronchial anastomoses. J Thorac Cardiovasc Surg 1995;110(5):1424–32 [discussion: 1432–3].
39. Shennib H, Massard G. Airway complications in lung transplantation. Ann Thorac Surg 1994;57(2):506–11.
40. Choong CK, Sweet SC, Zoole JB, et al. Bronchial airway anastomotic complications after pediatric lung transplantation: incidence, cause, management, and outcome. J Thorac Cardiovasc Surg 2006;131(1):198–203.
41. Meyers BF, de la Morena M, Sweet SC, et al. Primary graft dysfunction and other selected complications of lung transplantation: a single-center experience of 983 patients. J Thorac Cardiovasc Surg 2005;129(6):1421–9.
42. Stewart S, Fishbein MC, Snell GI, et al. Revision of the 1996 working formulation for the standardization of nomenclature in the diagnosis of lung rejection. J Heart Lung Transplant 2007;26(12):1229–42.
43. Elizur A, Faro A, Huddleston CB, et al. Lung transplantation in infants and toddlers from 1990 to 2004 at St. Louis Children's Hospital. Am J Transplant 2009;9(4):719–26.
44. Liu M, Worley S, Arrigain S, et al. Respiratory viral infections within one year after pediatric lung transplant. Transpl Infect Dis 2009;11(4):304–12.
45. Danziger-Isakov LA, Worley S, Michaels MG, et al. The risk, prevention, and outcome of cytomegalovirus after pediatric lung transplantation. Transplantation 2009;87(10):1541–8.
46. Danziger-Isakov LA, DelaMorena M, Hayashi RJ, et al. Cytomegalovirus viremia associated with death or retransplantation in pediatric lung-transplant recipients. Transplantation 2003;75(9):1538–43.
47. Duncan SR, Paradis IL, Dauber JH, et al. Ganciclovir prophylaxis for cytomegalovirus infections in pulmonary allograft recipients. Am Rev Respir Dis 1992;146(5 Pt 1):1213–5.
48. Danziger-Isakov LA, Worley S, Arrigain S, et al. Increased mortality after pulmonary fungal infection within the first year after pediatric lung transplantation. J Heart Lung Transplant 2008;27(6):655–61.
49. Tazelaar HD, Yousem SA. The pathology of combined heart-lung transplantation: an autopsy study. Hum Pathol 1988;19(12):1403–16.
50. Tamm M, Sharples LD, Higenbottam TW, et al. Bronchiolitis obliterans syndrome in heart-lung transplantation: surveillance biopsies. Am J Respir Crit Care Med 1997;155(5):1705–10.
51. Kramer MR, Stoehr C, Whang JL, et al. The diagnosis of obliterative bronchiolitis after heart-lung and lung transplantation: low yield of transbronchial lung biopsy. J Heart Lung Transplant 1993;12(4):675–81.
52. Estenne M, Maurer JR, Boehler A, et al. Bronchiolitis obliterans syndrome 2001: an update of the diagnostic criteria. J Heart Lung Transplant 2002; 21(3):297–310.
53. Sharples LD, McNeil K, Stewart S, et al. Risk factors for bronchiolitis obliterans: a systematic review of recent publications. J Heart Lung Transplant 2002;21(2): 271–81.
54. Glanville AR, Aboyoun CL, Havryk A, et al. Severity of lymphocytic bronchiolitis predicts long-term outcome after lung transplantation. Am J Respir Crit Care Med 2008;177:1033–40.
55. Chmiel C, Speich R, Hofer M, et al. Ganciclovir/valganciclovir prophylaxis decreases cytomegalovirus-related events and bronchiolitis obliterans syndrome after lung transplantation. Clin Infect Dis 2008;46:831–9.

56. Borro JM, Bravo C, Solé A, et al. Conversion from cyclosporine to tacrolimus stabilizes the course of lung function in lung transplant recipients with bronchiolitis obliterans syndrome. Transplant Proc 2007;39(7):2416–9.
57. Dusmet M, Maurer J, Winton T, et al. Methotrexate can halt the progression of bronchiolitis obliterans syndrome in lung transplant recipients. J Heart Lung Transplant 1996;15(9):948–54.
58. Verleden GM, Buyse B, Delcroix M, et al. Cyclophosphamide rescue therapy for chronic rejection after lung transplantation. J Heart Lung Transplant 1999;18(11):1139–42.
59. Date H, Lynch JP, Sundaresan S, et al. The impact of cytolytic therapy on bronchiolitis obliterans syndrome. J Heart Lung Transplant 1998;17(9):869–75.
60. Iacono AT, Johnson BA, Grgurich WF, et al. A randomized trial of inhaled cyclosporine in lung-transplant recipients. N Engl J Med 2006;354(2):141–50.
61. Fisher AJ, Rutherford RM, Bozzino J, et al. The safety and efficacy of total lymphoid irradiation in progressive bronchiolitis obliterans syndrome after lung transplantation. Am J Transplant 2005;5(3):537–43.
62. O'Hagan AR, Stillwell PC, Arroliga A, et al. Photopheresis in the treatment of refractory bronchiolitis obliterans complicating lung transplantation. Chest 1999;115(5):1459–62.
63. Benden C, Speich R, Hofbauer GF, et al. Extracorporeal photopheresis after lung transplantation: a 10-year single-center experience. Transplantation 2008;86(11):1625–7.
64. Gottlieb J, Szangolies J, Koehnlein T, et al. Long-term azithromycin for bronchiolitis obliterans syndrome after lung transplantation. Transplantation 2008;85:36–41.
65. Benden C, Kansra S, Ridout DA, et al. Chronic kidney disease in children following lung and heart-lung transplantation. Pediatr Transplant 2009;13(1):104–10.
66. Boyle GJ, Michaels MG, Webber SA, et al. Posttransplantation lymphoproliferative disorders in pediatric thoracic organ recipients. J Pediatr 1997;131(2):309–13.
67. Knoop C, Kentos A, Remmelink M, et al. Post-transplant lymphoproliferative disorders after lung transplantation: first-line treatment with rituximab may induce complete remission. Clin Transplant 2006;20(2):179–87.

Pediatric Kidney Transplantation

Ron Shapiro, MD[a],*, Minnie M. Sarwal, MD, PhD[b]

KEYWORDS

• Kidney transplantation • Pediatric • Evaluation • Outcomes

Kidney transplantation in pediatric patients has become a routinely successful procedure, with 1- and 5-year patient survival rates of 98% and 94%, and 1- and 5-year graft survival rates of 93% to 95% and 77% to 85% (the range takes into account differences between living and deceased donors). These good outcomes represent the cumulative effect of improvements in pre- and posttransplant patient care, operative techniques, immunosuppression, and infection prophylaxis, diagnosis, and treatment. This article provides a brief historical overview, discusses the indications for transplantation, describes the evaluation process for the recipient and the potential donor, outlines the operative details, reviews the various causes of and risk factors for graft dysfunction, and analyzes outcomes.

HISTORICAL NOTES

Pediatric kidney transplantation, like transplantation in general, is relatively young. Fifty years ago end-stage renal disease (ESRD) was a terminal illness, as neither dialysis nor transplantation were available. The first successful transplant took place in 1954 with an adult recipient and an identical twin donor; immunosuppression had not yet been developed (**Table 1**). The first immunosuppressive agent, azathioprine, was a failed anticancer agent found to be effective in dogs and then used with steroids in the first clinical experiences in the early 1960s. Unfortunately, early success rates for 1-year graft survival were in the 50% to 70% range, depending on the type of donor, and the high steroid dosages were associated with important and common side effects.

The advent of a failed antifungal agent, cyclosporine, in the late 1970s and early 1980s, transformed the field of transplantation, improving outcomes in kidney transplantation to 75% to 85% 1-year graft survival, and making routinely successful nonrenal abdominal and thoracic transplantation possible. The late 1980s and 1990s saw

[a] Thomas E. Starzl Transplantation Institute, University of Pittsburgh, 7 South, 3459 Fifth Avenue, Pittsburgh, PA 15213, USA
[b] Department of Pediatrics Nephrology, Stanford University Medical School, Stanford University, 300 Pasteur Drive, G 306, Stanford, CA 94305, USA
* Corresponding author.
E-mail address: shapiror@upmc.edu

Pediatr Clin N Am 57 (2010) 393–400
doi:10.1016/j.pcl.2010.01.016
0031-3955/10/$ – see front matter. Published by Elsevier Inc.

pediatric.theclinics.com

Table 1
Selected historical landmarks

	Adult	Pediatric
First identical twin transplant	1954	1959
Azathioprine/prednisone	1962	1962
Cyclosporine	1978	1982
Tacrolimus	1989	1989
Mycophenolate mofetil		
Sirolimus		
OKT3	1982	1987
Thymoglobulin	1997	1997
IL2 receptor antagonist	1997	1997
Alemtuzumab	1998	2005

the introduction of the currently used immunosuppressive agents including tacrolimus, mycophenolate mofetil (MMF), and more effective antibody induction agents. See the article by Dr Feng elsewhere in this issue for further explanation of immunosuppression.

Progress in pediatric kidney transplantation generally kept pace with that seen in adults, with some lag time related to technical issues and the slower introduction of newer immunosuppressive agents. Not surprisingly, clinical trials took place in adults before being conducted in children, as is true in most of medicine. In general, however, current progress in and outcomes of pediatric kidney transplantation are similar to those seen in adults.

Incidence and Trends in Pediatric Transplantation

Of the 1781 pediatric patients waitlisted for an organ transplant in the United States, 791 are awaiting a kidney transplant. To date, 10,762 renal transplants have been reported by the North American Pediatric Renal Transplant Cooperative Society (NAPRTCS) https://web.emmes.com/study/ped/registry for 9854 pediatric patients in North America. The United Network of Organ Sharing (UNOS) http://www.unos.org/ maintains a system of pediatric priority in kidney transplantation assigning additional points to recipients less than 11 years old waitlisted for a kidney from a deceased donor. In 2005, a revised allocation policy (Share 35) conferring preferential allocation of allografts from young deceased donors (<35 years old) to pediatric patients less than 18 years old was implemented (Organ Procurement and Transplant Network: Policies at http://www.optn.org/PoliciesandBylaws2/policies/). This policy change resulted in an overall increase in the mean number of pediatric kidney transplants per quarter from 188 to 211 ($P = .07$) with a reduction in the wait time after listing. The mean wait time for a deceased donor kidney before the rule change was 350 days compared with 119 days after the rule change ($P = .04$). The policy change also resulted in an increase in the number of HLA-mismatched allografts and more deceased donor transplants.[1] A reasonable question, given the historically longer half-lives with living donor kidneys compared with deceased donor kidneys, is whether the unanticipated consequence of the change in allocation (ie, an increased proportion of deceased donor kidney transplants in children) will lead to a higher rate of retransplantation in the future. However, the follow-up is too short for any meaningful data to have become available to answer this question, and, in any event, there is substantial selectivity in choosing deceased donor kidneys for children.

An analysis of the demographics of the pediatric transplants performed in the last decade, from the NAPRTCS database, reveals that approximately 20% of transplants are performed in young recipients less than 6 years old, and approximately 25% of primary transplants are performed preemptively. Thus, most pediatric kidney transplantation recipients are teenagers. For deceased donor transplantation, compared with adults, pediatric patients receive more poorly matched kidneys than adults, as only 5% of pediatric patients receive HLA antigen mismatched kidneys compared with almost 14% of adult recipients. This situation is probably a function of preferential allocation of kidneys from donors less than 35 years of age to children, without regard to HLA matching.

INDICATIONS FOR LISTING

The causes of ESRD in pediatric patients are different from those seen in adult patients. The important causes of ESRD in pediatric patients (**Table 2**) include obstructive uropathy secondary to posterior urethral valves; renal dysplasia; glomular diseases, such as focal segmental glomerulosclerosis (FSGS), hemolytic uremic syndrome (HUS), and membranoproliferative glomerulonephritis Type II (MPGN Type II); infantile polycystic kidney disease (PCK), and several less common diseases. In contrast to adults, where only 16% to 17% of the dialysis population is listed for transplant, most children with ESRD are referred for transplantation. The only circumstances in which a child would not be an appropriate candidate for renal transplantation would be in the setting of multiple medical issues and an overall poor prognosis for any meaningful recovery, untreated malignancy, or untreated infection. Isolated mild mental retardation is not per se a contraindication, and substantial intellectual catch-up can be seen routinely in pediatric patients.

RECIPIENT EVALUATION

In general, pediatric recipient evaluation is not that different from that used in adults. A thorough history and physical with routine comprehensive laboratory studies, chest radiograph and electrocardiogram are obvious starting points (**Box 1**). Urinalysis and urine culture, 24-hour urine collection, and occasional native renal biopsies are also routinely obtained. Pediatric urologic evaluation is performed as needed, particularly in patients with a history of posterior urethral valves, reflux, or other congenital

Table 2 Indications/causes of ESRD in pediatric patients	
	Percent
Obstructive uropathy	16
Dysplasia	16
FSGS	11
Reflux	5
GN	3.5
Prune belly	3
HUS	3
MPGN	3
PCK	3
Other	36.5

Box 1
Recipient evaluation

History and physical

Chest radiograph

Electrocardiogram

Routine chemistries, liver function tests, Ca, Mg, P, cytomegalovirus, Epstein-Barr virus (EBV), human immunodeficiency virus

Urine analysis, culture, protein

Additional studies as indicated

Urologic studies: voiding cystourethrography, urodynamic studies, postvoid residual volumes, as needed

---

problems. Most pediatric patients are reasonable medical candidates for transplantation. Social service and psychosocial evaluation are a particularly important part of the evaluation process, and represent poorly understood aspects of the care of pediatric (and for the matter, adult) renal transplant patients. Noncompliance, especially in teenagers, is an important source of graft loss and patient death after transplantation.[2]

DONOR SELECTION

Living donation confers superior outcomes for pediatric recipients, limits wait times, allows for preemptive transplantation, and thus should be recommended for pediatric patients. Parents comprise 80% of living donors. An analysis of the UNOS data over a decade[3] showed that transplantation of a pediatric recipient, with an excellent quality adult-sized kidney, without acute tubular necrosis, conferred a distinct and significant survival advantage, particularly for the young infant recipient less than 6 years old. The projected graft half-lives after the first year in the young recipients of living donors was even better (26.3 and 29.3 years for children aged 0–2.5 years and 2.5–5 years, respectively) than the gold standard transplant category (23.3-year graft half-lives of HLA-identical adult sibling recipients aged 19 to 45 years). Deceased donor kidneys tend to be from younger adults or teenagers, and there is fairly routine and obvious cherry-picking for good quality donors for pediatric recipients.

OPERATIVE PROCEDURE/TRANSPLANT SURGERY

In teenagers and in children weighing more then 30 kg, the technical details associated with kidney transplantation are similar to those in adults, with retroperitoneal exposure of, and anastomosis to the external iliac artery and vein. In smaller children and infants, anastomosis to larger vessels is necessary. Infants weighing 10 kg or less generally undergo a midline laparotomy with vascular anastomosis at the level of the vena cava and the aorta. For children between 10 and 30 kg, there is some variability in approach, with the common iliac vessels usually being used, and surgeon preference dictating a retroperitoneal versus an intraperitoneal approach. For young children with previous intra-abdominal procedures or vascular access issues, thrombosis of the major intra-abdominal vessels must be carefully evaluated for selection of an appropriately sized donor organ that can be accommodated to small collateral vessels in the abdomen.[4,5]

Ureteral reimplantation is perhaps the most variable part of the transplant proce-dure. Simple extravesical ureteroneocystostomy is generally the most common varia-tion, but formal open antireflux techniques are also used by some surgeons.[6] Pediatric patients with complex urologic issues may require more extensive pre- and peritrans-plant interventions, but this is beyond the scope of this article. Obviously, if the trans-plant surgeon is not a urologist, good planning and coordination among the different surgical members of the team is of great importance.

Important details of operative management include over hydration of the small recipient to ensure adequate perfusion. Adult kidneys in small infants can take up a huge percentage of the cardiac output, and appropriate volume loading is necessary to ensure a good perfusion pressure of the new kidney (generally a systolic blood pres-sure of 130 is adequate). Routine administration of mannitol 1 g/kg and furosemide 1 mg/kg during the performance of the vascular anastomoses is also useful to ensure prompt diuresis. Fluid management in the early postoperative period is governed by the urine output. Locally in Pittsburgh, the authors use a 1% glucose solution in half normal saline, to which 1 ampule of $NaHCO_3$ has been added, to replace the urine output. The authors replace 1 mL/1 mL for a urine output of 300 mL/h or less and 0.8 mL/1 mL for urine output greater than 300 mL/h.

Desensitization Strategies in Children

About 70% of children receiving a first transplant are unsensitized, but approximately 3% of children, mostly in the category of repeat transplants or blood transfusions, have prior allosensitization and thus have a panel reactive antibody (PRA) of more than 80%. Desensitizing patients to HLA antigens to allow for a negative cross match and transplantation is gaining momentum in adults and is now also being applied to children, so that children with long wait times on the sensitized lists can move toward successful transplantation. A recent open-label, phase 1/2, single-center study, building on a previous pilot trial (IG02; http://www.clinicaltrials.gov/, NCT00642655), provided encouraging results of desensitization in adults using the combination of high-dose immune globulin (IVIG) and rituximab, as the high rate of early rejection (50%) was reversible with excellent 1-year patient (100%) and graft survival (94%).[7] Other desensitization adaptations, applied primarily in adults, using low-dose IVIG, rit-uximab, and frequent plasmapheresis, with occasional splenectomy, have led to successful transplantation against a previously incompatible donor.[8,9] The recent reports of bortezomib for diminishing anti-HLA antibodies are encouraging for the additional use of this drug for desensitization strategies.[10] At Stanford University, the first pediatric randomized study for desensitization of highly sensitized pediatric recipients, testing the direct safety and efficacy of high-dose IVIG alone versus high-dose IVIG with rituximab, is actively enrolling highly sensitized pediatric patients.

GRAFT DYSFUNCTION

There are several causes of graft dysfunction, and they occur at different time points after transplantation. Initial delayed graft function (DGF), defined as the need for dial-ysis in the first week after transplantation, is related to ischemia-reperfusion injury. Deceased donor kidneys with long cold ischemia time (CITs) are at highest risk, and living donors kidneys with short CITs are at the lowest risk. Given the greater selec-tivity with which deceased donor kidneys are chosen for pediatric kidney transplanta-tion, the incidence of DGF in pediatric patients should be low.

Rejection is another important source of graft dysfunction. Rejection can occur early after transplantation, and is called acute rejection (which can be further subdivided into cellular or humoral), or it can occur late after transplantation, its nomenclature having evolved over time from chronic rejection, to chronic allograft nephropathy, to interstitial fibrosis/tubular atrophy. Rejection is a function of the immune system recognizing the transplanted organ as a foreign body and attempting to destroy it. It is a complex area of study and remains imperfectly understood. A variety of agents have been developed to prevent or treat rejection, and again this is discussed in a separate article in this issue.

Uniquely for the kidney, the most important immunosuppressive agents are nephrotoxic, and a great deal of graft loss can be associated with chronic nephrotoxicity related to immunosuppression, particularly the calcineurin inhibitors (CNIs) cyclosporine and tacrolimus. The CNIs can also cause renal failure of the native kidneys in nonrenal transplant patients. Acute graft dysfunction in kidney transplant patients related to elevated CNI levels is common and is generally reversible with dosage reduction.

Technical complications are fortunately uncommon after pediatric kidney transplantation, but do occur. They include arterial thrombosis or stenosis, venous thrombosis, ureteral leak, stenosis or reflux, and the development of fluid collections, including hematomas, seromas, or lymphoceles. Ultrasonography is a good screening test in the initial evaluation of these complications, with further diagnostic testing performed on an as-needed basis.

RISK FACTORS AND OUTCOMES

As stated at the outset, pediatric kidney transplantation at present is a generally successful procedure with high rates of short- and medium-term patient and graft survival. Different factors are associated with better or worse outcomes.

- Recipient age

The main effect of recipient age relates to poorer outcomes in teenagers, and this is largely related to noncompliance. Parenthetically, it is remarkable how little is known about compliance and how ineffective we are in preventing it. It is a dangerous problem and is associated with premature graft loss and death.

- Donor type

In general, living donor kidneys are associated with longer half-lives than deceased donor kidneys; this is almost assuredly related to better allograft quality and shorter CITs.

- DGF

DGF has remained an important risk factor for inferior graft survival throughout the history of kidney transplantation. There is also an association of DGF with acute rejection.

- Rejection

The effect of acute rejection has been somewhat controversial. Originally believed to be a negative prognostic factor, acute rejection has been subject to somewhat more nuanced analyses recently. Completely reversed acute rejection seems not to be associated with worse long-term outcomes. In addition, there are also registry data suggesting that a substantial reduction in the incidence of acute rejection has not led to improved long-term graft survival.

- Recipient race

Similar to registry data analyses in adults, African American race has been associated with more rejection and worse long-term outcomes. The reasons for this are not entirely clear.

- Recurrent disease

FSGS, MPGN Type II, and HUS all have the potential to recur in the transplanted kidney, but unpredictably. Our inability to predict or control these disease recurrences represents an important limitation of our understanding.

- Matching

There remains an advantage to O antigen mismatched kidneys from either deceased or living donors, but it is less clear that there are important differences at different levels of mismatching.

- Sensitization

As a group, sensitized patients have inferior outcomes after kidney transplantation, whether or not they have been subjected to trials of desensitization.

OUTCOMES AND LIMITATIONS

Although short- and medium-term outcomes have improved over the years, long-term (10 years) graft survival has not improved in 22 years. Chronic CNI toxicity and the side effects of immunosuppression, which can include diabetes, hypertension, and malignancy, have had important negative effects on graft survival, patient survival, and quality of life. The side effects of chronic corticosteroids have been particularly harmful to children, with an important effect on growth retardation. Thus, the field is still imperfect, and substantial progress remains to be made.

SPECIFIC AND INTEREST AREAS OF ACTIVE RESEARCH IN PEDIATRIC TRANSPLANTATION

Given the variations in the development of the immune response in the pediatric age group, the period of rapid linear growth in the child with age-dependent changes in drug pharmacokinetics and pharmacodynamics, and the clear discrepancy in size between the young recipient and the large adult-sized kidney, there are some specific issues that require further study in pediatric recipients of organ allografts. Some of these areas of interest are highlighted. Children, who are usually EBV naive, have a greater propensity for development of viral-driven lymphoproliferative disorders, which may differ in their prevalence under different immunosuppression protocols.[11] Understanding the development of viral and heterologous immunity in the young recipient, and its effect on skewing the immune response toward specific anergy or alloresponsiveness, is an important area of research. The molecular mechanisms that drive the extended survival of transplants from adult-sized kidney donors into infant recipients suggests the possibility of an accommodative response that requires further definition. Conversely, the rapid accrual of chronic tubular necrosis in kidneys of young pediatric recipients receiving adult-sized kidneys has highlighted the need for a better examination of the physiologic importance of vascular size discrepancy between the young recipient and the adult donor.[12,13] These issues, among others, are peculiar to pediatric transplantation, and deserve greater definition and study, with the aim of improving clinical and graft outcomes for this group of patients.

SUMMARY

Renal transplantation in pediatric patients is a successful therapy, with excellent short- and medium-term patient and graft survival rates. Pediatric patients with ESRD are generally candidates for kidney transplantation, and the technical issues involved have largely been resolved. Several factors can lead to short- or long-term graft dysfunction or even graft loss. Despite reasonable short- and medium-term outcomes, many factors can compromise long-term outcomes.

REFERENCES

1. Abraham EC, Wilson AC, Goebel J. Current kidney allocation rules and their impact on a pediatric transplant center. Am J Transplant 2009;9:404–8.
2. Shaw RJ, Palmer L, Blasey C, et al. A typology of non-adherence in pediatric renal transplant recipients. Pediatr Transplant 2003;7:489–93.
3. Sarwal MM, Cecka JM, Millan MT, et al. Adult-size kidneys without acute tubular necrosis provide exceedingly superior long-term graft outcomes for infants and small children: a single center and UNOS analysis. United Network for Organ Sharing. Transplantation 2000;70:1728–36.
4. Salvatierra O Jr, Concepcion W, Sarwal MM. Renal transplantation in children with thrombosis of the inferior vena cava requires careful assessment and planning. Pediatr Nephrol 2008;23:2107–9.
5. Eneriz-Wiemer M, Sarwal M, Donovan D, et al. Successful renal transplantation in high-risk small children with a completely thrombosed inferior vena cava. Transplantation 2006;82:1148–52.
6. Salvatierra O Jr, Sarwal M, Alexander S, et al. A new, unique and simple method for ureteral implantation in kidney recipients with small, defunctionalized bladders. Transplantation 1999;68:731–8.
7. Vo AA, Lukovsky M, Toyoda M, et al. Rituximab and intravenous immune globulin for desensitization during renal transplantation. N Engl J Med 2008;359:242–51.
8. Kraus ES, Parekh RS, Oberai P, et al. Subclinical rejection in stable positive cross-match kidney transplant patients: incidence and correlations. Am J Transplant 2009;9:1826–34.
9. Locke JE, Zachary AA, Haas M, et al. The utility of splenectomy as rescue treatment for severe acute antibody mediated rejection. Am J Transplant 2007;7:842–6.
10. Stegall MD, Dean PG, Gloor J. Mechanisms of alloantibody production in sensitized renal allograft recipients. Am J Transplant 2009;9:998–1005.
11. Li L, Chaudhuri A, Weintraub LA, et al. Subclinical cytomegalovirus and Epstein-Barr virus viremia are associated with adverse outcomes in pediatric renal transplantation. Pediatr Transplant 2007;11:187–95.
12. Gholami S, Sarwal MM, Naesens M, et al. Standardizing resistive indices in healthy pediatric transplant recipients of adult-sized kidneys. Pediatr Transplant 2010;14:126–31.
13. Naesens M, Kambham N, Concepcion W, et al. The evolution of nonimmune histological injury and its clinical relevance in adult-sized kidney grafts in pediatric recipients. Am J Transplant 2007;7:2504–14.

Liver Transplantation in Children: Update 2010

Binita M. Kamath, MBBChir, MRCP[a,b,*], Kim M. Olthoff, MD[c,d,e]

KEYWORDS

- Pediatric liver transplant • Liver disease
- Recipient • Donor

Pediatric liver transplantation is one of the most successful solid organ transplants.[1] According to the US Organ Procurement and Transplantation Network (OPTN)/Scientific Registry of Transplant Recipients (SRTR) data, the 1-year patient survival rate is 83% to 91%, depending on the age at transplant.[2] Five-year patient survival is also excellent, ranging from 82% to 84%. The number of pediatric liver transplants per year has remained steady in the last 10 years, averaging approximately 600 annually. Almost 12,000 pediatric liver transplants have been performed in the United States. The Studies in Pediatric Liver Transplantation (SPLIT) group is another important source of data regarding pediatric liver transplantation in North America. This group now represents 46 pediatric liver transplant centers across America and Canada and reflects the results of programs with a strong pediatric emphasis. This database has yielded valuable analyses on many of the issues surrounding pediatric liver transplantation. SPLIT survival data mirrors OPTN/SRTR results. The most recent review of the SPLIT database reveals patient survival rates of 91.4% and 86.5%, at 1 and 5 years following liver transplantation, respectively (R. Anand, personal communication, 2009).

Pediatric liver transplant recipients represent an important target population for primary care health professionals as well as transplant practitioners. With improving patient and graft survival, new concerns now face health care professionals caring for the transplant community, namely the long-term complications of immunosuppressive therapy and the potential for withdrawal of immunosuppression,

---

[a] Department of Pediatrics, University of Toronto, 27 King's College Circle, Toronto, ON M5S 1A1, Canada
[b] Division of Gastroenterology, Hepatology and Nutrition, The Hospital for Sick Children, 555 University Avenue, Toronto, ON M5G 1X8, Canada
[c] Department of Surgery, University of Pennsylvania, 3451 Walnut Street, Philadelphia, PA 19104, USA
[d] Transplant Center, The Children's Hospital of Philadelphia, 34th Civic Center Boulevard, Philadelphia, PA 19104, USA
[e] Liver Transplant Program, Penn Transplant Institute, 2 Dulles, 3400 Spruce Street, Philadelphia, PA, USA
* Corresponding author. Division of Gastroenterology, Hepatology and Nutrition, The Hospital for Sick Children, 555 University Avenue, Toronto, ON M5G 1X8, Canada.
E-mail address: binita.kamath@sickkids.ca.

Pediatr Clin N Am 57 (2010) 401–414
doi:10.1016/j.pcl.2010.01.012
0031-3955/10/$ – see front matter © 2010 Elsevier Inc. All rights reserved.

transplant recipients' quality of life, and the persistent shortage of donor organs leading to morbidity and mortality on the waiting list. These issues require constant collaboration between pediatricians, transplant hepatologists, transplant surgeons, nurses, dieticians, social workers, psychologists, and other supporting services.

HISTORICAL NOTES

Thomas E. Starzl performed the first liver transplantation in 1963 in a 3-year-old child with biliary atresia and thus pioneered a heroic journey through surgical refinement and improved immune suppression.[3] Although this first child died because of surgical difficulties and coagulopathy, Dr Starzl persisted and in the late 1960s performed another 8 pediatric liver transplants of which all the children survived surgery. Unfortunately, initial survival rates were poor because of inadequate immune suppression. The advent of cyclosporine A in 1978 transformed the field and dramatically improved rejection rates and outcomes. By 1983 pediatric liver transplantation was deemed the standard of care for hepatic failure or end-stage liver disease.[4] However, small infants had continued poor outcomes because of the technical challenges of creating and maintaining patent vascular anastomoses and waitlist mortality caused by the extreme shortage of appropriately sized small donors. The late 1980s was a period of surgical innovations that included reduced-sized grafts from adult deceased donors, split liver deceased donor grafts, and then live donor liver transplantation. These technical variants significantly reduced the waiting list mortality in children. In 2002 the implementation of the pediatric end-stage liver disease (PELD) and model for end-stage liver disease (MELD) scores designated priority for organ allocation to the sickest patients, rather than to those with the longest wait time, as had previously been the case. In addition, the PELD system conferred special status and protection to pediatric organs and recipients. Thus, in a mere 50 years this field has evolved from experimental conception to a successful, widespread, therapeutic strategy that benefits hundreds of children a year.

INDICATIONS FOR LISTING

There are 4 broad listing indications for evaluation and listing for pediatric liver transplantation (**Table 1**). The primary indication is the onset of life-threatening complications secondary to hepatic failure or chronic end-stage liver disease. Progressive primary liver disease refractory to maximal medical management is also an indication for liver transplantation, before the development of life-threatening complications. A smaller number of liver transplants are performed for metabolic disease, in which liver replacement is curative, and for unresectable primary liver tumors.

Chronic liver disease may lead to listing for liver transplantation either with a sudden deterioration, the so-called acute-on-chronic presentation, or with the progression of chronic disease leading to complications secondary to decompensation. Biliary atresia is the most common chronic disease leading to transplantation in children. The determination of the severity of liver disease requires an assessment of the life-sustaining functions of the liver. The major functions of the liver can be grouped into 4 general categories, namely protein synthesis (including clotting factors), bile formation and excretion, metabolic functions (including glucose homeostasis) and hemodynamic function (management of portal blood flow). A patient with chronic liver disease who has clinically significant abnormalities in 2 or more areas will likely benefit from liver transplantation. Children with only 1 area of dysfunction may be well sustained with medical therapies, although a severe abnormality in 1 area may still require

Table 1	
Underlying diagnoses of children undergoing liver transplantation	
Diagnosis	**Frequency (%)**
Cholestatic liver disease	48
Biliary atresia	15
Other: Alagille syndrome, sclerosing cholangitis, progressive familial intrahepatic cholestasis and so forth	
Fulminant hepatic failure	11
Metabolic liver disease	13
Primary hepatic disease: Wilson disease, α-1-antitrypsin deficiency, tyrosinemia, cystic fibrosis and so forth	
Primarily nonhepatic disease: ornithine transcarbamylase deficiency, primary hyperoxaluria type 1, organic acidemia	
Liver tumors	4
Other	9

Data from Ng VL, Fecteau A, Shepherd R, et al. Outcomes of 5-year survivors of pediatric liver transplantation: report on 461 children from a North American multicenter registry. Pediatrics 2008;122(6):e1128–35.

transplantation. A systematic evaluation according to these parameters may allow for a delay of liver transplantation, which can allow a child to grow, complete immunizations, and reduce the lifelong immune suppression load.

Fulminant hepatic failure (FHF) is the indication for liver transplantation in approximately 11% of pediatric cases.[5] Because these patients present with or rapidly develop life-threatening complications, the establishment of the underlying diagnosis is not always feasible and most cases are defined as secondary to unspecified viral etiology. Other important causes are drug and toxin exposures and previously unidentified metabolic diseases. Recent data suggest that many patients are designated as having indeterminate etiology and a presumed unspecified viral cause, but a significant number of these have undergone an incomplete evaluation, with more than half not having been tested for metabolic diseases and 20% not having been screened for autoimmune liver disease.[6] Although acetaminophen hepatotoxicity remains an important cause of FHF requiring immediate medical attention and transfer to a tertiary medical center with liver transplant team support, it is not a common reason for liver transplantation. A large retrospective analysis of United Network for Organ Sharing (UNOS) data showed that 5-year patient and graft survival in children with FHF was significantly lower than that of children transplanted for biliary atresia.[7] A study of FHF in the SPLIT database suggested that grade 4 encephalopathy, age less than 1 year and dialysis before transplantation were risk factors for poor outcomes.[8] In addition, this SPLIT analysis also showed that children with FHF have significantly higher pretransplant mortality compared with those with other liver diseases.[8]

In addition to transplantation for acute liver failure and end-stage chronic liver disease, a smaller number of children undergo liver transplantation because of metabolic diseases.[9–12] In children with urea cycle defects there is disruption of the conversion of ammonia into urea resulting in hyperammonemia and central nervous system toxicity. Although the liver is structurally normal in this condition, liver transplantation is offered as a curative procedure because the liver is the major site of ammonia metabolism. Similarly, in primary hyperoxaluria, there is systemic oxalate crystal deposition resulting in renal failure and cardiac arrhythmia, however liver transplantation restores normal oxalate metabolism. Children transplanted for metabolic diseases generally have excellent outcomes.[10,13]

Pediatric patients with liver tumors represent a growing group of transplant recipients. Hepatoblastoma is the most common pediatric primary liver tumor. Resection in combination with systemic chemotherapy is the preferred method of treatment. If the tumor is unresectable after appropriate chemotherapy, transplantation may be offered if there has been a demonstrated response to therapy, even in the face of pulmonary metastases.[14–16] Children with hepatoblastoma are granted special consideration in listing in that they are granted status 1B by exception within the PELD system. A similar mechanism exists in the Canadian listing system. Hepatocellular carcinoma is rare in children and when present, usually occurs in the setting of another chronic underlying disease such as tyrosinemia.

CONTRAINDICATIONS TO TRANSPLANTATION

It is important to identify contraindications to liver transplantation at the earliest stage of the evaluation process. In pediatric transplantation, there are very few absolute contraindications. These would include conditions in which liver transplantation is futile and will not improve overall survival or quality of life, and this list of conditions has shortened dramatically over the years (**Box 1**). These conditions are largely extrahepatic diseases in which liver transplantation cannot significantly change the devastating outcome. Relative contraindications to liver transplantation may only temporarily delay listing or require additional interventions before listing, such as malignancy and systemic infection requiring completion of therapy. An active alcohol or substance abuse problem in the candidate or a primary caregiver may also constitute a relative contraindication.

Box 1
Contraindications to pediatric liver transplantation

Absolute contraindications

1 Extrahepatic malignancy (considered incurable by standard oncologic criteria)

2. Sepsis

   - Uncontrolled systemic infection
   - Acquired immunodeficiency syndrome (AIDS)

3. Extrahepatic disease (incurable)

   - Irreversible massive brain injury
   - Uncorrectable congenital anomalies affecting major organs

Relative contraindications

1. Malignancy that is considered cured or curable by standard oncologic criteria

2. Sepsis

   - Treatable infection
   - Human immunodeficiency virus

3. Extrahepatic disease

   - Progressive extrahepatic disease
   - Substance abuse

EVALUATION OF RECIPIENT

The appropriate selection and evaluation of potential recipients is fundamental in achieving the level of liver transplant success described earlier. The initial purpose of detailed evaluation of a candidate is to determine that liver transplantation remains the best option and no other medical therapies could be life sustaining with adequate quality of life. Other goals of a complete evaluation are to maximize nutrition, finesse medical therapy, provide education and support to the patient and family, and attempt to optimize the timing of transplantation.

The medical evaluation of the recipient begins with recognition of the patient's original diagnosis and an assessment of any complications or comorbidities present. The process requires specific blood work, radiologic studies, and consultations with specialists. Potential contraindications are identified. The laboratory tests include exposures to viral infections (cytomegalovirus [CMV], Epstein-Barr virus [EBV]) that will affect posttransplant care. Radiologic evaluation includes a Doppler ultrasound at least, but may also require magnetic resonance imaging or computed tomography angiography to identify complex vascular anatomy or portal vein thrombosis that could alter operative care. Malnutrition should be considered a common and treatable comorbidity in transplant recipients, especially young children. Nutritional rehabilitation, sometimes in the guise of nasogastric tube feeds, is often necessary as optimizing nutrition improves postsurgical outcomes. Growth impairment has been associated with longer posttransplant hospital stays.[17] Nutrition support may also provide the opportunity for growth to lessen the technical difficulties seen in very small infants. The insertion of a nasogastric tube is not associated with esophageal variceal bleeding and is therefore not a concern in children with chronic liver disease. Evaluation of the recipient also addresses psychological and social factors in the family in terms of the child's and the parents' understanding of the process and also psychosocial and socioeconomic factors that may affect the posttransplant course.

Assessment for extrahepatic disease that might affect operative or postoperative management is an important part of the evaluation for transplantation and varies with the underlying liver disease. Children with Alagille syndrome, for example, require careful cardiac and renal assessment given the known involvement of those organs in this syndrome. Cardiac disease, even moderate, will clearly be an important factor during the prolonged transplant anesthesia and structural or medical renal disease affects immunosuppressive strategies. There are similar issues with syndromic biliary atresia and Wilson disease.

An important aspect of evaluation is preparation of the child for the transplant event. Every attempt is made to include the child in age-appropriate discussion of liver transplantation throughout the evaluation process. An older child may sign an assent form and is encouraged to ask the liver transplant team as many questions as possible. It may also be appropriate for the candidate to meet posttransplant patients during this time. The older child should be made aware of the need for medication compliance and alcohol avoidance.

Preparation of the recipient (and family) for liver transplantation is a key area in which the primary care practitioner has a vital role. Advocating for aggressive nutritional rehabilitation and supporting the notion of supplemental tube feedings can greatly assist the hospital transplant team in achieving this goal. It is also imperative that the primary practitioner complete and often accelerate immunization schedules before transplantation because immune suppression reduces the efficacy of vaccines. In general, live vaccines are not administered in immune suppressed patients for safety reasons and therefore the accelerated administration of these is particularly important. The primary pediatrician also has an important role in preparing the child and family for the transplantation from a psychosocial standpoint. The primary team is often best placed to identify and alert the specialist transplant team to risks such as potential financial issues, social concerns and other risks for medical nonadherence that may affect the posttransplant course.

DONOR OPTIONS

All potential options for transplantation should be discussed with the family at the time of evaluation, including deceased donor transplantation with appropriate size donor, split liver transplantation from a young adult donor, and living donor transplantation. The possibility of a living donor should be introduced during the evaluation process, if determined by the transplant team to be an appropriate option. It is important to provide an objective presentation of living donation with a clear outline of the risks (see discussion on Transplant Surgery later) and comparison with deceased donor transplantation. It is equally important for the family to have a realistic view of the current state of organ allocation, waiting times, and the possibility of their child deteriorating during the waiting time. Patients are most often listed for a deceased donor graft, regardless of whether a potential living donor exists.

Discussions surrounding living donor transplantation predominantly involve evaluation of the donor, however an assessment of the candidate's suitability is also important. Recipient size and age are important, because there is evidence that infants and small children do better than older children with living donor transplantation.[18] Special live donor considerations also exist for specific pediatric diseases. For example, potential related donors for a child with Alagille syndrome (and certain other inherited disorders) must be carefully assessed as individuals may be affected, even if apparently clinically healthy.[19]

Deceased donor offers and evaluation of the potential donor is often primarily the role of the transplant surgeon and involves dimensional matching for adequate parenchymal mass, and medical characteristics, namely donor age, hemodynamic stability, and comorbidities. In the live donor process there is usually more time for an extended evaluation involving an adult hepatologist, psychological and social work assessment, laboratory evaluation, and abdominal imaging. The live donor evaluation must be comprehensive in this fashion to avoid unnecessary risks to a healthy individual. Often a health care team separate to that of the recipient is allocated to the donor to avoid conflict of interest and undue pressure on the candidate to undergo live donation. At times, such as in the setting of FHF, the live donor evaluation is accelerated but should still contain all the key components, albeit in a contracted timeframe.

ORGAN ALLOCATION

Organ allocation is a complex process guided by principles of equity, justice, utility, and benefit, in an era when there is a persistent donor shortage. In most countries with an established liver transplantation network, similar concepts arise with an understanding that organs need to be allocated to the sickest patients. Thus, there are special considerations for patients with fulminant liver failure and malignancy. In addition, most systems preferentially allocate pediatric donors to pediatric recipients. However, some differences also remain globally. In the United Kingdom, organs are allocated on a center basis and in Canada time spent waiting on the list counts toward listing status.

In 2002 the PELD score was introduced in the United States to allocate deceased donor livers based on the severity of recipient liver disease and to ensure that the sickest individuals receive donor organs first.[20,21] The PELD score ranks children on a waiting list according to their probability of death and/or move to the intensive care unit (ICU) within 3 months of listing. The PELD score is calculated from a formula based on the following factors that are predictive of death or transfer to ICU: international normalized ratio (INR), total bilirubin, serum albumin, age less than 1 year, and height less than 2 standard deviations from the mean for age and gender.[22]

Although PELD (currently used for children up to 12 years old) and MELD scores rank children and adults on the same scale, certain provisions exist to benefit children. The same PELD and MELD scores indicate a greater mortality risk for adults, however the score is not adjusted for this, thus benefiting children. Pediatric candidates (<12 years) have priority to receive livers from pediatric donors (<18 years) over adults with the same score. Children can be listed outside their PELD score as Status 1 in fulminant liver failure, or be granted additional exception points in cases of chronic liver disease with significant complications that may not be reflected in a calculated PELD score. These exceptions are only granted after a formal request from the transplant team and approval by the UNOS regional review board.

Since the implementation of the PELD/MELD system, fewer patients are now dying on the waiting list for liver transplantation, including those children less than 2 years of age who previously had high death rates on the liver waiting list.[23] Patient and graft survival data are similar after introduction of PELD scores, suggesting that the system has not adversely affected children's access to donor livers. The PELD score does not accurately predict outcomes following transplantation.

Allocation of organs is undergoing constant monitoring and refinement. In 2005 a change in allocation policy was implemented that substituted the PELD score for the MELD for adolescents aged 12 to 17 years. Thus PELD became applicable only to children less than 12 years of age. At the time of this policy change 66% of PELD candidates had scores less than 11 and this number has fallen steadily to 60%. The fact remains, however, that most children on the liver transplant waiting list have relatively low PELD scores and very few (2%) have a score greater than 30 such that many continue to be transplanted by exception status, suggesting further modification of the allocation system is needed.[2]

TRANSPLANT SURGERY

It is not possible to review the details of liver transplant surgery here, however it is important for any health care professional caring for these children to have a basic understanding of the processes involved. Liver transplantation has 3 major phases beginning with the recipient hepatectomy. In pediatric patients at least half have previously undergone abdominal surgery (portoenterostomy or Kasai) and this is often the most difficult part of the transplant because of adhesions, and bleeding caused by coagulopathy and portal hypertension. The second phase is the anhepatic phase during which placement of the graft begins but the patient is functionally between livers. The vascular anastomoses (vena cava, portal vein, and hepatic artery) are performed during this period. The procedure concludes with the neohepatic phase as the liver graft undergoes reperfusion. Significant cardiovascular instability can result during reperfusion because of cold preservation techniques in the graft and an experienced anesthesia team is vital. The biliary anastomosis is done in this final phase. In biliary atresia patients the donor duct is implanted into a Roux-en-Y limb as there is no native biliary tree. This approach is also used in young children receiving a segmental graft, those with an abnormal native biliary tree, as in sclerosing cholangitis, or if the donor or recipient duct is very small. A duct-to-duct anastomosis is possible if there is relative parity in the size of the recipient and donor liver.

Technical Variants

The extreme shortage of pediatric donors has provided the transplant surgical community with the impetus to develop innovative techniques to address this issue. The first approach was reduced-size liver transplantation, which involved a right hepatectomy of the donor organ so that only the left lateral segment is transplanted, allowing a pediatric recipient to accept an organ from a much larger donor. However, this approach removes organs from the pool available to larger adults and has therefore largely been replaced by split liver and living related transplantation. Split liver transplantation involves dividing a whole deceased donor graft into a left lateral segment and a right trisegment, often in situ at the donor procurement, which can then be transplanted into a child and an adult.

Living related transplantation has greatly benefited the pediatric transplant population, particularly in countries in which there is limited availability of deceased donor grafts for cultural or even legal reasons.[24] In this procedure a left lateral segmentectomy (segments 2 and 3) is performed in the donor and transplanted in a similar fashion to the whole organ. Approximately 300 living donor liver transplants are performed annually and 20% of these are in child recipients.[2] This percentage has held steady for 7 years. Living donor transplantation typically occurs in relatively healthy recipients with a lower PELD score.

There have been several database studies comparing graft types and outcomes.[18,25–28] An earlier analysis of UNOS data revealed superior graft survival for live donor grafts compared with deceased donor whole, split, and reduced grafts in children less than 3 years.[18] There appeared to be a relative benefit of whole deceased donor grafts in older children. More recently UNOS data on pediatric liver transplant patients less than 12 years of age suggested better immediate postoperative survival in whole graft recipients but by 1 year, adjusted patient and allograft survivals were similar regardless of the type (whole liver, deceased donor segmental, or living donor).[26] In this cohort of more than 1200 pediatric recipients, 52% underwent whole liver transplantation, 33% underwent deceased donor segmental transplantation, and the remaining 15% had live donor liver transplantation. Single institution results also show much more comparable outcomes between deceased donor segmental and live donor grafts. This is likely related to the institution-specific experience. Thus, although live donor grafts may not show specific advantages in terms of graft survival, there are certainly some advantages in terms of being able to plan the transplant electively, although this has to be balanced with the risks and inconvenience to the donor.

Operative Complications

Early surgical complications of liver transplantation include primary nonfunction (PNF) of the hepatic graft, bleeding, hepatic artery thrombosis (HAT), and bile leak. PNF is a rare but catastrophic event of unknown etiology but most likely related to ischemia/reperfusion injury. It is characterized by high transaminase levels, coagulopathy, increased creatinine level, and progression to multisystem organ failure if the patient is not retransplanted. Pediatric liver transplant recipients are at particular risk of intra- and postoperative bleeding because of the high frequency of prior surgery, coagulopathy, and portal hypertension. HAT and other vascular complications result from the small vessels present in pediatric patients. HAT, which occurs in 5% to 8% of pediatric recipients, can present insidiously with a progressive increase in prothrombin time or rapid worsening of graft function, with increased transaminase levels and coagulopathy.[25,29] Suspected HAT requires prompt evaluation with duplex sonography, magnetic resonance angiography, or angiogram. If imaging is suspicious, immediate exploration and attempted thrombectomy is mandatory. If significant graft dysfunction and biliary necrosis ensue, the only option is retransplantation. HAT can also occur as a late complication and can manifest as biliary strictures, bilomas, or sepsis. Portal vein thrombosis can occur months or years after a liver transplantation in an infant and results in varices at the Roux-en-Y limb and presentation with gastrointestinal bleeding.

Biliary complications with either duct-to-duct or Roux-en-Y anastomoses occur in 10% to 30% of pediatric liver transplant recipients, particularly small infants.[30,31] Early biliary leaks are manifested by bile-leak fluid in abdominal drains. Most biliary leaks resolve on their own just with simple drainage, particularly with cut surface leaks, but sometimes require decompression via endoscopic retrograde cholangiopancreatography or a percutaneous transhepatic approach. Surgical exploration and revision of the anastomosis is also sometimes required. HAT should always be considered when leaks occur, because it may be to the result of ischemic necrosis of the distal donor duct. Biliary strictures present later, even years after transplant, with bile duct dilatation on ultrasound, increased γ-glutamyltransferase level and/or recurrent cholangitis. Often these can be definitively diagnosed and treated with percutaneous transhepatic cholangiography with stenting and dilatation, but surgical revision may be necessary.

Retransplantation

Retransplantation in the pediatric liver population is not an uncommon event, occurring with a frequency of approximately 10% to 20%.[32,33] Hepatic retransplantation can be classified as occurring early (<30 days) or late (>30 days) from the original transplant. Early retransplantation is usually because of PNF or HAT. Late retransplantation usually results from chronic rejection or biliary complications. Retransplantation results in decreased survival compared with primary liver transplantation.[33]

GRAFT DYSFUNCTION

There are multiple causes of graft dysfunction after liver transplantation and the relative likelihood of each of these varies according to the time since surgery and the clinical context. An exhaustive discussion of graft dysfunction is not possible here and the following is intended as a simple overview.

Rejection

Rejection is the primary cause of graft dysfunction following liver transplantation. Despite prophylactic therapy, rejection is seen in approximately 60% of children following transplantation.[5,34] Although most common in the first 3 to 6 months following the transplant, it can occur years later, and is often associated with immune suppressant noncompliance. Rejection is generally suspected because of increasing liver enzymes, often with aspartate aminotransferase level higher than alanine aminotransferase and increase in γ-glutamyltranspeptidase level. At times it is an increase only in the bilirubin level. These laboratory abnormalities develop before the onset of symptoms such as fever, malaise, and jaundice. Liver biopsy is indicated for histologic confirmation and characteristic pathologic findings of acute cellular rejection (ACR) include portal tract inflammation with a mixed cellular infiltrate, bile duct injury, and endothelialitis. ACR usually responds well to pulsed steroid therapy, increasing calcineurin inhibitor drug levels, and possibly the addition of another immunosuppressant such as mycophenolate mofetiel. Rejection that is unresponsive to this approach, which is uncommon, may be treated with anti-T-cell antibody preparations. Chronic rejection, an uncommon event in compliant pediatric patients, is characterized by cholestasis and typical arterial injury and bile duct paucity (vanishing bile ducts) on liver biopsy. Chronic rejection is less responsive to medical therapies and severe allograft dysfunction from this cause may require retransplantation.

Infection

Infectious causes of graft dysfunction are an important group of problems and this area is covered in detail in another article by Allen and Green elsewhere in this issue. Children with chronic debilitating underlying disease and complicated intensive care courses are at particular risk of bacterial and fungal infections in the immediate posttransplant period. Infants and young children are also susceptible to viral infections, especially CMV and EBV. Fever in a young child in the first 12 months after liver transplantation warrants an evaluation for sepsis including physical examination, chest radiograph, complete blood count and differential, blood chemistry, serum EBV and CMV, blood and urine cultures, and probable duplex ultrasonography. The management depends on the degree of immune suppression but may include hospitalization and administration of intravenous broad-spectrum antibiotics awaiting results of blood cultures.

De Novo Autoimmune Hepatitis and Primary Sclerosing Cholangitis

In general, recurrence of the primary liver disease in the graft is uncommon in pediatrics, generally because liver diseases requiring transplantation in children are usually congenital or developmental and therefore transplantation is curative. This is in contrast to the situation in adults. Primary sclerosing cholangitis can recur and the disease is almost identical to the original disease. De novo autoimmune hepatitis can occur in any graft, regardless of the original disease, and is therefore not considered recurrence of disease, but a new phenomenon.[35,36] De novo autoimmune hepatitis presents with increased transaminase levels, positive autoantibodies, and interface hepatitis on liver biopsy. This condition usually requires the addition of a second-line immunosuppressant and can be difficult to treat.

Vascular and Biliary Complications

Vascular and biliary complications after liver transplantation can occur early within the first few weeks of surgery or much later and both events can present with graft dysfunction. These issues are described in detail in the section on Transplant Surgery. Unfortunately, the late occurrence of a vascular or biliary complications is often difficult to correct and may warrant consideration for retransplantation, or other surgical intervention.

Chronic Hepatitis

Chronic hepatitis has been recently recognized as a prevalent problem in late allografts.[37] This condition is defined by portal inflammation without bile duct or vascular changes on liver biopsy, in the setting of normal serum aminotransferase levels. Therefore, this condition is largely diagnosed by protocol biopsies, which are not standard of care in many centers. The treatment of this condition is also not yet clear.

RISK FACTORS AND OUTCOMES

The overall results from pediatric liver transplantation are exemplary. OPTN data reveal 1- and 5-year patient survival rates of 83% to 91% and 82% to 84%, respectively. These survival rates vary according to the age at transplantation. Although survival for children less than 1 year old has improved dramatically, they still represent the lower end of the range. The underlying diagnosis at transplantation also has an effect on outcomes. Patients with acute liver failure have worse early and long-term survival rates.[7,8,38]

Neonates represent a special population and their outcomes from liver transplantation are worthy of consideration. Traditionally liver transplantation for babies weighing less than 5 kg has been viewed as technically too difficult. However, in recent years these medical and surgical challenges have been met with success. Although small babies have higher complication rates and longer hospital stays following transplantation, neonatal liver transplant recipients now have similar patient and graft survival rates compared with older children.[39,40] In addition, these neonates have also been reported as having good neurodevelopmental outcomes.[39]

Death following pediatric liver transplantation most commonly occurs as a result of recurrent malignancy, sepsis, multisystem organ failure, and posttransplant lymphoproliferative disorder.[41] Because survival rates are so good and these deaths are uncommon, the focus of posttransplant care has now shifted to encompass outcomes beyond life or death. Renal dysfunction has been noted in more than 30% of long-term survivors[5,42] and this has modified immunosuppressive practices in at-risk transplant recipients and shaped screening practices (see the article by Choquette, Goebel, and Campbell elsewhere in this issue for further explanation of this topic). Similarly, current immunosuppressants are associated with an increased risk for diabetes, dyslipidemia, and obesity.[5,43-45] Lifestyle modification and minimization of immune suppressants can be effective in reducing these risks. Persistent linear growth impairment is also common in the pediatric liver transplant population, despite evidence of some catch-up growth.[46] In an analysis of the SPLIT database, more than 30% of pediatric liver transplant recipients were less than the 10th percentile for height at 24 months following liver transplantation.[46] Avoiding advanced pretransplant growth failure is 1 mechanism to minimize posttransplant linear growth impairment and one in which in the primary care team has an essential role, as described earlier (see the article by Mohammad and Alonso elsewhere in this issue for further explanation of this topic). Optimizing outcomes in pediatric liver transplant recipients also involves giving them the tools to transition to adulthood. An awareness of the changing needs of adolescents is vital to tackle primary care issues surrounding birth control, smoking, and drug use (see the article by Kaufman, Shemesh, and Benton elsewhere in this issue for futher explanation of this topic). Effective transition strategies are also important during this period when nonadherence is more common[47] (see the article by Bell and Sawyer elsewhere in this issue for further explanation of this topic). Many of the issues facing adolescents transitioning to adulthood are common across the transplant population.[48]

SUMMARY

Pediatric liver transplantation is a well-established and successful strategy. Much of the discussion in this article has focused on the management of peri- and posttransplant patients. Another area of concern for the transplant community is the supply of available donors. In 2006 there were more than 350 children waiting for a liver transplant and children less than 6 years old have the highest death rate of all candidates.[49] Surgical advances to split organs and living related donation has clearly helped but not eliminated this problem. The total number of pediatric liver donors has decreased in the last 10 years (from 20% to 12%).[49] One of the efforts aimed at increasing the donor supply has been the consideration of donation after cardiac death (DCD), that is death based on cardiopulmonary rather than neurologic criteria.[50,51] DCD expands the donor pool by allowing the use of organs from donors who have irreversible brain injury and are ventilator dependent, but do not meet the criteria for brain death. This is not yet a widespread strategy in children, with less than 30 DCD livers having been transplanted into pediatric recipients between 2000 and 2007.[2]

Thus pediatric liver transplantation in 2010 has evolved into one of the most successful solid organ transplants. The future outcomes of pediatric liver transplantation will require broad efforts to tackle donor organ shortage and collaborative care by transplant specialists and primary care practitioners to improve patients' overall health and long-term survival, psychosocial well-being, and transition to adulthood.

REFERENCES

1. Kelly DA. Current issues in pediatric transplantation. Pediatr Transplant 2006; 10(6):712–20.
2. Berg CL, Steffick DE, Edwards EB, et al. Liver and intestine transplantation in the United States 1998–2007. Am J Transplant 2009;9(4 Pt 2):907–31.
3. Otte JB. History of pediatric liver transplantation. Where are we coming from? Where do we stand? Pediatr Transplant 2002;6(5):378–87.
4. National Institutes of Health Consensus Development Conference Statement: liver transplantation–June 20–23, 1983. Hepatology 1984;4(1 Suppl):107S–10S.
5. Ng VL, Fecteau A, Shepherd R, et al. Outcomes of 5-year survivors of pediatric liver transplantation: report on 461 children from a North American multicenter registry. Pediatrics 2008;122(6):e1128–35.
6. Narkewicz MR, Dell Olio D, Karpen SJ, et al. Pattern of diagnostic evaluation for the causes of pediatric acute liver failure: an opportunity for quality improvement. J Pediatr 2009;155(6):801–6 e801.
7. Futagawa Y, Terasaki PI. An analysis of the OPTN/UNOS Liver Transplant Registry. Clin Transplant 2004;315–29.
8. Baliga P, Alvarez S, Lindblad A, et al. Posttransplant survival in pediatric fulminant hepatic failure: the SPLIT experience. Liver Transpl 2004;10(11):1364–71.
9. Florman S, Shneider B. Living-related liver transplantation in inherited metabolic liver disease: feasibility and cautions. J Pediatr Gastroenterol Nutr 2001;33(4):520–1.
10. Kayler LK, Rasmussen CS, Dykstra DM, et al. Liver transplantation in children with metabolic disorders in the United States. Am J Transplant 2003;3(3):334–9.
11. Treem WR. Liver transplantation for non-hepatotoxic inborn errors of metabolism. Curr Gastroenterol Rep 2006;8(3):215–23.
12. Hansen K, Horslen S. Metabolic liver disease in children. Liver Transpl 2008; 14(5):713–33.
13. Sze YK, Dhawan A, Taylor RM, et al. Pediatric liver transplantation for metabolic liver disease: experience at King's College Hospital. Transplantation 2009;87(1):87–93.
14. Austin MT, Leys CM, Feurer ID, et al. Liver transplantation for childhood hepatic malignancy: a review of the United Network for Organ Sharing (UNOS) database. J Pediatr Surg 2006;41(1):182–6.
15. Avila LF, Luis AL, Hernandez F, et al. Liver transplantation for malignant tumours in children. Eur J Pediatr Surg 2006;16(6):411–4.
16. Faraj W, Dar F, Marangoni G, et al. Liver transplantation for hepatoblastoma. Liver Transpl 2008;14(11):1614–9.
17. Barshes NR, Chang IF, Karpen SJ, et al. Impact of pretransplant growth retardation in pediatric liver transplantation. J Pediatr Gastroenterol Nutr 2006;43(1):89–94.

18. Abt PL, Rapaport-Kelz R, Desai NM, et al. Survival among pediatric liver trans-plant recipients: impact of segmental grafts. Liver Transpl 2004;10(10):1287–93.
19. Gurkan A, Emre S, Fishbein TM, et al. Unsuspected bile duct paucity in donors for living-related liver transplantation: two case reports. Transplantation 1999; 67(3):416–8.
20. Wiesner RH, McDiarmid SV, Kamath PS, et al. MELD and PELD: application of survival models to liver allocation. Liver Transpl 2001;7(7):567–80.
21. Freeman RB Jr, Wiesner RH, Harper A, et al. The new liver allocation system: moving toward evidence-based transplantation policy. Liver Transpl 2002;8(9): 851–8.
22. McDiarmid SV, Anand R, Lindblad AS. Development of a pediatric end-stage liver disease score to predict poor outcome in children awaiting liver transplantation. Transplantation 2002;74(2):173–81.
23. McDiarmid SV, Merion RM, Dykstra DM, et al. Selection of pediatric candidates under the PELD system. Liver Transpl 2004;10(10 Suppl 2):S23–30.
24. Strong RW, Lynch SV, Ong TH, et al. Successful liver transplantation from a living donor to her son. N Engl J Med 1990;322(21):1505–7.
25. Martin SR, Atkison P, Anand R, et al. Studies of pediatric liver transplantation 2002: patient and graft survival and rejection in pediatric recipients of a first liver transplant in the United States and Canada. Pediatr Transplant 2004;8(3):273–83.
26. Becker NS, Barshes NR, Aloia TA, et al. Analysis of recent pediatric orthotopic liver transplantation outcomes indicates that allograft type is no longer a predictor of survivals. Liver Transpl 2008;14(8):1125–32.
27. Roberts JP, Hulbert-Shearon TE, Merion RM, et al. Influence of graft type on outcomes after pediatric liver transplantation. Am J Transplant 2004;4(3):373–7.
28. Diamond IR, Fecteau A, Millis JM, et al. Impact of graft type on outcome in pedi-atric liver transplantation: a report from Studies of Pediatric Liver Transplantation (SPLIT). Ann Surg 2007;246(2):301–10.
29. Tiao GM, Alonso M, Bezerra J, et al. Liver transplantation in children younger than 1 year–the Cincinnati experience. J Pediatr Surg 2005;40(1):268–73.
30. Peclet MH, Ryckman FC, Pedersen SH, et al. The spectrum of bile duct compli-cations in pediatric liver transplantation. J Pediatr Surg 1994;29(2):214–9 [discussion: 219–20].
31. Sunku B, Salvalaggio PR, Donaldson JS, et al. Outcomes and risk factors for failure of radiologic treatment of biliary strictures in pediatric liver transplantation recipients. Liver Transpl 2006;12(5):821–6.
32. Bourdeaux C, Brunati A, Janssen M, et al. Liver retransplantation in children. A 21-year single-center experience. Transpl Int 2009;22(4):416–22.
33. Ng V, Anand R, Martz K, et al. Liver retransplantation in children: a SPLIT data-base analysis of outcome and predictive factors for survival. Am J Transplant 2008;8(2):386–95.
34. Tiao GM, Alonso MH, Ryckman FC. Pediatric liver transplantation. Semin Pediatr Surg 2006;15(3):218–27.
35. Hubscher S. What does the long-term liver allograft look like for the pediatric recipient? Liver Transpl 2009;15(Suppl 2):S19–24.
36. Venick RS, McDiarmid SV, Farmer DG, et al. Rejection and steroid dependence: unique risk factors in the development of pediatric posttransplant de novo auto-immune hepatitis. Am J Transplant 2007;7(4):955–63.
37. Evans HM, Kelly DA, McKiernan PJ, et al. Progressive histological damage in liver allografts following pediatric liver transplantation. Hepatology 2006;43(5): 1109–17.

38. Squires RH Jr, Shneider BL, Bucuvalas J, et al. Acute liver failure in children: the first 348 patients in the pediatric acute liver failure study group. J Pediatr 2006; 148(5):652–8.
39. Grabhorn E, Richter A, Fischer L, et al. Emergency liver transplantation in neonates with acute liver failure: long-term follow-up. Transplantation 2008; 86(7):932–6.
40. Sundaram SS, Alonso EM, Anand R. Outcomes after liver transplantation in young infants. J Pediatr Gastroenterol Nutr 2008;47(4):486–92.
41. Soltys KA, Mazariegos GV, Squires RH, et al. Late graft loss or death in pediatric liver transplantation: an analysis of the SPLIT database. Am J Transplant 2007; 7(9):2165–71.
42. Campbell KM, Yazigi N, Ryckman FC, et al. High prevalence of renal dysfunction in long-term survivors after pediatric liver transplantation. J Pediatr 2006;148(4): 475–80.
43. Everhart JE, Lombardero M, Lake JR, et al. Weight change and obesity after liver transplantation: incidence and risk factors. Liver Transpl Surg 1998;4(4):285–96.
44. Varo E, Padin E, Otero E, et al. Cardiovascular risk factors in liver allograft recipients: relationship with immunosuppressive therapy. Transplant Proc 2002;34(5): 1553–4.
45. Hathout E, Alonso E, Anand R, et al. Post-transplant diabetes mellitus in pediatric liver transplantation. Pediatr Transplant 2009;13(5):599–605.
46. Alonso EM, Shepherd R, Martz KL, et al. Linear growth patterns in prepubertal children following liver transplantation. Am J Transplant 2009;9(6):1389–97.
47. Shemesh E. Non-adherence to medications following pediatric liver transplantation. Pediatr Transplant 2004;8(6):600–5.
48. Bell LE, Bartosh SM, Davis CL, et al. Adolescent transition to adult care in solid organ transplantation: a consensus conference report. Am J Transplant 2008; 8(11):2230–42.
49. Magee JC, Krishnan SM, Benfield MR, et al. Pediatric transplantation in the United States, 1997–2006. Am J Transplant 2008;8(4 Pt 2):935–45.
50. Abt PL, Fisher CA, Singhal AK. Donation after cardiac death in the US: history and use. J Am Coll Surg 2006;203(2):208–25.
51. Naim MY, Hoehn KS, Hasz RD, et al. The Children's Hospital of Philadelphia's experience with donation after cardiac death. Crit Care Med 2008;36(6):1729–33.

Intestine Transplantation in Children: Update 2010

Yaron Avitzur, MD[a,b,*], David Grant, MD[b,c]

KEYWORDS

- Intestine transplantation • Children • Outcome
- Complications • Treatment • Surgical techniques

The treatment of chronic intestinal failure has made remarkable strides in the past 2 decades. The establishment of multidisciplinary teams at leading centers specialized in the treatment of intestinal failure and the introduction of innovative surgical and medical treatments such as the serial transverse enteroplasty (STEP) procedure,[1,2] omega-3-based lipid emulsions,[3,4] and novel gut trophic factors have provided major advances. Survival has improved and the morbidity associated with parenteral nutrition (PN) therapy has significantly declined.[5–7]

In parallel with the advances in other therapies for intestine failure, intestine transplantation (IT) has progressed in the last 20 years from an experimental treatment to become the accepted treatment of children and adults who develop life-threatening complications associated with the standard therapies for intestinal failure. The improved short- and long-term survival in the last decade can be attributed to better surgical techniques, improved use of immunosuppressive (IS) medications, comprehensive infection control with careful monitoring of viral pathogens such as Epstein-Barr virus (EBV), cytomegalovirus (CMV), and adenovirus, and a better understanding of IT pathophysiology and the recipient's needs. As of 2009, more than 2000 IT and multivisceral transplants (MVTx) have been performed worldwide; 50% of the recipients are alive and most are independent of PN (Intestinal Registry Report, Bologna, 2009).

[a] Division of Gastroenterology, Hepatology and Nutrition, The Hospital for Sick Children, 555 University Avenue, Toronto, ON M5G 1X8, Canada
[b] Transplant Centre, SickKids, The Hospital for Sick Children, 555 University Avenue, Toronto, ON M5G 1X8, Canada
[c] Division of General Surgery, SickKids, The Hospital for Sick Children, 555 University Avenue, Toronto, ON M5G 1X8, Canada
* Corresponding author. Division of Gastroenterology, Hepatology and Nutrition, The Hospital for Sick Children, 555 University Avenue, Toronto, ON M5G 1X8, Canada
E-mail address: yaron.avitzur@sickkids.ca

Pediatr Clin N Am 57 (2010) 415–431
doi:10.1016/j.pcl.2010.01.019
0031-3955/10/$ – see front matter © 2010 Elsevier Inc. All rights reserved.

INTESTINAL FAILURE

Intestinal failure in children is defined as the reduction of functional gut mass below the minimum needed for digestion and absorption of nutrients and fluids required for growth.[8] Causes of intestinal failure that lead to IT are outlined in **Box 1**, with short bowel syndrome as the leading cause, followed by motility and mucosal disorders. The important role of dedicated multidisciplinary and professional gut failure programs has become evident in the last decade. Children who are treated by such programs have improved survival rates, expedited intestinal adaptation, faster weaning from PN, a lower incidence and severity of intestinal failure-associated complications, and a reduced requirement for IT.[5–7]

A combined medical and surgical treatment is a key factor in successful intestinal adaptation. Surgical interventions include early stoma closure and lengthening procedures that can improve the absorptive capacity of the failing gut and shorten the duration of PN. Reports on the novel STEP bowel lengthening procedure have shown a 50% to 60% increase in small bowel length and a significant improvement in oral tolerance.[1,2] Medical strategies to improve intestinal adaptation include prevention of infections by careful central line care and control of bacterial overgrowth; early and continuous enteral feeding; use of elemental formulas; optimization of PN treatment; and prevention of intestinal failure-associated liver disease (IFALD). Uncontrolled studies suggest that treatment with a fish oil-based lipid emulsion often corrects the hyperbilirubinemia associated with soy-based lipid emulsions.[3,4] Although more studies are needed to define the efficacy and optimal balance of lipid sources, it seems that fish oil-based emulsions have the potential to substantially reduce the frequency of IFALD. Although most patients with chronic intestine failure do well with these treatments, a small proportion are refractory to standard therapies and this is where IT plays a role.

HISTORICAL NOTES

IT has had a slower genesis than other solid-organ transplants. In 1959, Richard Lillehei and coworkers[9] published a landmark paper describing the techniques for orthotopic IT in dogs, which demonstrated absorptive function for up to 7 days before the grafts were lost to rejection. Subsequent early attempts at clinical IT using

---

Box 1
Common causes of intestine failure in children leading to IT

Short gut syndrome (68%)

- Volvulus 15%

- Gastroschisis 24%

- Necrotizing enterocolitis 16%

- Atresia 9%

- Other 4%

Motility disorders 14%

Mucosal defects (eg, microvillus inclusion disease, tufting enteropathy) 10%

Retransplantation 5%

Other 3%

antilymphocyte products, azathioprine, and steroids failed because of graft rejection. In 1989, Goulet's group, at the Hôpital Necker-Enfants Malades, Paris, performed the first deceased-donor clinical isolated IT to achieve long-term survival in an infant who was initially treated with cyclosporine.[10] Around the same time, Grant and colleagues[11] (London, Ontario, Canada) reported the first successful combined liver and intestine transplant. The techniques for IT and MVTx using tacrolimus were subsequently developed, refined, and reported by Sudan and colleagues (Omaha, NA), Abu-Almagd and colleagues (Pittsburgh, PA), and Selvaggi and Tzakis (Miami, FL).[12–14] In the early 1990s, the results of live-donor IT with tacrolimus were reported by Benedetti and colleagues[15] and Gruessner and Sharp.[16] From the late 1990s until today, these groups along with Beath and colleagues (Birmingham, AL), Venick and colleagues (Los Angeles, CA), Fishbein (Washington, DC), and others have continued to advance the field through a reemphasis on the development of multidisciplinary teams to treat intestine failure; earlier referral and listing for transplantation; the use of anti-interleukin 2 (anti-IL-2) agents for induction immune suppression; the use of more aggressive methods to prevent and preemptively treat viral infections; the introduction of rapamycin for IT; and early detection and treatment of acute rejection (AR).[17–19]

REFERRAL CRITERIA AND INDICATIONS FOR LISTING

Despite optimal treatment of intestinal failure, about 10% to 15% of patients develop life-threatening complications. Early and timely referral of these patients for a pretransplant assessment is a crucial determinant for their survival because (1) the waiting list mortality is higher for IT than for other solid-organ transplants; and (2) patients who are transplanted while waiting at home have an approximately 15% higher survival rate than those who are transplanted while waiting in hospital (Intestinal Registry Report, Bologna 2009). Early reports assessing the mortality of patients on the waiting list for IT during the late 1990s showed a significantly higher mortality compared with other solid-organ recipients,[20] with mortality of 50% in some series.[21] A variety of reasons contribute to this high incidence, including late referrals of patients for transplant, scarcity of size-matched donors in the young age group, and allocation criteria (United Network for Organ Sharing [UNOS] and others) that did not account for the unique risk factors of IT candidates. To reduce waiting list mortality, UNOS criteria were recently revised, adding 23 points to the MELD (Model for End-stage Liver Disease) or PELD (Pediatric End-stage Liver Disease) score of patients needing liver transplantation and IT.[20]

Criteria for referral for pretransplant assessment are provided in **Table 1**.[22] Unlike the restricted listing criteria, the referral criteria are more inclusive to ensure timely referral and listing with better patient outcome. Many patients who are referred for transplant assessment can be treated by other means and do not necessarily require listing for IT.

Listing for transplant based on the following criteria is considered only when all treatment options directed to achieve intestinal adaptation have failed. The American Society of Transplantation (AST) recommends that listing should be considered for the complications outlined in **Table 1**.[23] When considering listing for IT, intestinal adaptation is not simply length dependent, and under some circumstances adaptation can be achieved in children with intestinal length as short as 10 to 15 cm. In addition, there is a wide spectrum of disease severity with many of the congenital causes of gut failure, and expert management can significantly improve the outcome in these cases. Thus, each child requires an individualized assessment to evaluate the unique circumstances of their disease with judicious use of the listing criteria.

Table 1
Recommended criteria for consultation or referral for IT assessment and for listing for IT

Referral Criteria	Listing Criteria
Children with massive intestine resection	Small bowel length of <25 cm without an ileocecal valve
Children with severely diseased bowel and unacceptable morbidity	Intestinal failure with high morbidity and poor QOL
Microvillous inclusion disease or intestinal epithelial dysplasia	Congenital intractable mucosal disorder such as microvillous inclusion disease or tufting enteropathy
Persistent hyperbilirubinemia (>6 mg/dL)	Persistent hyperbilirubinemia (>3–6 mg/dL) and signs of portal hypertension, or synthetic liver dysfunction with coagulopathy
Thrombosis of 2 of 4 upper body central veins	Loss of more than 50% of the standard central venous access sites
Continuing prognostic or diagnostic uncertainty	Recurrent life-threatening episodes of sepsis resulting in multiorgan failure, metastatic infectious foci, or acquisition of flora with limited antibiotic sensitivities
Request of the patient or family	

Data from Beath S, Pironi L, Gabe S, et al. Collaborative strategies to reduce mortality and morbidity in patients with chronic intestinal failure including those who are referred for small bowel transplantation. Transplantation 2008;85:1378; with permission; Kaufman SS, Atkinson JB, Bianchi A, et al. Indications for pediatric intestinal transplantation: a position paper of the American Society of Transplantation. Pediatr Transplant 2001;5:80.

The survival advantage of IT for patients with liver failure as a result of PN has recently been confirmed by Pironi and colleagues.[24] This group conducted a 3-year prospective European multicenter study to assess the validity of the AST listing criteria by comparing the 3-year outcome of adults (n = 357) and children (n = 114) with intestinal failure who were either candidates (n = 153) or noncandidates (n = 320) for IT. Three-year survival was lower in candidates without transplantation compared with noncandidates (87% vs 94%, respectively), supporting the view that IT is the standard of care for children and adults with chronic intestine failure who are doing poorly on PN. However, unlike patients who were listed for liver failure or central line-related complications, patients who were listed for QOL reasons alone or for high-risk disease (microvillus inclusion disease, tufting enteropathy) had a higher mortality after transplantation than those patients who were not transplanted. Thus, great caution should be exercised when considering IT for treatment of a poor QOL on PN or high-risk disease.

The contraindications to IT are similar to other solid-organ transplants: severe neurologic disabilities, life-threatening systemic diseases, severe immunologic deficiencies, nonresectable malignancies, and specifically for IT, multisystem autoimmune disease and insufficient vascular patency to guarantee vascular access for up to 6 months after transplant.[23]

PRETRANSPLANT EVALUATION OF RECIPIENT

As in other solid-organ recipients, the goals of the pretransplant assessment are to achieve a comprehensive evaluation of the patient's clinical status before transplant; to exclude patients with contraindication for transplant; to stabilize and improve the candidate's nutritional and clinical status to improve their posttransplant outcome; and to ensure that the child and family understand and are able to manage the requirements after transplant.

In the authors' center, pretransplant assessment includes viral serology (hepatitis A virus, hepatitis B virus, hepatitis C virus, herpes simplex virus, CMV, EBV, human immunodeficiency virus, varicella-zoster virus, measles, rubella) and toxoplasmosis; anthropometric and laboratory nutritional assessment with optimization of pretransplant nutrition; cardiology and nephrology assessment including glomerular filtration rate (GFR) measurement to assess kidney reserve before transplant and the need for renal transplantation; imaging studies (Doppler survey of central veins, abdominal ultrasound, and for selected patients gastrointestinal follow-through, gastric emptying studies, and abdominal computed tomography scan); and assessments by an oral therapist for eating behavior, by a physiotherapist for motor skills, and by a social worker for the family and the child's ability to cope with the challenges after transplant. During the assessment process the candidate and the family are informed by the medical and surgical team about the pre- and posttransplant process, the related risks, and the possible outcome of IT. Further studies and consultations are tailored to the specific patient according to their medical history and clinical status. In addition to this comprehensive assessment the patient is followed routinely every 3 to 6 months by the transplant team until transplantation.

TRANSPLANT SURGERY AND TECHNIQUES

There are 3 major types of grafts: isolated intestine transplants; intestine plus liver transplants, which usually include the duodenum and head of pancreas to avoid the need for a biliary anastomosis; and MVTx, which can include any of the abdominal organs along with the small intestine (**Fig. 1**). Partial intestine and liver grafts can be procured from living donors, although these techniques are not routinely used as in liver or kidney transplantation.

Isolated intestine grafting is indicated for patients with limited venous access, recurrent line infections, reversible liver dysfunction as a result of PN, and unmanageable fluid and electrolyte problems associated with PN. An isolated intestine graft is the preferred surgical option because there is no shortage of deceased-donor organs and the graft can be removed, if necessary, without compromising the function of other intra-abdominal organs.

The liver should be added to an intestine graft when the recipient has irreversible liver damage as a result of PN, usually manifested by severe fibrosis with or without portal hypertension and liver dysfunction.

MVTx are indicated for children with severe motility disorders; locally aggressive but nonmetastazing tumors; or patients with extensive abdominal pathology that cannot be safely removed without an evisceration or reconstruction with multiple organs (eg, children with multiple previous operations and severe portal hypertension). Inclusion of colon in the graft is controversial. The allografted colon has been shown experimentally to slow intestinal transit time and improve absorption. However, early clinical studies suggest that it may also increase the bacterial load in the terminal ileum, leading to bacterial translocation and an increased rate of sepsis.[25] A recent report by Kato and colleagues[26] has shown that inclusion of colon had no additional effect on morbidity or on poor graft survival.

With isolated intestinal grafts, the donor superior mesenteric artery (SMA) is anastamosed to the recipient's SMA or native aorta. It does not seem to matter whether the portal venous drainage of the graft is directed to the inferior vena cava or into

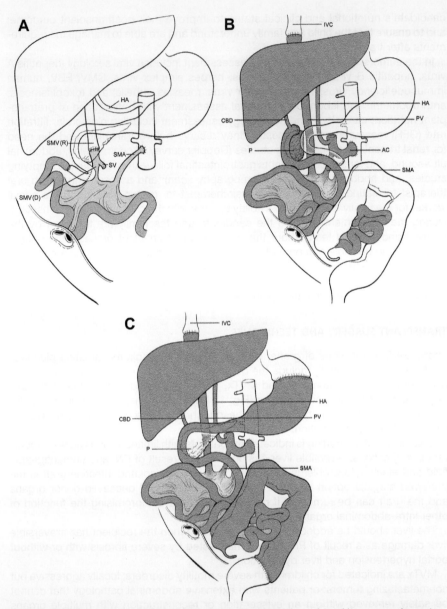

Fig. 1. Surgical techniques of IT and MVTx: (*A*) Isolated IT, (*B*) combined liver transplantation and IT, (*C*) MVTx including the colon. AC, aortic conduit; CBD, common bile duct; D, donor; HA, hepatic artery; IVC, inferior vena cava; P, pancreas; PV, portal vein; R, recipient; SMA, superior mesenteric artery; SMV, superior mesenteric vein; SV, splenic vein.

the portal system of the recipient. For composite grafts, a donor aortic conduit is usually anastomosed to the recipient's infrarenal aorta. The proximal bowel is anastamosed to the native bowel. The distal bowel is brought out as an end ileostomy or anastamosed end to end with the recipient bowel, with creation of a proximal, diverting loop ileostomy.

GRAFT DYSFUNCTION
IS Treatment

Intestine graft rejection has been more difficult to prevent and treat than rejection of other solid organs. Moreover, intestine rejection carries significant morbidity because it leads to a breakdown of gut barrier function, which results in bacterial translocation and severe infections. Patients with a nucleotide oligomerization domain 2 polymorphism, a gene associated with Crohn disease,[27] have a higher rate of graft rejection, suggesting a role for innate immunity in the pathophysiology of this complication.

Aggressive maintenance IS protocols used in the early era of IT failed to consistently prevent rejection and resulted in high death rates because of infection and posttransplant lymphoproliferative disease (PTLD). Results have improved in the modern era by using high-dose induction therapy followed by rapid tapering to conventional levels of immune suppression paired with aggressive protocols for early detection and treatment of rejection and infections.[28–30]

The history and current trends of IS treatment have been extensively reviewed recently.[28,30] Although IS protocols vary between centers, all protocols seem to achieve similar long-term outcomes in expert hands. Most centers use induction therapy with thymoglobulin or IL-2 blockers and maintenance treatment with tacrolimus and prednisone with initial trough blood levels of tacrolimus at 10 to 18 ng/mL. With these protocols the rates of AR are now about 30% to 50%.[28,31,32] Attempts to use alemtuzumab as induction therapy in children by the Miami group failed because of a high rate of posttransplant complications (mainly respiratory related) in children younger than 4 years.[29]

Two recent innovative protocols aimed at minimizing IS and promotion of partial tolerance have been reported by the Pittsburgh and Leuven groups.[28,30] A total of 206 adults and children in Pittsburgh were induced with thymoglobulin and 2 steroid boluses followed by maintenance monotherapy with tacrolimus with slow withdrawal of immune suppression starting at 6 months after transplant. Steroids were added to the posttransplant treatment in cases of AR or adrenal insufficiency. Partial tapering of tacrolimus was successful in 57% of patients in whom it was attempted (66% of the patients). However, the rate of AR reached 50% and the rate of chronic rejection (CR) is unknown because of short follow-up.[28] Thus, the long-term effect of the high AR rate is unknown as yet.

The Leuven protocol was designed to enhance the generation of regulatory T cells. The protocol includes careful selection of healthy donors, maintaining short cold and warm ischemia times; donor intestine decontamination; administration of glutamine to donor and recipient; a donor-specific blood transfusion at the time of transplantation; induction with either IL-2 blockers or thymoglobulin; avoidance of high-dose steroids; and maintenance immune suppression with tacrolimus and azathioprine.[30] Only 7 patients have been treated according to this protocol so far, with AR in 1 case only and 100% survival. Firm conclusions cannot be drawn because of the small sample size; however, the initial experience is promising and merits consideration of larger-scale studies for confirmation.

NUTRITION AFTER TRANSPLANT

Discontinuation of PN and oral autonomy are major goals of IT. The optimal nutritional treatment after transplant has not been studied in large randomized studies and is currently based on expert opinion and individual center experience. Key management questions such as polymeric versus elemental diet, timing of introduction and type of solid foods to be used after transplant, and rate of PN weaning have not been fully answered yet.

Tolerance of tube feeding or solids in the early phase after transplant is frequently hampered by graft malfunction as a result of infection, rejection, or PTLD and by the physiologic changes in the intestine after transplant, including extrinsic denervation, dysmotility, lymphatic disruption, and fat malabsorption. Prevention of these post-transplant complications promotes PN weaning and oral tolerance. PN is commonly initiated 1 to 3 days after transplant and enteral feeding is started at postoperative day 5 to 7 following resolution of the postsurgical ileus. Some centers start feeding with an elemental, low-fat, low-osmolality formula,[33] whereas others use polymeric formula.[34] Introduction of solids, which can be started as early as 2 weeks after transplant, is often challenging in children who have been dependent on PN for years, have not acquired eating habits, or suffer from food aversion. Solids are usually limited initially to low-fat, low-osmolarity, low-sugar, and low-lactose feeds to avoid high stoma output. The diet is advanced as tolerated.[35] Augmentation of solid-food diet with overnight tube feeding and extra fluids is frequently required in young children to avoid dehydration and to promote growth.

SURVEILLANCE FOR GRAFT REJECTION AND INFECTIONS

Early detection and prompt treatment of graft rejection and infections has been a major factor contributing to the improved results of IT. Unlike other solid-organ grafts such as liver or kidney there is no simple laboratory marker to monitor graft function and screen for new pathology of the graft. Thus, protocol ileoscopies with intestinal biopsies are the recommended method to monitor the intestine graft after transplant. The required and optimal frequency of protocol endoscopies is unknown but 1 to 2 per week is usual for the first month after transplant, followed by a gradual reduction in the frequency until stoma closure.

Diarrhea is a nonspecific finding that can be a result of rejection but can also have many other causes, ranging from infection to drug reactions (**Table 2**), and thus requires prompt investigation. Urgent endoscopy is indicated for increased stoma output, change in stool habits, gastrointestinal symptoms, fever, and abnormal laboratory findings such as hypoalbuminemia or anemia. The endoscopic findings of AR include blunted and short villi, edematous and friable mucosa, superficial or deep ulcers, and diffuse mucosal exfoliation; these findings can be mimicked by infection. Measures that may improve the sensitivity of surveillance endoscopies include the use of zoom endoscopy[36] and capsule endoscopy[37] but their use in small pediatric recipients is challenging because of size limitations.

Table 2 Possible causes of diarrhea after IT	
	Cause
Immune	AR, ischemia reperfusion injury, GVHD
Infectious	Viral, bacterial, fungal
Medications	IS medications, antibiotic
Surgical related	Dysmotility, lymphatic disruption
Neoplastic	PTLD, lymphoma
Other	Mild degree of fat malabsorption, nonrestricted diet

Two markers have been assessed in the ongoing search for reliable laboratory indicators to screen for AR and infections. Plasma citrulline is produced primarily by enterocytes and thus blood levels reflect intestinal cell mass. Acute intestine rejection or infections are associated with low citrulline levels.[38–40] However, citrulline levels have a wide normal range, are age dependent, correlate with bowel length, are increased in patients with chronic renal failure, and are unstable in the first months after transplant,[39] characteristics that limit the usefulness of this measure as a screening test.

Calprotectin is a cytosolic protein of enterocytes and neutrophils and can be detected in stool during active inflammation. Sudan and colleagues[41] have shown that stool calprotectin levels are significantly higher in patients with AR compared with viral enteritis or normal biopsies, with specificity of 77% and sensitivity of 83%. A similarly designed study from the Miami group using a cut-off point of calprotectin level of more than 100 ng/kg showed a significant difference between patients with normal intestinal biopsy and abnormal biopsy without the ability to discriminate between various intestinal pathologies such as rejection, infection, or nonspecific inflammation.[42] These findings suggest that stool calprotectin levels may be a useful method to screen for early intestinal disease that requires prompt investigation with ileoscopy and intestinal biopsy.

Surveillance of graft function should be a combined effort of the primary care pediatrician in the community and the hospital-based transplant team. Careful follow-up of the patient and detection of subtle symptoms and signs of early and late complications can have a substantial effect on long-term outcome. The primary care practitioner will be the first to observe and react to these changes. The community pediatrician should be able to identify concerning clinical symptoms that deserve attention and in many cases requires referral to the transplant center. Fever, weight loss, poor growth, diarrhea or increased stoma output, bloody diarrhea, abdominal pain, vomiting, or general reduction in clinical status require further work-up and assessment. As described in **Table 2** diarrhea is the most common clinical abnormality after transplant and frequently requires a referral for further work-up in the transplant center. Lymphadenopathy, abdominal distension, ascites and edema, discolorization or prolapse of stoma, and hepatomegaly or splenomegaly should always trigger a careful medical assessment. Side effects of IS medications are a common occurrence after transplant and should be looked for in any routine clinic visit. The most common are renal failure, PTLD, infections, hypertension, hyperlipidemia, and occasionally neurologic symptoms. A close follow-up in the community with ongoing communication between the primary care pediatrician and the patient and their family can lead to early detection of compliance problems and appropriate intervention to prevent any damage to the graft. A combined follow-up with shared responsibility between the community and hospital pediatricians can lead to improved long-term outcome of solid-organ recipients and is a desirable care model.

MANAGEMENT AND OUTCOME OF AR AND CR

AR is the leading cause for graft loss and death after intestinal transplantation; thus, early detection and treatment of AR are crucial to achieve good patient outcomes. Patients with AR can be asymptomatic or can present with an increased stoma output, diarrhea, intestinal obstruction, or bleeding in severe exfoliative rejection. The accurate diagnosis of graft rejection relies on biopsies that should be taken from a minimum of 3 locations because of the patchy nature of intestinal rejection. In MVTx, the most common site of AR is the intestine; however, AR can be detected in any organ of the composite graft and even isolated liver rejection can be found occasionally.[43] Higher rates of AR are reported in isolated IT compared with composite grafts containing the liver,[44] probably as a result of the poorly immunologically defined tolerogenic effect of the liver. Even subclinical asymptomatic rejection in the initial postoperative period is also associated with lower graft survival at 5 years and higher risk for death as a result of infection.[45]

Criteria for pathologic definition and grading of AR were published in 2004.[46] The characteristic histologic findings include crypt epithelial cell apoptosis, crypt injury, inflammation with mixed cell population (primarily mononuclear cells), villus blunting with architectural distortion, and edema with vascular congestion. With severe AR, the changes mentioned earlier are accompanied by diffuse mucosal ulceration and erosion up to a complete loss of the bowel morphology and mucosal sloughing. Exfoliative rejection is associated with a high graft loss and mortality so it is important to treat AR before patients are symptomatic or during its early stages to ensure an improved outcome.[47] Initial therapy includes methylprednisolone pulse or thymoglobulin or alemtuzumab for moderate to severe AR. Sporadic case reports suggested a favorable outcome for patients with AR resistant to steroid- or lympho-cyte-depleting agents who were treated with infliximab, an antitumor necrosis factor α antagonist.[48,49]

CR is the most common cause of late graft dysfunction. Typical symptoms include chronic diarrhea, abdominal pain, chronic bleeding, and graft malfunction with weight loss. The pathophysiologic process of CR involves intimal hyperplasia and obliterative arteriopathy in the submucosal layers. Endoscopic biopsies may show mucosal and submucosal fibrosis and atrophy, distorted villi, crypt damage, and occasionally arte-riopathy of small arterioles.[50] However, a full thickness biopsy is needed to confirm this diagnosis, which is manifested by atherosclerotic-type lesions with eccentric intimal hyperplasia and concentric fibrous intimal thickening in the large and medium-size arteries. Patients with recurrent, early, and severe AR and recipients of isolated IT are more susceptible for CR[50] and should be carefully monitored to ensure optimal IS treatment and avoid further episodes of AR. In an analysis of explanted composite grafts, the liver and pancreas had a similar incidence of CR compared with the intestine, unlike the differential susceptibility to AR of composite organs.[43] There is no definite treatment of CR because of poor understanding of the mechanism of this type of rejection, and retransplantation is usually the only solution.[51]

RISK FACTORS AND OUTCOME
Infection

Infections remain a common complication after transplant. The use of intense immune suppression, breakdown of the gut barrier as a result of AR and ischemia reperfusion injury, and PTLD contribute to the high incidence of infection after IT.[52] The Miami group[29] reported that 91% of the children after IT or MVTx (n = 112) had at least 1 episode of infection, with a median of 5 infectious episodes per child. Bacterial infec-tions usually present as sepsis, bacteremia, pneumonia, intra-abdominal infection, or wound infection and are the most common cause for infection.[53] Cicalese and colleagues[54] reported that 44% of their patients had an episode of bacterial translo-cation with pathogens such as Klebsiella, Enterococcus, Staphylococcus and Enter-obacter. However, there is a poor correlation between the stool culture isolates and the bacterial pathogens identified in blood or peritoneal fluid.[55] Most bacterial infec-tion can be controlled with appropriate antibiotic treatment but sepsis remains a leading cause of death and accounts for approximately 50% of the causes of death, according to the international intestinal transplant registry results (Intestinal Registry Report, Bologna, 2009).

Viral pathogens that usually induce self-limited diarrhea in an immune-competent child can lead to severe and prolonged diarrhea in IT recipients. Patients with enteric viral infections usually require supplemental intravenous fluid infusion for a prolonged time until the infection resolves. Clinical symptoms and endoscopic findings of viral infection and AR overlap, and thus differentiation between the 2 is often challenging. Correct interpretation of biopsies in these cases demands an experienced pathologist. Subtle histologic changes that support the diagnosis of viral enteritis include superficial apoptosis, thicker mononuclear infiltrate adjacent to the gut lumen, and pathologic abnormalities in the graft and the native bowel.[56–58] In addition to hematoxylin and eosin stains, immunohistochemistry and use of the polymerase chain reaction may facilitate the identification of the viruses. Besides common and known viral pathogens such as CMV, EBV, and rotavirus, other less common enteric viral infection such as adenovirus and calicivirus have emerged in the last decade as important pathogens in IT recipients.[59,60] Adenovirus infection is common after IT, affecting up to 21% of IT recipients.[60] Occasionally viral infection can precede AR, and careful follow-up of signs and symptoms of rejection at the time or immediately after infection is advisable.[19,61] Routine surveillance of CMV, EBV, and adenovirus in blood and intestinal biopsies is recommended to ensure early and timely detection of infection. These strategies plus routine prophylaxis treatment of CMV with ganciclovir and cytogam have reduced mortality and morbidity related to infections after transplant.[62]

OTHER COMPLICATIONS

PTLD, an EBV-driven B-cell lymphoproliferation, continues to plague IT recipients. The use of antibody-depleting agents and high levels of maintenance immune suppression have led to the highest incidence of PTLD among solid-organ recipients. The initial reported PTLD rates were 20% to 32% among IT recipients but these rates have decreased to less than 10% as a result of the use of lower levels of maintenance immune suppression and careful monitoring for EBV with the use of preemptive therapy.[17,29,62,63] Reyes and colleagues[62] have shown that the odds ratio for development of PTLD decreased to 0.39 following the implementation of preemptive therapy with IS reduction, ganciclovir, and cytogam. Although a reduction in IS is an effective method to reduce EBV proliferation, AR is an occasional sequela of this strategy and thus careful graft monitoring for early signs of AR is needed. Other treatment modalities for advanced PTLD include the use of rituximab, monoclonal anti-CD20 antibodies, and chemotherapy. Non-EBV-related lymphoma presenting as non-Hodgkin B-cell or T-cell lymphoma should also be considered in patients with suspected malignancy.[64]

The large inoculum of donor lymphoid cells within the graft occasionally results in graft-versus-host disease (GVHD). GVHD occurs in 5% of IT recipients, a rate that is much higher than the rate associated with other solid organs.[29,65] Donor-derived lymphocytes damage skin, native gastrointestinal tract, native liver, and bone marrow. Children with MVTx have the highest risk of GVHD.[65] Recent reports have shown that mycophenolate mofetil (MMF) induces GVHD-like histologic changes in the duodenum and colon.[66,67] Hence, careful assessment is warranted in IT recipients who present with gastrointestinal symptoms and are treated with MMF, before establishing the diagnosis of GVHD. Mild cases of skin rash often resolve spontaneously but occasionally treatment is needed. Most patients respond to high-dose prednisone; despite treatment, mortality is high in severe cases.[29,65]

Chronic renal failure (CRF) is common after solid-organ transplantation and is a leading cause of posttransplant morbidity and mortality.[68] In the study by Ojo and colleagues,[68] 21% of 5-year survivors of IT had CRF (defined as GFR < 29 mL/min/1.73 m^2), the highest incidence among nonrenal transplant recipients. Data assessing renal function in children after IT are limited. Ueno and colleagues[69] calculated GFR in 44 children who survived more than 2 years after transplantation. Mean GFR at 2 years after transplant was 102 mL/min/1.73 m^{2,28}, 81% of the pretransplant GFR. Kato and colleagues[29] reported GFR less than 90 mL/min/1.73 m^2 in 35% of their patients at 2 years after transplant. Because calculated GFR was used in these studies, it is reasonable to assume that the actual number of patients with CRF is higher because the calculated GFR usually overestimates measured GFR. Risk factors for CRF include high tacrolimus levels, low preoperative GFR, and admission to the intensive care unit before transplant.[69,70] These concerning numbers call for better management of renal function after transplant, with careful monitoring of nephrotoxic medications, especially calcineurin inhibitors.

OUTCOME

A preliminary report on the world experience with IT was presented in September 2009 at the XI International Intestine Transplant Symposium in Bologna. Experience with more than 2000 cases (an estimated 95% of the world experience) was reviewed. About half of these transplants were performed at 3 US centers. Children accounted for more than 50% of the recipients. In the previous 5 years the 1-year patient survival was close to 80% and the 3-year survival was 65%. This finding is in contrast to the outcome 10 years previously, with 1- and 5-year survival of 60% to 65% and 45%, respectively. However, mortality continues beyond the first year after transplant and the 5- and 10-year patient survival rates in the last decade are 50% and 45%, respectively. Unlike the short-term outcome, the long-term outcome has not improved significantly in the last decade. The main cause of death has not changed and is a result of sepsis in 50% of cases.

Survival in high-volume centers in the United States and Europe is even better. Children transplanted in the last 5 to 10 years have a 70% to 84% 3-year survival rate at the major transplant centers.[71–73] The 1-, 3- and 5-year patient survival of 199 children who were transplanted in Pittsburgh in the new era is 95%, 84%, and 77%, respectively. Graft survival is 88%, 74%, and 58%, respectively.[73] Poor prognostic markers include children younger than 1 year, no induction therapy with IL-2 blockers, waiting in hospital before transplant, and recipients of isolated IT or combined liver-intestine transplantation.[29] As time passes, the number of retransplants is slowly increasing as a result of graft loss for AR or CR, PTLD, and graft dysfunction. Mazariegos and colleagues[51] reported that 8.1% of their pediatric transplants are now retransplants, with 71% overall patient survival. It seems that the number of retransplants will continue to increase in the near future because of the current results of long-term graft survival.

GROWTH AND NUTRITION

The ultimate goal of IT is to achieve full enteral feeding and to ensure normal growth after transplant. Of the survivors of pediatric IT, 80% to 100% are weaned from PN and are maintained on full enteral feeding by either oral or tube feeding.[74–76] Discontinuation of PN is achieved in most patients in the first 1 to 3 months after transplant, but many children require tube feeding for prolonged periods of time. Despite consumption of the recommended caloric needs for age and normal weight for height after transplant, catch-up growth is often not achieved in the first 2 to 5 years after transplant[74–78] and may not occur even in longer periods. Ueno and colleagues[78] recorded catch-up growth in a subpopulation of recipients with severe growth delay before transplant (z score < 2), but this finding has not been confirmed by others.

A comprehensive assessment of nutritional status and growth after IT was published recently by Lacaille and colleagues.[77] In addition to abnormal growth pattern as described earlier, about 50% of the patients had lower levels of biologic markers of nutrition such as retinol binding protein, cholesterol, and vitamin A. Despite high energy and protein intake, energy absorption was less than 90% because of persistent fat malabsorption. Carbohydrate and protein absorption were normal. These findings highlight the need to monitor nutrition carefully before and after transplantation and possibly provide 20% to 30% more calories than the recommended amount for age to ensure adequate growth after transplant.

QOL

There are limited data on health-related QOL (HRQOL) after IT, particularly in children. A general assessment of QOL by means of oral tolerance and Karnofsky score, a general performance status tool, showed that most surviving recipients tolerate enteral feeding and are capable of normal activities as recorded in the Intestinal Registry Report, Bologna, 2009. A limited assessment of QOL in the early era of IT reported a similar QOL in adults on home PN compared with recipients of IT.[79] A similar comparison using the short-form 36-item questionnaire that examines 8 specific domains of QOL[80] showed that adults after IT tended to score better than patients on home PN, but these differences did not reach statistical significance in 7 domains. An assessment of adults before and after IT using a self-administered questionnaire originally designed for liver transplantation showed an overall improvement in HRQOL after transplant, including domains dealing with coping, social relations, optimism, and energy.[81] The only pediatric assessment of HRQOL, conducted by Sudan and colleagues,[82] evaluated recipients and their parents (n = 22) with the Child Health Questionnaire, which measured 14 health domains. IT recipients reported the same scores as normal children but their parents perceived their QOL as lower in general health, physical functioning, and the effect of illness on family life. Thus, although preliminary results confirm that it is possible to achieve an excellent HRQOL with a well-functioning intestine graft, more studies are needed to learn how to optimize long-term results.

SUMMARY

The short-term survival of pediatric IT recipients has significantly improved in the last decade, and reached 90% at the end of the first year after transplant in high-volume IT centers. Measures to reduce short- and long-term morbidity and to improve long-term outcome and QOL constitute the next challenges of IT.

REFERENCES

1. Modi BP, Javid PJ, Jaksic T, et al. First report of the international serial transverse enteroplasty data registry: indications, efficacy, and complications. J Am Coll Surg 2007;204:365.
2. Wales PW, de Silva N, Langer JC, et al. Intermediate outcomes after serial transverse enteroplasty in children with short bowel syndrome. J Pediatr Surg 2007;42:1804.

3. Diamond IR, Sterescu A, Pencharz PB, et al. Changing the paradigm: omegaven for the treatment of liver failure in pediatric short bowel syndrome. J Pediatr Gastroenterol Nutr 2009;48:209.
4. Gura KM, Lee S, Valim C, et al. Safety and efficacy of a fish-oil-based fat emulsion in the treatment of parenteral nutrition-associated liver disease. Pediatrics 2008; 121:e678.
5. Diamond IR, de Silva N, Pencharz PB, et al. Neonatal short bowel syndrome outcomes after the establishment of the first Canadian multidisciplinary intestinal rehabilitation program: preliminary experience. J Pediatr Surg 2007; 42:806.
6. Nucci A, Burns RC, Armah T, et al. Interdisciplinary management of pediatric intestinal failure: a 10-year review of rehabilitation and transplantation. J Gastrointest Surg 2008;12:429.
7. Torres C, Sudan D, Vanderhoof J, et al. Role of an intestinal rehabilitation program in the treatment of advanced intestinal failure. J Pediatr Gastroenterol Nutr 2007; 45:204.
8. Goulet O, Ruemmele F, Lacaille F, et al. Irreversible intestinal failure. J Pediatr Gastroenterol Nutr 2004;38:250.
9. Lillehei RC, Goott B, Miller FA. The physiological response of the small bowel of the dog to ischemia including prolonged in vitro preservation of the bowel with successful replacement and survival. Ann Surg 1959;150:543.
10. Ruemmele FM, Sauvat F, Colomb V, et al. Seventeen years after successful small bowel transplantation: long term graft acceptance without immune tolerance. Gut 2006;55:903.
11. Grant D, Wall W, Mimeault R, et al. Successful small-bowel/liver transplantation. Lancet 1990;335:181.
12. Abu-Elmagd KM, Costa G, Bond GJ, et al. Five hundred intestinal and multivisceral transplantations at a single center: major advances with new challenges. Ann Surg 2009. [Epub ahead of print].
13. Selvaggi G, Tzakis AG. Small bowel transplantation: technical advances/updates. Curr Opin Organ Transplant 2009;14:262.
14. Sudan DL, Iyer KR, Deroover A, et al. A new technique for combined liver/small intestinal transplantation. Transplantation 1846;72:2001.
15. Benedetti E, Holterman M, Asolati M, et al. Living related segmental bowel transplantation: from experimental to standardized procedure. Ann Surg 2006; 244:694.
16. Gruessner RW, Sharp HL. Living-related intestinal transplantation: first report of a standardized surgical technique. Transplantation 1997;64:1605.
17. Fishbein TM. Intestinal transplantation. N Engl J Med 2009;361:998.
18. Grant D, Abu-Elmagd K, Reyes J, et al. 2003 report of the intestine transplant registry: a new era has dawned. Ann Surg 2005;241:607.
19. Ziring D, Tran R, Edelstein S, et al. Infectious enteritis after intestinal transplantation: incidence, timing, and outcome. Transplant Proc 2004;36:379.
20. Magee JC, Krishnan SM, Benfield MR, et al. Pediatric transplantation in the United States, 1997–2006. Am J Transplant 2008;8:935.
21. Fecteau A, Atkinson P, Grant D. Early referral is essential for successful pediatric small bowel transplantation: the Canadian experience. J Pediatr Surg 2001;36:681.
22. Beath S, Pironi L, Gabe S, et al. Collaborative strategies to reduce mortality and morbidity in patients with chronic intestinal failure including those who are referred for small bowel transplantation. Transplantation 2008;85:1378.

23. Kaufman SS, Atkinson JB, Bianchi A, et al. Indications for pediatric intestinal transplantation: a position paper of the American Society of Transplantation. Pediatr Transplant 2001;5:80.
24. Pironi L, Forbes A, Joly F, et al. Survival of patients identified as candidates for intestinal transplantation: a 3-year prospective follow-up. Gastroenterology 2008;135:61.
25. Todo S, Tzakis A, Reyes J, et al. Small intestinal transplantation in humans with or without the colon. Transplantation 1994;57:840.
26. Kato T, Selvaggi G, Gaynor JJ, et al. Inclusion of donor colon and ileocecal valve in intestinal transplantation. Transplantation 2008;86:293.
27. Fishbein T, Novitskiy G, Mishra L, et al. NOD2-expressing bone marrow-derived cells appear to regulate epithelial innate immunity of the transplanted human small intestine. Gut 2008;57:323.
28. Abu-Elmagd KM, Costa G, Bond GJ, et al. Evolution of the immunosuppressive strategies for the intestinal and multivisceral recipients with special reference to allograft immunity and achievement of partial tolerance. Transpl Int 2009;22:96.
29. Kato T, Tzakis AG, Selvaggi G, et al. Intestinal and multivisceral transplantation in children. Ann Surg 2006;243:756.
30. Pirenne J, Kawai M. Intestinal transplantation: evolution in immunosuppression protocols. Curr Opin Organ Transplant 2009;14:250.
31. Nishida S, Levi DM, Moon JI, et al. Intestinal transplantation with alemtuzumab (Campath-1H) induction for adult patients. Transplant Proc 2006;38:1747.
32. Sudan DL, Chinnakotla S, Horslen S, et al. Basiliximab decreases the incidence of acute rejection after intestinal transplantation. Transplant Proc 2002;34:940.
33. Silver HJ, Castellanos VH. Nutritional complications and management of intestinal transplant. J Am Diet Assoc 2000;100:680.
34. Matarese LE, Costa G, Bond G, et al. Therapeutic efficacy of intestinal and multivisceral transplantation: survival and nutrition outcome. Nutr Clin Pract 2007;22:474.
35. Weseman RA, Gilroy R. Nutrition management of small bowel transplant patients. Nutr Clin Pract 2005;20:509.
36. Kato T, Gaynor JJ, Nishida S, et al. Zoom endoscopic monitoring of small bowel allograft rejection. Surg Endosc 2006;20:773.
37. de Franchis R, Rondonotti E, Abbiati C, et al. Capsule enteroscopy in small bowel transplantation. Dig Liver Dis 2003;35:728.
38. David AI, Gaynor JJ, Zis PP, et al. An association of lower serum citrulline levels within 30 days of acute rejection in patients following small intestine transplantation. Transplant Proc 2006;38:1731.
39. Gondolesi GE, Kaufman SS, Sansaricq C, et al. Defining normal plasma citrulline in intestinal transplant recipients. Am J Transplant 2004;4:414.
40. Pappas PA, Tzakis GA, Gaynor JJ, et al. An analysis of the association between serum citrulline and acute rejection among 26 recipients of intestinal transplant. Am J Transplant 2004;4:1124.
41. Sudan D, Vargas L, Sun Y, et al. Calprotectin: a novel noninvasive marker for intestinal allograft monitoring. Ann Surg 2007;246:311.
42. Akpinar E, Vargas J, Kato T, et al. Fecal calprotectin level measurements in small bowel allograft monitoring: a pilot study. Transplantation 2008;85:1281.
43. Takahashi H, Kato T, Delacruz V, et al. Analysis of acute and chronic rejection in multiple organ allografts from retransplantation and autopsy cases of multivisceral transplantation. Transplantation 2008;85:1610.

44. Jugie M, Canioni D, Le Bihan C, et al. Study of the impact of liver transplantation on the outcome of intestinal grafts in children. Transplantation 2006;81:992.

45. Takahashi H, Kato T, Selvaggi G, et al. Subclinical rejection in the initial postoperative period in small intestinal transplantation: a negative influence on graft survival. Transplantation 2007;84:689.

46. Ruiz P, Bagni A, Brown R, et al. Histological criteria for the identification of acute cellular rejection in human small bowel allografts: results of the pathology workshop at the VIII International Small Bowel Transplant Symposium. Transplant Proc 2004;36:335.

47. Ishii T, Mazariegos GV, Bueno J, et al. Exfoliative rejection after intestinal transplantation in children. Pediatr Transplant 2003;7:185.

48. De Greef E, Grant D, Ng V, et al. Infliximab as salvage therapy for steroid and thymoglobulin resistant late acute intestinal rejection in pediatric intestinal transplant recipients. In: XIth International Small Bowel Transplant Symposium. Bologna, Italy; September 9–12, 2009. p. 65.

49. Pascher A, Klupp J, Langrehr JM, et al. Anti-TNF-alpha therapy for acute rejection in intestinal transplantation. Transplant Proc 2005;37:1635.

50. Parizhskaya M, Redondo C, Demetris A, et al. Chronic rejection of small bowel grafts: pediatric and adult study of risk factors and morphologic progression. Pediatr Dev Pathol 2003;6:240.

51. Mazariegos GV, Soltys K, Bond G, et al. Pediatric intestinal retransplantation: techniques, management, and outcomes. Transplantation 2008;86:1777.

52. Sigurdsson L, Reyes J, Kocoshis SA, et al. Bacteremia after intestinal transplantation in children correlates temporally with rejection or gastrointestinal lymphoproliferative disease. Transplantation 2000;70:302.

53. Loinaz C, Kato T, Nishida S, et al. Bacterial infections after intestine and multivisceral transplantation. The experience of the University of Miami (1994–2001). Hepatogastroenterology 2006;53:234.

54. Cicalese L, Sileri P, Green M, et al. Bacterial translocation in clinical intestinal transplantation. Transplantation 2001;71:1414.

55. John M, Gondolesi G, Herold BC, et al. Impact of surveillance stool culture guided selection of antibiotics in the management of pediatric small bowel transplant recipients. Pediatr Transplant 2006;10:198.

56. Eisengart LJ, Chou PM, Iyer K, et al. Rotavirus infection in small bowel transplant: a histologic comparison with acute cellular rejection. Pediatr Dev Pathol 2009;12:85.

57. Morotti RA, Kaufman SS, Fishbein TM, et al. Calicivirus infection in pediatric small intestine transplant recipients: pathological considerations. Hum Pathol 2004;35:1236.

58. Parizhskaya M, Walpusk J, Mazariegos G, et al. Enteric adenovirus infection in pediatric small bowel transplant recipients. Pediatr Dev Pathol 2001;4:122.

59. Kaufman SS, Chatterjee NK, Fuschino ME, et al. Characteristics of human calicivirus enteritis in intestinal transplant recipients. J Pediatr Gastroenterol Nutr 2005;40:328.

60. McLaughlin GE, Delis S, Kashimawo L, et al. Adenovirus infection in pediatric liver and intestinal transplant recipients: utility of DNA detection by PCR. Am J Transplant 2003;3:224.

61. Pascher A, Klupp J, Schulz RJ, et al. CMV, EBV, HHV6, and HHV7 infections after intestinal transplantation without specific antiviral prophylaxis. Transplant Proc 2004;36:381.

62. Reyes J, Mazariegos GV, Bond GM, et al. Pediatric intestinal transplantation: historical notes, principles and controversies. Pediatr Transplant 2002;6:193.

63. Finn L, Reyes J, Bueno J, et al. Epstein-Barr virus infections in children after transplantation of the small intestine. Am J Surg Pathol 1998;22:299.
64. Berho M, Viciana A, Weppler D, et al. T cell lymphoma involving the graft of a multivisceral organ recipient. Transplantation 1999;68:1135.
65. Mazariegos GV, Abu-Elmagd K, Jaffe R, et al. Graft versus host disease in intestinal transplantation. Am J Transplant 2004;4:1459.
66. Papadimitriou JC, Cangro CB, Lustberg A, et al. Histologic features of mycophenolate mofetil-related colitis: a graft-versus-host disease-like pattern. Int J Surg Pathol 2003;11:295.
67. Parfitt JR, Jayakumar S, Driman DK. Mycophenolate mofetil-related gastrointestinal mucosal injury: variable injury patterns, including graft-versus-host disease-like changes. Am J Surg Pathol 2008;32:1367.
68. Ojo AO, Held PJ, Port FK, et al. Chronic renal failure after transplantation of a non-renal organ. N Engl J Med 2003;349:931.
69. Ueno T, Kato T, Gaynor J, et al. Renal function after pediatric intestinal transplant. Transplant Proc 2006;38:1759.
70. Watson MJ, Venick RS, Kaldas F, et al. Renal function impacts outcomes after intestinal transplantation. Transplantation 2008;86:117.
71. Grant W, Botha J, Mercer D, et al. 19 years of experience with intestinal transplantation at a single institution. In XIth International Small Bowel Transplant Symposium. Bologna, Italy; September 9–12, 2009. p. 94.
72. Gupte GL, Sharif K, Mayer AD, et al. Strategies, complications and learning experiences of a national intestinal transplant programme (1993–2009). In XIth International Small Bowel Transplant Symposium. Bologna, Italy; September 9–12, 2009. p. 53.
73. Mazariegos GV, Squires RH, Sindhi RK. Current perspectives on pediatric intestinal transplantation. Curr Gastroenterol Rep 2009;11:226.
74. Iyer K, Horslen S, Iverson A, et al. Nutritional outcome and growth of children after intestinal transplantation. J Pediatr Surg 2002;37:464.
75. Nucci AM, Barksdale EM Jr, Beserock N, et al. Long-term nutritional outcome after pediatric intestinal transplantation. J Pediatr Surg 2002;37:460.
76. Venick RS, Farmer DG, Saikali D, et al. Nutritional outcomes following pediatric intestinal transplantation. Transplant Proc 2006;38:1718.
77. Lacaille F, Vass N, Sauvat F, et al. Long-term outcome, growth and digestive function in children 2 to 18 years after intestinal transplantation. Gut 2008;57:455.
78. Ueno T, Kato T, Revas K, et al. Growth after intestinal transplant in children. Transplant Proc 2006;38:1702.
79. Rovera GM, DiMartini A, Schoen RE, et al. Quality of life of patients after intestinal transplantation. Transplantation 1998;66:1141.
80. Pironi L, Paganelli F, Lauro A, et al. Quality of life on home parenteral nutrition or after intestinal transplantation. Transplant Proc 2006;38:1673.
81. O'Keefe SJ, Emerling M, Koritsky D, et al. Nutrition and quality of life following small intestinal transplantation. Am J Gastroenterol 2007;102:1093.
82. Sudan D, Horslen S, Botha J, et al. Quality of life after pediatric intestinal transplantation: the perception of pediatric recipients and their parents. Am J Transplant 2004;4:407.

Immunosuppression Armamentarium in 2010: Mechanistic and Clinical Considerations

Simon Urschel, MD[a,b],
Luis A. Altamirano-Diaz, Medico-Cirujano, FRCP[b],
Lori J. West, MD, DPhil[a,b],*

KEYWORDS

- Immunosuppressive treatment • Pediatric transplantation
- Solid-organ transplantation • Induction
- Maintenance immunosuppression
- Mechanism of action • Side effects

Effective immunosuppression is the key to successful organ transplantation, with success being defined as minimal rejection risk with concomitant minimal drug toxicities. Despite the general recognition of this fact, there is a lack of standardization of clinical management regimens, with an extensive diversity of favored approaches, particularly in pediatric transplantation. Although differences associated with the transplanted organ are obvious, even single organ transplant groups are far from consensus on the ideal approach to immunosuppression.

Current strategies in pediatric solid-organ transplantation are different amongst the organs. Induction treatment as an early first strike on the immune system during the perioperative period has become more common, but is not universally accepted as a mandatory part of organ transplantation. With improved pretransplant identification of high-risk patients such as patients with preformed anti-HLA antibodies, different desensitization protocols have been proposed, which require further evaluation.

Strategies used for maintenance immunosuppression also vary amongst the organ transplant groups, illustrated in the various registry reports. In kidney transplantation the North American Pediatric Renal Trials and Collaborative Studies (NAPRTCS) annual report 2008 showed that more than 50% of patients now receive a combination

[a] Cardiac Transplant Research, University of Alberta, Alberta Diabetes Institute, Room-6-002 HRIF East, Edmonton, AB T6G 2E1, Canada
[b] Department of Pediatrics, Division of Pediatric Cardiology, University of Alberta, 4C2 WMC, Edmonton, AB T6G 2R7, Canada
* Corresponding author. Department of Pediatrics, Division of Pediatric Cardiology, University of Alberta, 4C2 WMC, Edmonton, AB T6G 2R7, Canada.
E-mail address: ljwest@ualberta.ca

Pediatr Clin N Am 57 (2010) 433–457
doi:10.1016/j.pcl.2010.01.018
0031-3955/10/$ – see front matter © 2010 Elsevier Inc. All rights reserved.

of calcineurin inhibitors (CNI), cell cycle inhibitors and steroids, with tacrolimus (TAC) being used more commonly than cyclosporine A (CSA).[1] The International Society of Heart and Lung Transplantation (ISHLT) 2009 Registry Pediatric Report showed that heart transplant immunosuppression is mainly based on a combination of CNI with cell cycle inhibitors.[2] TAC/mycophenolate (mycophenolic acid; MPA) is the most common combination in current use followed by CSA/MPA. Steroids are continued beyond the first year in nearly half of the patients and mTOR (mammalian target of rapamycin) inhibitors are used in 8% of patients.[2] For pediatric lung transplant recipients, the maintenance immunosuppression used is usually a combination of CNI and cell cycle inhibitors. The most commonly used CNI is TAC, which is used almost twice as often as CSA, with the most frequent combination regimen being TAC/MPA. Nearly all patients remain on steroids at 5 years after transplant.[3]

A study from the Studies of Pediatric Liver Transplantation (SPLIT) database registry examining 5-year liver transplant survivors showed that 64% are on CNI-based monotherapy immunosuppression. Of those patients, 74% are receiving TAC. Steroids are still used at 5 years after transplant in 24%.[4]

Fig. 1 illustrates the options for immunosuppression in a time line. Most transplant patients require some kind of indefinite maintenance immunosuppression, with the exception of weaning from immunosuppression late after transplantation, which has been successful in up to 20% of pediatric liver transplant recipients.[5] Single cases of pediatric patients weaned from immunosuppression have also been reported after kidney transplantation,[6] and, although anecdotal cases exist, there have not been published reports of successful weaning from immunosuppression in pediatric recipients of thoracic organ transplants. Perioperative high-dose steroid treatment is also accepted as a general approach amongst all organs, although the role of steroids in maintenance treatment is currently under vigorous discussion.

Fig. 2 illustrates the cellular targets of immunosuppressive drugs. The drugs in most common current usage, including dosage and specific side effects, are shown in **Table 1** and discussed in the following sections. The later sections provide a future outlook and discussion of current investigative approaches.

INDUCTION THERAPY

The use of induction immunotherapy is defined as intense immunosuppression in the immediate perioperative phase of organ implantation and has become more common in the last decade in all areas of solid-organ transplantation. The initial rationale for the use of induction treatment was the expected lower incidence of acute rejection in the early posttransplant phase. This finding was proven for several different agents for 1-year posttransplant outcomes of several organs.[5,7–16] As chronic graft failure and decreased long-term survival correlate with the frequency of acute rejection, induction treatment will likely bring advantages in these aspects as well. However, it is recognized that associated adverse events such as higher incidence of (opportunistic) infections, lymphoproliferative disorders, and hypersensitivity reactions may outweigh the benefits. A more recent approach uses the immunosuppressive potential of induction treatment to facilitate a delayed and more careful initiation of maintenance therapy. The avoidance of nephrotoxic effects of high doses of CNI, TAC, and CSA is especially beneficial to avoid early graft failure in kidney transplant patients[17] and prolonged kidney dysfunction following heart transplantation.[18,19]

Although various transplant registries generally show an increasing use of induction therapy in adult and pediatric transplantation in the last 5 to 10 years,[2,5,13,20,21] the frequency of induction treatment and the agents used vary widely amongst centers

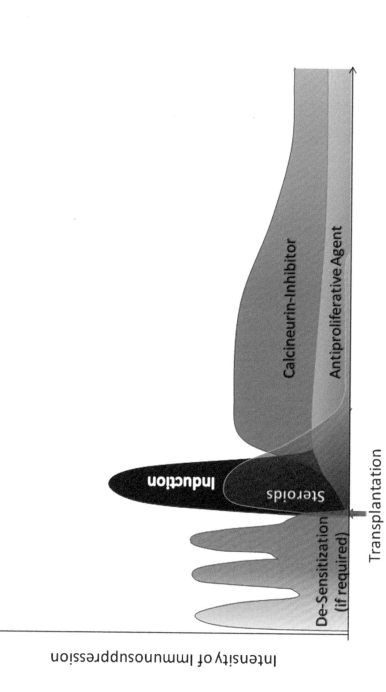

Fig. 1. Time line showing the different approaches for immunosuppression in relation to the time of transplant. Pre-transplant protocols are reserved for patients with specific risk factors (eg, HLA-sensitization or ABO-incompatible transplantation). Depending on the transplanted organ and center, the use of induction may or may not be part of the protocol. Furthermore, low-dose steroids may remain part of the maintenance therapy, supporting a regimen of 1 or 2 drugs of different classes. Additional treatments are used for treatment of rejection.

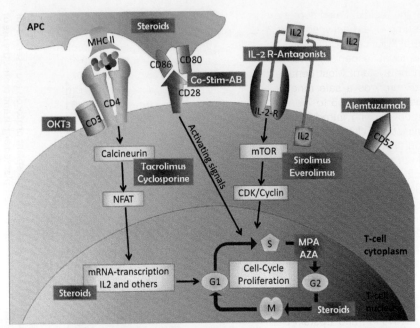

Fig. 2. The mechanisms of action of the different immunosuppressive agents. Beside the presentation of a peptide fragment of the antigen in the MHC II complex of the antigen-presenting cell (APC) a cosignal is required over interaction from CD80/CD86 and CD28. This interaction is targeted by specific antibodies (Co-stim-AB) abatacept and belatacept. Basiliximab and Daclizumab (IL-2R antagonists) target the receptor for IL-2, required for cell activation via target of rapamycin (TOR), which is targeted by sirolimus and everolimus and the cyclin-dependent kinase (CDK). TAC and CSA interfere in the signal transduction from the T-cell receptor by inhibiting calcineurin nuclear factor of activated T-cells (NFAT). MPA and AZA interfere in the cell cycle, preventing the T cell as well as the B cell from proliferation. Steroids target multiple sites in the interaction. ATM and muronomab target specific lymphocytic surface structures to induce cytolysis; a similar principle is used from antithymocte globulins but with multiple targets on the surface.

and transplanted organs. Some protocols generally include induction in any immunosuppressive regimen, whereas others choose an individualized approach using induction only for special indications (eg, accompanying renal failure or presensitization), or modify the agents and doses according to the individual indication. The use of high initial doses of steroids, which could be classified as induction, is discussed together with maintenance steroids in a later section.

Polyclonal Cytolytic Sera and Antithymocyte Globulin

This group contains the initially custom-made polyclonal antibody sera (often referred to as antilymphocyte globulin) as well as the currently commercially available drugs, equine antithymocyte globulin (ATG) and rabbit ATG. Polyclonal sera are prepared by injection of human thymocytes into animals that subsequently produce antibodies against a variety of human antigens including HLA and surface receptors of immune cells (eg, CD3, CD4). As thymocytes are used for sensitization of the animals, the main targets of the antibodies are T lymphocytes, but other lymphocytes and antigen-presenting cells are also targeted. After processing and purification these sera can be administered intravenously to patients. The antibodies coat the recipient's immune cells, inducing a variety of mechanisms to deplete them via complement activation, opsonization to optimize phagocytosis, and activation of natural killer cells. Sufficient dosage leads to a rapid drop in the circulating lymphocyte count, especially T cells, resulting in profound suppression of the adaptive immune system. Most centers define a target threshold of 0.1 to 0.3 lymphocytes $(\times 10^3/\text{mm}^3)$ as a safe range of sufficient immunosuppression and maintain these values for the first 5 to 7 days after transplant. This approach allows renal function to recover, with introduction of CNI therapy by either intravenous (IV) or enteral administration later after the operative procedure. In the setting of cardiac transplantation, this process allows smoother recovery of hemodynamic stability before initiation of agents that impair renal function. Comparative studies have shown that the rabbit-derived preparation Thymoglobulin provides a more profound and more easily adjustable lymphocyte reduction than the equine-derived ATG without increasing side effects.[7,8]

Side effects of polyclonal lymphocyte depleting sera may be severe, including fever, rash, weakness, hypotension, and allergic-type reactions such as anaphylactic shock. The reduction in immune cell numbers may exceed the duration of therapy for weeks and in some cases even months, associated with an increased risk of infectious complications. The available literature analyzing this is not unanimous, however.[12,22] Opportunistic infections have been reported, and most studies have attributed a higher probability of cytomegalovirus (CMV) infection or reactivation and Epstein-Barr virus (EBV)-associated posttransplant lymphoproliferative disorder (PTLD) to the use of ATG, when compared with no induction or to use of monoclonal CD25-directed antibodies.[23] Increased incidence of opportunistic infections was mainly found when ATG was used as a rejection treatment, most likely because of lower surveillance and absence of prophylaxis later after transplant.[23]

Monoclonal Antibodies

Muronomab

The first available commonly used monoclonal antibody used for transplant induction therapy was muronomab, a murine antibody that targets CD3, a cell-surface molecule present on all T cells, and reduces their number.[24] Because of severe systemic side effects including rapid sensitization[25] and a cytokine release syndrome[10,26,27] as well as absence of proven long-term benefits,[28] this substance has almost disappeared from clinical use[13] and therefore is not discussed further.

Anti-interleukin 2 receptor (CD25) antibodies (daclizumab, basiliximab)

CD25, the interleukin 2 (IL-2) receptor α chain, is expressed on activated and regulatory CD4+ T cells and provides transduction of the most powerful signal for T-cell proliferation.[29] Therefore, monoclonal antibodies to CD25 specifically target these T-cell subsets. In contrast to polyclonal antibodies, the monoclonal anti-CD25 antibodies do not necessarily cause depletion of target cells but mainly inactivate the function of the IL-2 receptor (IL-2R).[30] This prevents T lymphocytes from becoming activated and actively engaging in the immune response toward the donor organ. Despite expression of CD25, regulatory T cells seem to be less targeted by anti-CD25 antibodies than activated T cells and are more likely to persist beyond resolution of the receptor blockade.[30] This finding explains why it is crucial to administer the antibodies before the implantation of the graft (typically infusion starts about 2 hours before transplant operation). Thus the blockade of massive early T-cell activation outweighs the theoretic disadvantages of inactivation of immune-suppressing

Table 1
Immunosuppressive options in pediatric transplantation

Drug Name	Mechanism	Pediatric Dose	Side Effects	Comments
Induction Therapy				
Polyclonal Antibodies				
• Rabbit ATG (thymoglobulin)	Antibodies against thymus-derived human epitopes	1.5 mg/kg/d	Anaphylaxis and increased risk of (opportunistic) infections	Aim for lymphocyte count of 0.1–0.3 lymphocytes/mL
• Equine ATG		10–25 mg/kg/d		
Monoclonal Antibodies				
• Basiliximab	IL-2 receptor (CD25) blocking antibodies	2 doses 12 mg/m^2 day 0 and 4	Hypersensitivity	Start before transplant
• Daclizumab	Inhibit T-cell activation	5 doses 1 mg/kg every 14 days	Hypersensitivity	Start before transplant
Induction and Maintenance Therapy				
Steroids				
• Methylprednisolone	Inhibition of activator protein-1 and nuclear factor κ-B	Induction 5–10 mg IV pre-/intraoperative IV or oral steroids are weaned to maintenance dose 0.1–0.3 mg/kg/d	Hypertension, diabetes, salt/water, retention, osteopenia, hyperlipidemia, Cushingoid habitus, hirsutism, acne, growth retardation	Can be discontinued in liver, heart and kidney Usually continues in lung
• Prednisone				

Maintenance Therapy

Calcineurin Inhibitors

Drug	Mechanism	Dose	Side effects	Comments
• Cyclosporin	Inhibit expansion and differentiation of T cells	IV starting dose 1–3 μg/kg/d Oral maintenance 3–8 mg/kg/d in 2 divided doses	CSA: Hypertrichosis, gingival hyperplasia and hypertension	Choice and aimed level of CSA or TAC depend on type of organ, time after transplant and individual variables eg, renal impairment
• TAC	Inhibit expansion and differentiation of T cells	IV starting dose 0.01–0.05 mg/kg/d Oral maintenance 0.15–0.2 mg/kg/d divided in 2 doses	TAC: Hyperglycemia, tremor, alopecia, dose-dependent neurotoxicity All CNI: Nephrotoxicity and hypertention	

Antiproliferative Drugs

Drug	Mechanism	Dose	Side effects	Comments
• MMF • ecMPA	Inhibit de novo DNA synthesis	25–50 mg/kg/d divided in 2 doses	Myelosuppression, leucopenia, gastrointestinal symptoms	Doses for MMF and ecMPA equal Change from one to the other formulation may relieve gastrointestinal problems. Avoid MMF/ecMPA use in pregnancy.
• AZA		1–2 mg/kg/d divided in 2 doses	Myelosuppression, leucopenia, UV-dependent increase in skin cancer	Limit sun exposure on AZA

mTOR Inhibitors

Drug	Mechanism	Dose	Side effects	Comments
• Sirolimus • Everolimus	Arrest in cell cycle and differentiation	1 mg/m² daily 0.8–1.5 mg/m² daily	Delayed wound healing, aphthous ulcers, hyperlipidemia, edema, bone marrow suppression, pneumonitis	May be protective against coronary allograft vasculopathy

regulatory T cells.[30] Administration of IL-2R blockade after transplant has been found to be clinically less beneficial.[31]

Basiliximab is a chimeric (mouse/human) antibody. It is generally administered in 2 doses of 12 mg/m^2 with the first infusion starting about 2 hours before transplant and the second on day 4 after transplant. With a half-life of approximately 7 days, this regimen in pediatric kidney transplant patients has been found to provide IL-2R saturation for 5 weeks when used without mycophenolate mofetil (MMF) and 10 weeks when used in combination with MMF.[32] A shorter saturation interval has been found to be associated with higher rates of early acute rejection.[32]

Daclizumab is a humanized antibody (<10% mouse and more than 90% human). Although the general aim of humanizing an antibody is a lower likelihood of sensitization in the recipient, this is not clinically proven for daclizumab. The recommended dosing of 5 doses of 1 mg/kg at intervals of 14 days starting shortly before transplant provides complete saturation of CD25 for at least 3 months, but regimens of only 2 doses have also been used and lead to saturation for 10 to 12 weeks.[33] Daclizumab was withdrawn by the marketing authorization holder from the European market for commercial reasons in January 2009, but is still licensed and distributed in North America.

Several multicenter studies in adults have shown a significant reduction in the occurrence of acute rejection in the first year following kidney transplantation using basiliximab[34,35] or daclizumab.[36,37] Occurrence of side effects was comparable to the placebo groups, and long-term follow-up studies showed no increased incidence of infectious complications or PTLD.[12] However, induction with either IL-2R antagonist failed to show long-term increased graft or patient survival in studies in kidney transplantation,[38] confirmed by a Cochrane meta-analysis.[39] The observations in adult heart transplantation are similar, showing low occurrence of side effects and reduction of early acute rejection but failing to prove long-term benefit for patient or graft.[40] Few studies have been performed in pediatric patients.

Use of Induction: When and Which?

Currently available data do not allow a definitive recommendation as to whether the use of induction therapy in general is beneficial to pediatric transplant patients. Moreover, the question of which type of induction to use remains unresolved. Although the immediate benefits of induction treatment are undisputed in terms of reduction of acute rejection and improved early renal function, none of the available agents has shown a significant improvement in long-term outcomes in follow-up studies and registry reports.[2,20,39] This finding, however, needs to be interpreted with caution as it is subject to confounding factors. With general improvement in the management of transplanted children, there has been a tendency to offer organ transplantation to more critically ill patients. Some centers use induction preferentially in the sickest patients and therefore generate a negative selection bias in registry data. Furthermore, actuarial survival analysis (eg, from the ISHLT Registry[2]) sometimes focuses on conditional survival of patients who were still alive at various time points after transplantation and therefore may not capture deaths associated with severe infections or overwhelming immune activation in the perioperative period immediately after induction therapy.

Across the different organ groups in pediatric transplantation, the use of induction therapy remains controversial and highly variable. Only about 20% of pediatric liver transplant patients receive any induction.[5] In pediatric heart transplantation, the use of induction treatment has consistently increased in recent years except for a slight decline for the first time in 2008, with a reported use of CD25-directed antibodies in about 22% and polyclonal cytolytic agents in 38% of patients.[2] In the last 10 years 10% to 15% of pediatric lung transplant recipients received polyclonal induction and 30% to 50% received CD25-directed antibodies.[3] In pediatric kidney transplantation, the frequency of polyclonal induction declined until the beginning of the century, with a slight increase to 16% in deceased-donor and living-donor transplant recipients in the 2008 NAPRTC report.[1] The use of monoclonal antibodies has consistently increased in the last 10 years to 50% in living-donor and 51% in deceased-donor pediatric kidney transplant recipients. Within this group muronomab has nearly disappeared and been replaced with basiliximab or daclizumab.[1]

Overall it is appropriate that the use and type of induction treatment is tailored to the individual situation and the specific needs of a transplant candidate considering the benefits and risks. More recently developed drugs such as alemtuzumab (ATM) and costimulator targeting agents such as belatacept are discussed in the section about new developments.

MAINTENANCE THERAPY
Steroids

Corticosteroids have been used in solid-organ transplantation since the late 1950s, and are still used in most solid-organ transplant protocols from induction and maintenance to the treatment of acute rejection. They have a potent nonspecific immunosuppressive action, affecting all leukocytes. Lymphocyte concentration distribution and function are altered, in particular, by the inhibition of 2 transcription factors, the activator protein-1 and nuclear factor κ-B, which have an important role in the production of cytokines, including IL-1 and IL-2, γ interferon, tumor necrosis factor α, and granulocyte-macrophage colony-stimulating factor,[41] as well as CD40 ligand.

Steroids have an extensive side-effect profile, including hypertension, diabetes mellitus, osteopenia, poor wound healing, cataracts, emotional lability, hyperlipidemia, salt and water retention, and cosmetic effects, including Cushingoid habitus, weight gain, hirsutism, acne, and in pediatric patients, in addition, growth impairment.

Steroid withdrawal as reported in the different pediatric transplant registries is successfully accomplished in many organ transplant regimens.[1–3,5] Only about 25% of liver transplant recipients are still receiving steroids by 5 years after transplant,[5] whereas steroids are successfully withdrawn in more than 45% of heart transplant patients after the first year.[2] The percentage of kidney transplant recipients on steroids by 1 month after transplant declined from 95% in 1996 to 61% in 2007.[1] In contrast virtually 100% of lung[3] transplant recipients remain on a maintenance protocol that includes low-dose steroids. Results of steroid withdrawal and steroid avoidance trials have been published in adults and children. In adult liver transplantation, a recent meta-analysis[42] showed no difference in rejection rate or reduction in frequency of CMV infection and development of posttransplant diabetes mellitus in patients treated with a steroid-free regimen (steroids replaced by another immunosuppressant) compared with a steroid-based regimen. Both arms had a CNI as primary immunosuppressant. In adult kidney transplantation, a Cochrane review[43] showed increased acute rejection in patients withdrawn from steroids (after 3–6 months) without increasing the risk of early graft failure in patients receiving CSA or TAC with MPA; the rate of acute rejection was higher in patients receiving CSA when compared with those receiving TAC in the steroid withdrawal studies. The observed benefits of steroid-sparing strategies included reduction in new-onset diabetes and in serum cholesterol levels. In pediatric studies, steroid withdrawal has also been shown to have important benefits. Reports in pediatric liver[44] and kidney[45] and kidney transplant populations showed that steroid-free protocols were safe, with no increased rejection episodes and important catch-up growth when compared with steroid-based induction. Random controlled trials are needed to establish this practice definitively as safe and effective in pediatric solid-organ transplantation.

Calcineurin-inhibitors

Calcineurin is a calcium/calmodulin-dependent serine and threonine phosphatase. When activated it directly dephosphorylates the nuclear factor of activated T cells transcription factors within the cytoplasm, promoting their translocation into the nucleus, regulating IL-2 gene expression and cellular activation after antigen challenge.

First isolated from bovine neuronal tissue (hence its name), calcineurin was shown to inhibit phosphodiesterase activity[46]; later it was discovered to be the target of the immunosuppressants CSA and TAC.[47]

CSA was discovered in the early 1970s in Basel, Switzerland. The compound was isolated from a Norwegian soil sample produced by an aerobic filamentous fungus *Tolypocladium inflatum*. It was introduced to the clinical arena by Sir Roy Calne and first used in a solid-organ transplant patient in the late 1970s. CSA revolutionized transplantation. It was the first immunosuppressive drug to target T-lymphocyte function[48] and dramatically improved 1-year survival in cadaveric renal transplant recipients.[49]

TAC is a macrolide discovered in the mid-1980s. It is produced by the bacterium *Streptomyces tsukubaensis,* initially found in a soil sample obtained in Mount Tsukuba in Tokyo.[50]

Mechanism of action

CNI inhibit the phosphatase activity of calcineurin after binding to intracellular proteins with high affinity for immunosuppressive drugs called immunophilins (cyclophilin for CSA and FK-binding protein-12 [FKBP12] for TAC). Inhibition of this pathway decreases formation and secretion of several cytokines including IL-2 by the T lymphocyte, resulting in inhibition of expansion of CD4+ and CD8+. Furthermore, CNI inhibit the differentiation of Th1 and Th2 CD4+ T-cell subsets.

Pharmacokinetics

CSA and TAC share the same variability in absorption and pathways for metabolism, distribution, and excretion. The cytochrome P450 system (isoenzymes CYP3A4 and CYP3A5) and the efflux pump P-glycoprotein, which are expressed in the gastrointestinal tract and liver, are involved in oral bioavailability and systemic clearance of CNI.[51] There is significant interindividual variability in CNI pharmacokinetics, which change further during childhood maturation.[52] Pharmacogenomic variables (gene polymorphisms in the P450 CYP3A family and in the gene *ABCB1* encoding PGp) can also alter pharmacokinetic and pharmacodynamic profiles of CNI. Patients with the CYP3A5*3 allele have higher TAC area under the curve (AUC) when compared with patients with CYP3A5*1 allele, who need a higher TAC dose (**Box 1**).[53]

Drug monitoring

Optimal methods of CSA therapeutic drug monitoring are still under debate. The AUC of plasma drug concentration versus time after dose correlates better with levels measured 2 hours after dosing (C_2) than trough levels (C_0). However, there is not compelling published evidence that monitoring C_2 levels improves clinical outcomes when compared with monitoring C_0 levels.[54] CSA monitoring using C_0 is currently the method most commonly used in most centers.

In contrast to CSA drug monitoring, TAC levels measured at the C_0 trough correlate well with the AUC. High performance liquid chromatography (HPLC) is the preferred method of analysis as it measures only the parent TAC compound. In contrast, the immunoassay, in which the detection antibody cross-reacts with TAC metabolites (some biologically inactive), results in higher TAC levels when compared with HPLC.

Drug interactions
Drugs inducing or inhibiting the CYP3A enzymes may reduce or increase concentrations of CSA and TAC; therefore these drugs should be avoided when possible. If such drugs must be used, close monitoring of CNI levels and appropriate dose adjustments are necessary.[55]

Side effects
Nephrotoxicity is an adverse side effect common to CSA and TAC and is a major concern in pediatric solid-organ transplant patients. Acute toxicity is dose dependent, characterized by vasoconstriction of kidney arterioles and arteries. Chronic renal damage is characterized by progressive high-grade arteriolar hyalinosis with vessel narrowing, glomerulosclerosis, and tubule-interstitial injury.[56]

Although the side-effect profiles of the CNI generally overlap, certain effects are observed more commonly with 1 or the other drug. Adverse side effects that predominate with CSA include hirsutism, gingival hyperplasia, hypertension, and hyperlipidemia.[57] Patients receiving TAC are, in general, more likely to develop diabetes, tremor, peripheral neuropathy, alopecia, and gastrointestinal symptoms.[57] Autoimmune hemolytic anemia and leucopenia have been reported with both CNI drugs, but may improve by switching to the other CNI.

Efficacy
Many studies have compared the CNI used most commonly in organ transplantation. Two Cochrane reviews in adult kidney and liver transplant patients showed that TAC improved graft survival and prevented acute rejection more effectively when compared with CSA.[57,58] Two recent meta-analyses showed similar trends. One study of heart transplant patients showed a reduction in biopsy-proven acute rejection episodes at 6 and 12 months with TAC-based immunosuppression. The other in lung transplant patients again showed reduced rejection with TAC and a trend toward reduction of bronchiolitis obliterans syndrome.[59,60]

Renal-sparing Strategies
In patients receiving CNI-based immunosuppression, renal-sparing strategies include several approaches. Late initiation of CNI using induction therapy has been used in patients with perioperative renal dysfunction. CNI reduction in combination with MPA or mTOR inhibitors can be used with or without steroids. CNI-free regimens have also been used, again generally with a combination of MPA and mTOR inhibitors. The strategies used are different between the organ groups and there is little consensus on overall effectiveness. Few published studies have included children.[61,62]

Common Pediatric Issues
Infections are common in pediatric transplant patients, including diarrhea and respiratory tract infections. Plasma TAC levels can increase substantially with diarrhea. The mechanism has not been clearly defined, but theories include inflammation in the intestinal wall, which reduces function of P-glycoprotein (drug efflux pump) and metabolism by CYP450 3A4, increasing TAC bioavailability.[63] Another possible

Box 1
Cytochrome p450 drug interactions for TAC, CSA, sirolimus, and everolimus

Inducers (Decrease Levels of the Drug by Inducing Metabolism)

Antiepileptics

- Phenobarbitone
- Phenytoin
- Fosphenytoin
- Carbamazepine
- Oxcarbazepine

Antibiotics

- Caspofungin
- Nafcillin
- Rigabutin
- Rifampicine
- Rifapentine

Antivirals

- Efavirenz
- Etravirine
- Nevirapine

Others

- Antacids (containing magnesium, calcium or aluminium)
- Dererazirox
- Modafinil
- St John's wort
- Thalidomide
- Ticlopidine
- Troglitazone

Inhibitors (Increase Levels of the Drug by Inhibiting Metabolism)

Antibiotics

- Clarithromycin
- Erythromycin (Not azithromycin)
- Metronidazole
- Tinidazole
- Levofloxacin

Antifungals

- Clotrimazole
- Fluconazole
- Ketoconazole
- Itraconazole
- Voriconazole

Antivirals
- Indinavir
- Nelfinavir
- Ritonavir

Cardiovascular
- Amiodarone
- Lidocaine
- Diltiazem
- Verapamil

Others
- Grapefruit juice
- Nefazodone

mechanism is related to a shifting in the site of TAC absorption from the duodenum and jejunum to ileum and colon, where metabolism is weaker. Close monitoring of TAC levels is particularly important when diarrhea is present.

The use of antibiotics is another potential problem in pediatric patients after transplant. One example is the commonly used macrolides erythromycin and clarithromycin, which increase TAC blood levels. This finding is not seen with azithromycin. Other drugs commonly used in pediatrics include omeprazole, which can also increase serum TAC levels (see **Table 1**).

ANTIPROLIFERATIVE AGENTS
Azathioprine

Azathioprine (AZA) was invented as the first immunosuppressive maintenance therapy after steroids and before the invention of CNI. It is a prodrug of the active metabolite 6-thioguanine, which is converted into a purine analog that competes with inosine monophosphate. The result is inhibition of de novo DNA synthesis. It is also incorporated into DNA, replacing guanosine. This process leads to reduced numbers of circulating bone marrow-derived leukocytes, particularly monocytes and granulocytes. AZA specifically impairs the capability of activated lymphocytes to proliferate, leading to reduced adaptive immune responses.[64] The mechanism of action explains the main side effect: impaired proliferation of all bone marrow-derived cells, resulting in leucopenia, thrombocytopenia, and megaloblastic anemia.[64] Like all immunosuppressive agents, the impaired immune response is not limited to graft immunity; thus AZA increases the risk of infections and neoplasms. Increased rates of neoplastic disease were found, especially for skin cancer as a result of an enhancing effect of ultraviolet (UV) light.[65] Therefore sun exposure should be limited in patients treated with AZA. Rarer side effects include pancreatitis, alopecia, and hepatotoxicity.

Early studies showed superiority of triple drug therapies combining AZA with CSA and steroids compared with dual drug regimens without AZA.[66] However, with the development of MPA drugs claiming higher potency with a similar mechanism of action, AZA was widely replaced by these drugs and is currently used less often in organ transplantation. The main purpose for AZA use in current immunosuppressive regimens is persistent intolerance and severe side effects of one of the more modern antiprolifera-tive agents. The recommended dose of AZA for children is 1 to 2 mg/kg/d.

MMF and MPA

MPA has a similar mechanism of action to AZA. It noncompetitively inhibits inosine monophosphate dehydrogenase in eukaryotic cells and therefore the conversion of ino-sine monophosphate to guanosine monophosphate.[67] This process leads to impaired de novo purine synthesis, a mechanism on which proliferating leucocytes rely more than other proliferating cells, and which results in a potent inhibition of lymphocyte proliferation without relevant effect on other cells (eg, fibroblasts or epithelial cells).[68] This mechanism of action targeting different aspects of the cellular immune response than CNI makes MPA an ideal partner for a synergistic combination with these agents, even more so as it also affects B cells and therefore antibody development.[68]

There are currently 2 drugs available containing MPA: MMF (CellCept, Roche Labo-ratories, NJ, USA, licensed in 1995) is a prodrug that is rapidly metabolized in vivo to the active metabolite, and the more recently invented enterocoated MPA (ecMPA) (Myfortic, Novartis Pharmaceuticals Corporation, NJ, USA). Most clinical trials were performed with the older formulation MMF, and showed reduction of acute rejection episodes compared with AZA in combination with a CNI in (adult) recipients of various organ transplants.[69–72] This finding has been confirmed in a recent systematic review, suggesting that beyond the reduction of rejection episodes, long-term graft survival may also be improved with use of MMF in kidney transplantation.[73] However, it should be noted that other groups did not find a benefit in kidney and liver transplantation that would justify the higher cost (up to 16-fold) of MPA therapy compared with AZA.[74–76]

The largest datasets in pediatric transplantation are available for kidney transplant patients. A European study found significantly improved survival of patients treated with MPA compared with AZA at 1, 3, and 5 years after transplant.[77–79] The reason, however, was a massive difference in graft rejection early after transplantation, although conditional survival later after transplant was not different between the 2 groups.[78] This finding did not correspond to findings of an earlier United States-based study in 67 patients that detected no difference in early rejection rates.[80] In heart trans-plantation, benefits of MPA therapy were identified especially in regards to chronic graft vasculopathy.[81] However, more recent data have revealed further improvement of this problem when using mTOR inhibitors in combination with CNI.[82]

The 2 main side effects of MPA are gastrointestinal problems, mainly diarrhea and abdominal pain, and bone marrow depression, leading to severe leucopenia and specifically lymphopenia. Both side effects are common and occur in approximately one-third of patients, often recurring and leading finally to discontinuation of the drug as part of the immunosuppressive regimen. The invention of ecMPA aimed for a reduced frequency of gastrointestinal problems but comparative studies failed to prove this benefit.[83,84] In an individual patient, however, a switch from one substance to the other may lead to improvement of this side effect.[85,86] The problem of lympho-penia often leads to dose adjustments and treatment interruptions, which sometimes allow titration of an optimized individual dose. Lymphopenia can also be addressed with a switch to either AZA or, in some patients, to an mTOR inhibitor. As MPA therapy has revealed a teratogenic potential, it should not be given during and in cases of planned pregnancy.[87]

The dose recommendation for MPA in children is 1200 mg/m^2/d or 20 to 40 (or 50) mg/kg/d in 2 to 4 doses; both available enteral formulations offer identical bioavailability.[88] IV administration is also effective, with the same dosage range.

Separation to more doses may improve gastrointestinal side effects in individual patients.

Monitoring of drug levels in the plasma is problematic for MPA, especially in pediatric patients. Trough levels have not proven to be a reliable or useful tool for dose adjustment except for recognition of severe overdosing.[89] Determination of pharmacokinetics requires several time points of blood drawing and is therefore not practical in children. Calculation of the pharmacokinetics using a Bayesian approach seems to provide reliable results with only 2 measurements.[90] In comparative studies, adjustment of the MPA dose in response to plasma levels did not show clinical improvement in several adult organ transplant groups.[91,92] Therefore MPA dose measurements should be limited to occasional determination of the trough level or evaluation of clinically suspected side effects such as severe lymphopenia. There is no evidence that drastically subtherapeutic dosing has any therapeutic effect. The bioavailability of MPA is increased when combined with CNI, although the CNI plasma levels also increase in this combination; therefore CNI dose adjustments may be necessary.

mTOR INHIBITORS

mTOR is a serine/threonine protein kinase. It has direct control of protein synthesis; it also controls cell cycle progression from G1 into S phase. In cytokine-stimulated T cells, mTOR is activated, leading to proliferation and differentiation of CD4+ T lymphocytes.[93,94]

Our understanding of mTOR function continues to grow. It is part of numerous complex intracellular and extracellular signaling pathways. When bound to different proteins, mTOR forms distinctive complexes with different physiologic functions. mTOR inhibitors such as sirolimus (RAPA, rapamycin) and everolimus bind to FKBP12, forming a complex that blocks mTOR activity[94] and leads to arrest in cell cycle and cell differentiation. RAPA inhibits vascular smooth muscle proliferation and hence may have a protective effect against coronary artery vasculopathy in cardiac allografts.[95]

RAPA, isolated from the fungus *Streptomyces hygroscopicus*, was found in soil collected in Rapa Nui (Easter Island) in 1975. Initially it was found to have antifungal and antitumor activity. It took 13 years for its immunosuppressive action to be described.[96]

Pharmacokinetics

CYP450 and P-glycoprotein are important in the bioavailability and systemic clearance of the mTOR inhibitors. RAPA metabolites are believed to have minimal immunosuppressive effects. Of the parent compound, 90% is excreted in the feces with little urinary excretion. The half-life of RAPA is shorter in children (14 hours) when compared with adults (60 hours), therefore some children may need twice daily dosing.[97] Everolimus has a shorter half-life and greater bioavailability than RAPA.

Interactions with other drugs metabolized by CYP3A4 are important because they can either increase or decrease RAPA plasma concentration. When administered with CSA microemulsion, the plasma levels of both drugs increase, therefore administration of the drugs should be 4 hours apart.[98] This interaction is not seen with TAC.

Therapeutic drug monitoring of mTor inhibitors is recommended to assess efficacy and toxicity. Trough (C_0) levels correlate well with AUC. Drug monitoring using HPLC is preferred as immunoassays will also measure RAPA metabolites, giving approximately 23% higher levels.

Side Effects

Adverse side effects of mTOR inhibitors include renal dysfunction, mostly secondary to enhancement of CNI-induced nephrotoxicity, but there are also reports suggesting that RAPA alone is nephrotoxic. Hyperlipidemia is also commonly observed, and typically responds to 3-hydroxy-3-methylglutaryl coenzyme A (statins) treatment. Delayed wound healing, leucopenia, and thrombocytopenia are common and correlate with trough levels. Inflammatory manifestations are less common side effects of mTOR inhibitors, including pneumonitis, glomerulonephritis, systemic inflammatory response syndrome, and anemia of chronic disease. Altered sex hormone levels and impaired spermatogenesis have also been described,[99] which are important side effects in young adults.

IMMUNOSUPPRESSIVE MEDICATION IN ACUTE REJECTION

The most common frontline treatment of acute organ rejection is a pulse of IV steroids, usually methylprednisolone (10 to 20 mg/kg/d for 3 to 5 days), or in mild rejection an oral course of prednisone (5 mg/kg/d). In more severe grades of rejection, or in cardiac transplantation with hemodynamic compromise, a 3- to 5-day course of polyclonal lymphocyte depleting antibodies (ATG) is most commonly used. A Cochrane review and a systematic review by the same investigators in kidney transplantation showed that ATG is better than steroids in reversing the first episode of rejection and preventing graft loss.[100,101] If rejection does not respond to pulse steroids, lymphocyte-depleting antibodies may overcome the therapy resistance. Most centers transiently increase the intensity of maintenance immunosuppression to achieve sustained absence of rejection. Maintenance immunosuppression can also be altered by changing CSA to TAC to reduce the risk or treat recurrent rejection.[57,58,102,103]

The treatment of antibody-mediated rejection (AMR) is one of the major challenges of current posttransplant therapy. Different antibody removal strategies have been used, including plasmapheresis, plasma exchange, and antigen-specific and nonspecific immunoadsorption columns, as well as immunomodulatory approaches with IV immunoglobulin. The depletion of all mature B cells by the use of the anti-CD20 monoclonal antibody rituximab shows a delayed effect in the decrease of (donor-specific) HLA antibodies, but lacks an immediate effect. Plasma cells, which are the terminally differentiated antibody-secreting cells, are not depleted by rituximab. New approaches are being explored for depletion of plasma cells, such as the proteasome inhibitor bortezomib, which is currently licensed for treatment of multiple myeloma. One recent study has shown encouraging results in treatment of AMR with bortezomib in renal transplant recipients[104]; however, it must be noted that the drug was added to numerous ongoing therapies. Another promising new strategy blocks the damaging effects of activated complement using the C5 inhibitor eculizumab. Success with this approach for treatment of AMR was also recently reported in renal transplant patients[105]; however, in the face of ongoing antibody production, expected duration of this expensive therapy is unclear.

NEW AND INVESTIGATIONAL APPROACHES
Anti-CD52 Antibodies (ATM)

Antibodies against the CD52 molecule were invented in 1987 and used in a variety of autoimmune and lymphatic neoplastic disorders.[106] The currently available formulation is the humanized antibody ATM, which was engineered from the earlier used murine antibodies to achieve less sensitization. The target molecule CD52 is present on virtually all lymphocytes, thus these agents result in profound lymphocyte deple-tion. The lytic capacity of the antibody depends on, amongst other factors, the strength of cell-surface CD52 expression. T cells have been found to be the most profoundly depleted lymphocyte subset, with some reduction found also in B cells, natural killer cells, and monocytes (in descending order).[11] ATM is currently licensed for B-cell chronic lymphatic leukemia and not for transplantation and is therefore avail-able only for off-label use for transplantation.

ATM was aggressively promoted initially as a tolerance-inducing substance. However, all clinical trials to date, most of which were not prospective, randomized, or controlled, have failed to support this concept.[11] Several trials and retrospective analyses aimed at reduction of maintenance therapy following ATM induction. A recent report of a retrospec-tive uncontrolled study of 42 pediatric kidney transplant recipients who had received ATM induction followed by TAC monotherapy showed 85.4% 4-year patient and graft survival, similar to historical data. A spaced-dose TAC regimen was tried in 16 of the patients, leading to trough levels less than 3 to 3.5 ng/dL, which was maintained in 12 of these chil-dren without consequent graft loss.[15] A randomized study in adult kidney recipients compared 2 groups with standard dose maintenance immunosuppression (TAC trough level 8–10 ng/mL and MMF 1 g/d) with either ATG or daclizumab induction versus reduced maintenance therapy (TAC trough level 4–7 ng/mL and MMF 500 mg/d) following ATM induction. Although acute rejection episodes were similar in the 3 groups, incidence of chronic allograft nephropathy was significantly higher in the ATM group after 27 months.[107] One-year results from an observational uncontrolled study in heart transplan-tation compared more recent patients induced with ATM to earlier transplanted patients from the same center. All patients were treated with TAC, but the target trough level following induction was 10 to 12 ng/mL compared with 12 to 15 ng/mL in the noninduced group, and the induced patients received half the MMF dose (750 mg vs 1500 mg twice a day). Both groups received identical steroid regimens. The incidence of acute rejection was significantly lower in the first year after transplant in the ATM group; however, 1-year survival was lower in the induced patients (85.1% vs 93.6% in the noninduced patients), but without statistical significance ($P = .09$). The renal function after 6 and 12 months was significantly better in the noninduced patients despite higher CNI trough levels.[108]

In summary, ATM has so far failed not only to prove a positive role in development of tolerance in the clinical setting but also lacks compelling data showing equal or more potent effectiveness as induction treatment compared with the currently established agents. An increasing number of studies instead suggest that reduction of mainte-nance therapy following ATM induction may be inferior in terms of long-term results to conventional immunosuppressive strategies.[107,108] Off-label use should therefore be limited until randomized controlled clinical trials can confirm improvement compared with current immunosuppressive regimens.

Costimulation Blockade (Abatacept, Belatacept)

Interactions between antigen-presenting cells and T cells occur at several contact sites. Besides presentation of antigen fragments by major histocompatibility complex (MHC) molecules to T-cell receptors, cosignals are induced by, amongst others, binding of the CD28 receptor on the T cell to CD80/CD86 on the antigen-presenting cell,[109] resulting in the expression of the receptor CTLA4 on the T cell. CD28 blockade with the preclinical antibody TGN1412 in a pilot study led to cytokine storm and multi-organ failure in 6 volunteers in a phase I trial,[110] and is therefore not under further clin-ical investigation. Abatacept is a dimeric fusion protein functioning as an inhibitor of CTLA4, and showed some efficacy in preclinical trials in transplantation as well as in autoimmune disorders. In primate studies with solid-organ transplantation the immunosuppressive effect was not persistent enough to move forward toward clinical use. Therefore the agent was modified to increase the affinity against CD86. The result was the development of the compound belatacept, which shows a 10-fold more potent inhibition of T-cell activation compared with abatacept.[111] An initial clinical study in adults compared 3 groups receiving more intensive or less intensive continuous belatacept treatment or CSA following kidney transplantation, with identical adjunct immunosuppression (induction with basiliximab, maintenance with 2 g/d MPA and a steroid-tapering regimen).[112] The belatacept groups were found to preserve a better glomerular filtration rate after 12 months as well as a lower incidence of chronic allograft nephropathy than the CSA-treated patients, likely because of avoidance of CSA nephrotoxic effects. The rate of acute rejection was similar in all groups. However, in the more intensified belatacept group 3 patients developed PTLD and another 2 within the 3-year follow-up of 102 of the initial patients (BENEFIT-Ext-study) compared with none in the CNI group. It is important that the PTLD occurred in the central nervous system in 2 of these patients,[113] which implies a poorer prognosis. All patients who developed PTLD were EBV negative at the time of transplant. This finding needs to be taken into account when use of belatacept is considered in pediatric transplantation, in which there is a much higher incidence of EBV-negative recipients and PTLD overall. To the authors' knowledge there are currently no published data on the use of belatacept in pediatric transplantation.

SUMMARY

The evolution of sophisticated immunosuppressive therapies in the past 3 decades has led to profound improvements in graft and patient outcomes in organ transplantation. Safe and effective application of these therapies to infants and children has been, and continues to be, hampered by lack of sufficient appropriately powered and controlled clinical trials. Thus, transplant physicians and colleagues involved in the management of these complex pediatric patients are faced with using powerful and complicated drug regimens with incomplete data. This situation needs to be remedied by support of appropriate research into use of these therapies in these vulnerable populations, specifically aimed at the advantages and disadvantages of the developing individual. The lifetime burden of immunosuppression beginning in infancy is unknown. Despite these caveats, outcomes of organ transplantation in infants and children continue to improve, and pediatric organ transplant recipients generally face a reasonable likelihood of excellent survival with good quality of life.

ACKNOWLEDGMENTS

Research of Dr Lori West's group is supported by the National Institute of Health (Grant # HL79067), the Canadian Institutes for Health Research, the Heart and Stroke Foundation, the Alberta Heritage Foundation for Medical Research and the Women's and Children's Health Research Institute. Dr Simon Urschel is supported by The Transplantation Society and the German Research Foundation (Deutsche Forschungsgemeinschaft).

REFERENCES

1. Martz K, Stablein DM. NAPRTCS 2008 Annual Report. In: North American Pediatric Renal Trials and Collaborative Studies; 2008.

2. Kirk R, Edwards LB, Aurora P, et al. Registry of the International Society for Heart and Lung Transplantation: Twelfth Official Pediatric Heart Transplantation Report-2009. J Heart Lung Transplant 2009;28(10):993–1006.
3. Aurora P, Edwards LB, Christie JD, et al. Registry of the International Society for Heart and Lung Transplantation: Twelfth Official Pediatric Lung and Heart/Lung Transplantation Report-2009. J Heart Lung Transplant 2009;28(10):1023–30.
4. Ng VL, Fecteau A, Shepherd R, et al. Outcomes of 5-year survivors of pediatric liver transplantation: report on 461 children from a North American multicenter registry. Pediatrics 2008;122(6):e1128–35.
5. Pillai AA, Levitsky J. Overview of immunosuppression in liver transplantation. World J Gastroenterol 2009;15(34):4225–33.
6. Kawai T, Cosimi AB, Spitzer TR, et al. HLA-mismatched renal transplantation without maintenance immunosuppression. N Engl J Med 2008;358(4):353–61.
7. Brennan DC, Flavin K, Lowell JA, et al. A randomized, double-blinded comparison of Thymoglobulin versus Atgam for induction immunosuppressive therapy in adult renal transplant recipients. Transplantation 1999;67(7):1011–8.
8. Brophy PD, Thomas SE, McBryde KD, et al. Comparison of polyclonal induction agents in pediatric renal transplantation. Pediatr Transplant 2001;5(3):174–8.
9. Carlsen J, Johansen M, Boesgaard S, et al. Induction therapy after cardiac transplantation: a comparison of anti-thymocyte globulin and daclizumab in the prevention of acute rejection. J Heart Lung Transplant 2005;24(3):296–302.
10. Chin C, Pittson S, Luikart H, et al. Induction therapy for pediatric and adult heart transplantation: comparison between OKT3 and daclizumab. Transplantation 2005;80(4):477–81.
11. Ciancio G, Burke GW 3rd. Alemtuzumab (Campath-1H) in kidney transplantation. Am J Transplant 2008;8(1):15–20.
12. Kirk AD, Cherikh WS, Ring M, et al. Dissociation of depletional induction and posttransplant lymphoproliferative disease in kidney recipients treated with alemtuzumab. Am J Transplant 2007;7(11):2619–25.
13. Pescovitz MD. Use of antibody induction in pediatric renal transplantation. Curr Opin Organ Transplant 2008;13(5):495–9.
14. Pollock-BarZiv SM, Allain-Rooney T, Manlhiot C, et al. Continuous infusion of thymoglobulin for induction therapy in pediatric heart transplant recipients; experience and outcomes with a novel strategy for administration. Pediatr Transplant 2009;13(5):585–9.
15. Tan HP, Donaldson J, Ellis D, et al. Pediatric living donor kidney transplantation under alemtuzumab pretreatment and tacrolimus monotherapy: 4-year experience. Transplantation 2008;86(12):1725–31.
16. Yamani MH, Taylor DO, Czerr J, et al. Thymoglobulin induction and steroid avoidance in cardiac transplantation: results of a prospective, randomized, controlled study. Clin Transplant 2008;22(1):76–81.
17. Vilalta R, Lara E, Madrid A, et al. Delayed graft function is reduced with antithymocyte globulin induction in pediatric kidney transplantation. Transplant Proc 2009;41(6):2373–5.
18. Delgado DH, Miriuka SG, Cusimano RJ, et al. Use of basiliximab and cyclosporine in heart transplant patients with pre-operative renal dysfunction. J Heart Lung Transplant 2005;24(2):166–9.
19. Gustafsson F, Ross HJ. Renal-sparing strategies in cardiac transplantation. Curr Opin Organ Transplant 2009;14(5):566–70.

20. Smith JM, Stablein DM, Munoz R, et al. Contributions of the Transplant Registry: the 2006 Annual Report of the North American Pediatric Renal Trials and Collaborative Studies (NAPRTCS). Pediatr Transplant 2007;11(4):366–73.

21. Christie JD, Edwards LB, Aurora P, et al. The Registry of the International Society for Heart and Lung Transplantation: Twenty-Sixth Official Adult Lung and Heart-Lung Transplantation Report-2009. J Heart Lung Transplant 2009;28(10): 1031–49.

22. Goland S, Czer LS, Coleman B, et al. Induction therapy with thymoglobulin after heart transplantation: impact of therapy duration on lymphocyte depletion and recovery, rejection, and cytomegalovirus infection rates. J Heart Lung Transplant 2008;27(10):1115–21.

23. Issa NC, Fishman JA. Infectious complications of antilymphocyte therapies in solid organ transplantation. Clin Infect Dis 2009;48(6):772–86.

24. Bonnefoy-Berard N, Revillard JP. Mechanisms of immunosuppression induced by antithymocyte globulins and OKT3. J Heart Lung Transplant 1996;15(5): 435–42.

25. Mayes JT, Thistlethwaite JR Jr, Stuart JK, et al. Reexposure to OKT3 in renal allograft recipients. Transplantation 1988;45(2):349–53.

26. Sgro C. Side-effects of a monoclonal antibody, muromonab CD3/orthoclone OKT3: bibliographic review. Toxicology 1995;105(1):23–9.

27. Lindenfeld J, Miller GG, Shakar SF, et al. Drug therapy in the heart transplant recipient: part I: cardiac rejection and immunosuppressive drugs. Circulation 2004;110(24):3734–40.

28. Benfield MR, Tejani A, Harmon WE, et al. A randomized multicenter trial of OKT3 mAbs induction compared with intravenous cyclosporine in pediatric renal transplantation. Pediatr Transplant 2005;9(3):282–92.

29. Lan RY, Selmi C, Gershwin ME. The regulatory, inflammatory, and T cell programming roles of interleukin-2 (IL-2). J Autoimmun 2008;31(1):7–12.

30. Wang Z, Shi BY, Qian YY, et al. Short-term anti-CD25 monoclonal antibody administration down-regulated CD25 expression without eliminating the neogenetic functional regulatory T cells in kidney transplantation. Clin Exp Immunol 2009;155(3):496–503.

31. Grundy N, Simmonds J, Dawkins H, et al. Pre-implantation basiliximab reduces incidence of early acute rejection in pediatric heart transplantation. J Heart Lung Transplant 2009;28(12):1279–84.

32. Hocker B, Kovarik JM, Daniel V, et al. Pharmacokinetics and immunodynamics of basiliximab in pediatric renal transplant recipients on mycophenolate mofetil comedication. Transplantation 2008;86(9):1234–40.

33. Praditpornsilpa K, Avihingsanon Y, Kupatawintu P, et al. Monitoring of T-cell subsets in patients treated with anti-CD 25 antibody. Transplant Proc 2004; 36(2 Suppl 1):S487–91.

34. Nashan B, Moore R, Amlot P, et al. Randomised trial of basiliximab versus placebo for control of acute cellular rejection in renal allograft recipients. CHIB 201 International Study Group. Lancet 1997;350(9086):1193–8.

35. Kahan BD, Rajagopalan PR, Hall M. Reduction of the occurrence of acute cellular rejection among renal allograft recipients treated with basiliximab, a chimeric anti-interleukin-2-receptor monoclonal antibody. United States Simulect Renal Study Group. Transplantation 1999;67(2):276–84.

36. Nashan B, Light S, Hardie IR, et al. Reduction of acute renal allograft rejection by daclizumab. Daclizumab Double Therapy Study Group. Transplantation 1999;67(1):110–5.

37. Bumgardner GL, Hardie I, Johnson RW, et al. Results of 3-year phase III clinical trials with daclizumab prophylaxis for prevention of acute rejection after renal transplantation. Transplantation 2001;72(5):839–45.
38. Sheashaa HA, Bakr MA, Ismail AM, et al. Basiliximab induction therapy for live donor kidney transplantation: a long-term follow-up of prospective randomized controlled study. Clin Exp Nephrol 2008;12(5):376–81.
39. Webster AC, Playford EG, Higgins G, et al. Interleukin 2 receptor antagonists for kidney transplant recipients. Cochrane Database Syst Rev 2004;(1):CD003897.
40. Moller CH, Gustafsson F, Gluud C, et al. Interleukin-2 receptor antagonists as induction therapy after heart transplantation: systematic review with meta-analysis of randomized trials. J Heart Lung Transplant 2008;27(8):835–42.
41. Auphan N, DiDonato JA, Rosette C, et al. Immunosuppression by glucocorticoids: inhibition of NF-kappa B activity through induction of I kappa B synthesis. Science 1995;270(5234):286–90.
42. Sgourakis G, Radtke A, Fouzas I, et al. Corticosteroid-free immunosuppression in liver transplantation: a meta-analysis and meta-regression of outcomes. Transpl Int 2009;22(9):892–905.
43. Pascual J, Zamora J, Galeano C, et al. Steroid avoidance or withdrawal for kidney transplant recipients. Cochrane Database Syst Rev 2009;(1):CD005632.
44. Gras JM, Gerkens S, Beguin C, et al. Steroid-free, tacrolimus-basiliximab immunosuppression in pediatric liver transplantation: clinical and pharmacoeconomic study in 50 children. Liver Transpl 2008;14(4):469–77.
45. Sarwal MM, Vidhun JR, Alexander SR, et al. Continued superior outcomes with modification and lengthened follow-up of a steroid-avoidance pilot with extended daclizumab induction in pediatric renal transplantation. Transplantation 2003;76(9):1331–9.
46. Klee CB, Crouch TH, Krinks MH. Calcineurin: a calcium- and calmodulin-binding protein of the nervous system. Proc Natl Acad Sci U S A 1979;76(12):6270–3.
47. Liu J, Farmer JD Jr, Lane WS, et al. Calcineurin is a common target of cyclophilin-cyclosporin A and FKBP-FK506 complexes. Cell 1991;66(4):807–15.
48. Borel JF, Feurer C, Gubler HU, et al. Biological effects of cyclosporin A: a new antilymphocytic agent. Agents Actions 1976;6(4):468–75.
49. Calne RY, White DJ, Evans DB, et al. Cyclosporin A in cadaveric organ transplantation. Br Med J (Clin Res Ed) 1981;282(6268):934–6.
50. Kino T, Hatanaka H, Miyata S, et al. FK-506, a novel immunosuppressant isolated from a streptomyces. II. Immunosuppressive effect of FK-506 in vitro. J Antibiot (Tokyo) 1987;40(9):1256–65.
51. Cummins CL, Jacobsen W, Benet LZ. Unmasking the dynamic interplay between intestinal P-glycoprotein and CYP3A4. J Pharmacol Exp Ther 2002; 300(3):1036–45.
52. de Jonge H, Naesens M, Kuypers DR. New insights into the pharmacokinetics and pharmacodynamics of the calcineurin inhibitors and mycophenolic acid: possible consequences for therapeutic drug monitoring in solid organ transplantation. Ther Drug Monit 2009;31(4):416–35.
53. Cattaneo D, Baldelli S, Perico N. Pharmacogenetics of immunosuppressants: progress, pitfalls and promises. Am J Transplant 2008;8(7):1374–83.
54. Knight SR, Morris PJ. The clinical benefits of cyclosporine C2-level monitoring: a systematic review. Transplantation 2007;83(12):1525–35.
55. Christians U, Jacobsen W, Benet LZ, et al. Mechanisms of clinically relevant drug interactions associated with tacrolimus. Clin Pharmacokinet 2002;41(11): 813–51.

56. Tonshoff B, Hocker B. Treatment strategies in pediatric solid organ transplant recipients with calcineurin inhibitor-induced nephrotoxicity. Pediatr Transplant 2006;10(6):721–9.

57. Webster A, Woodroffe RC, Taylor RS, et al. Tacrolimus versus cyclosporin as primary immunosuppression for kidney transplant recipients. Cochrane Database Syst Rev 2005;(4):CD003961.

58. Haddad EM, McAlister VC, Renouf E, et al. Cyclosporin versus tacrolimus for liver transplanted patients. Cochrane Database Syst Rev 2006;(4): CD005161.

59. Ye F, Ying-Bin X, Yu-Guo W, et al. Tacrolimus versus cyclosporine microemulsion for heart transplant recipients: a meta-analysis. J Heart Lung Transplant 2009; 28(1):58–66.

60. Fan Y, Xiao YB, Weng YG. Tacrolimus versus cyclosporine for adult lung transplant recipients: a meta-analysis. Transplant Proc 2009;41(5):1821–4.

61. Nankivell BJ, Borrows RJ, Fung CL, et al. The natural history of chronic allograft nephropathy. N Engl J Med 2003;349(24):2326–33.

62. Groetzner J, Kaczmarek I, Schulz U, et al. Mycophenolate and sirolimus as calcineurin inhibitor-free immunosuppression improves renal function better than calcineurin inhibitor-reduction in late cardiac transplant recipients with chronic renal failure. Transplantation 2009;87(5):726–33.

63. Sato K, Amada N, Sato T, et al. Severe elevations of FK506 blood concentration due to diarrhea in renal transplant recipients. Clin Transplant 2004;18(5): 585–90.

64. Krensky AM, Clayberger C. Transplantation immunology. Pediatr Clin North Am 1994;41(4):819–39.

65. Terhorst D, Drecoll U, Stockfleth E, et al. Organ transplant recipients and skin cancer: assessment of risk factors with focus on sun exposure. Br J Dermatol 2009;161(Suppl 3):85–9.

66. Copeland JG, Mammana RB, Fuller JK, et al. Heart transplantation. Four years' experience with conventional immunosuppression. JAMA 1984;251(12):1563–6.

67. Young CJ, Sollinger HW. RS-61443: a new immunosuppressive agent. Transplant Proc 1994;26(6):3144–6.

68. Allison AC, Eugui EM. Mycophenolate mofetil and its mechanisms of action. Immunopharmacology 2000;47(2–3):85–118.

69. Kobashigawa JA, Meiser BM. Review of major clinical trials with mycophenolate mofetil in cardiac transplantation. Transplantation 2005;80(2 Suppl):S235–43.

70. Sollinger HW. Mycophenolate mofetil for the prevention of acute rejection in primary cadaveric renal allograft recipients. U.S. Renal Transplant Mycophenolate Mofetil Study Group. Transplantation 1995;60(3):225–32.

71. A blinded, randomized clinical trial of mycophenolate mofetil for the prevention of acute rejection in cadaveric renal transplantation. The Tricontinental Mycophenolate Mofetil Renal Transplantation Study Group. Transplantation 1996;61(7):1029–37.

72. Mathew TH. A blinded, long-term, randomized multicenter study of mycophenolate mofetil in cadaveric renal transplantation: results at three years. Tricontinental Mycophenolate Mofetil Renal Transplantation Study Group. Transplantation 1998;65(11):1450–4.

73. Knight SR, Russell NK, Barcena L, et al. Mycophenolate mofetil decreases acute rejection and may improve graft survival in renal transplant recipients when compared with azathioprine: a systematic review. Transplantation 2009; 87(6):785–94.

74. Germani G, Pleguezuelo M, Villamil F, et al. Azathioprine in liver transplantation: a reevaluation of its use and a comparison with mycophenolate mofetil. Am J Transplant 2009;9(8):1725–31.

75. Remuzzi G, Cravedi P, Costantini M, et al. Mycophenolate mofetil versus azathioprine for prevention of chronic allograft dysfunction in renal transplantation: the MYSS follow-up randomized, controlled clinical trial. J Am Soc Nephrol 2007; 18(6):1973–85.

76. Cravedi P, Perna A, Ruggenenti P, et al. Mycophenolate mofetil versus azathioprine in organ transplantation. Am J Transplant 2009;9(12):2856–7.

77. Jungraithmayr T, Staskewitz A, Kirste G, et al. Pediatric renal transplantation with mycophenolate mofetil-based immunosuppression without induction: results after three years. Transplantation 2003;75(4):454–61.

78. Jungraithmayr TC, Wiesmayr S, Staskewitz A, et al. Five-year outcome in pediatric patients with mycophenolate mofetil-based renal transplantation. Transplantation 2007;83(7):900–5.

79. Staskewitz A, Kirste G, Tonshoff B, et al. Mycophenolate mofetil in pediatric renal transplantation without induction therapy: results after 12 months of treatment. German Pediatric Renal Transplantation Study Group. Transplantation 2001; 71(5):638–44.

80. Benfield MR, Symons JM, Bynon S, et al. Mycophenolate mofetil in pediatric renal transplantation. Pediatr Transplant 1999;3(1):33–7.

81. Kaczmarek I, Ertl B, Schmauss D, et al. Preventing cardiac allograft vasculopathy: long-term beneficial effects of mycophenolate mofetil. J Heart Lung Transplant 2006;25(5):550–6.

82. Meiser B, Kaczmarek I, Mueller M, et al. Low-dose tacrolimus/sirolimus and steroid withdrawal in heart recipients is highly efficacious. J Heart Lung Transplant 2007;26(6):598–603.

83. Budde K, Knoll G, Curtis J, et al. Long-term safety and efficacy after conversion of maintenance renal transplant recipients from mycophenolate mofetil (MMF) to enteric-coated mycophenolate sodium (EC-MPA, myfortic). Clin Nephrol 2006; 66(2):103–11.

84. Kobashigawa JA, Renlund DG, Gerosa G, et al. Similar efficacy and safety of enteric-coated mycophenolate sodium (EC-MPS, myfortic) compared with mycophenolate mofetil (MMF) in de novo heart transplant recipients: results of a 12-month, single-blind, randomized, parallel-group, multicenter study. J Heart Lung Transplant 2006;25(8):935–41.

85. Robaeys G, Cassiman D, Verslype C, et al. Successful conversion from mycophenolate mofetil to enteric-coated mycophenolate sodium (myfortic) in liver transplant patients with gastrointestinal side effects. Transplant Proc 2009; 41(2):610–3.

86. Darji P, Vijayaraghavan R, Thiagarajan CM, et al. Conversion from mycophenolate mofetil to enteric-coated mycophenolate sodium in renal transplant recipients with gastrointestinal tract disorders. Transplant Proc 2008;40(7): 2262–7.

87. Merlob P, Stahl B, Klinger G. Tetrada of the possible mycophenolate mofetil embryopathy: a review. Reprod Toxicol 2009;28(1):105–8.

88. Johnston A, He X, Holt DW. Bioequivalence of enteric-coated mycophenolate sodium and mycophenolate mofetil: a meta-analysis of three studies in stable renal transplant recipients. Transplantation 2006;82(11):1413–8.

89. Kuypers DR, Claes K, Evenepoel P, et al. Long-term changes in mycophenolic acid exposure in combination with tacrolimus and corticosteroids are dose

dependent and not reflected by trough plasma concentration: a prospective study in 100 de novo renal allograft recipients. J Clin Pharmacol 2003;43(8): 866–80.

90. Payen S, Zhang D, Maisin A, et al. Population pharmacokinetics of mycophenolic acid in kidney transplant pediatric and adolescent patients. Ther Drug Monit 2005;27(3):378–88.

91. van Gelder T, Silva HT, de Fijter JW, et al. Comparing mycophenolate mofetil regimens for de novo renal transplant recipients: the fixed-dose concentration-controlled trial. Transplantation 2008;86(8):1043–51.

92. Kamar N, Marquet P, Gandia P, et al. Mycophenolic acid 12-hour area under the curve in de novo liver transplant patients given mycophenolate mofetil at fixed versus concentration-controlled doses. Ther Drug Monit 2009;31(4):451–6.

93. Yang Q, Guan KL. Expanding mTOR signaling. Cell Res 2007;17(8):666–81.

94. Saemann MD, Haidinger M, Hecking M, et al. The multifunctional role of mTOR in innate immunity: implications for transplant immunity. Am J Transplant 2009; 9(12):2655–61.

95. Keogh A, Richardson M, Ruygrok P, et al. Sirolimus in de novo heart transplant recipients reduces acute rejection and prevents coronary artery disease at 2 years: a randomized clinical trial. Circulation 2004;110(17):2694–700.

96. Vezina C, Kudelski A, Sehgal SN. Rapamycin (AY-22,989), a new antifungal antibiotic. I. Taxonomy of the producing streptomycete and isolation of the active principle. J Antibiot (Tokyo) 1975;28(10):721–6.

97. Schachter AD, Benfield MR, Wyatt RJ, et al. Sirolimus pharmacokinetics in pediatric renal transplant recipients receiving calcineurin inhibitor co-therapy. Pediatr Transplant 2006;10(8):914–9.

98. Kaplan B, Meier-Kriesche HU, Napoli KL, et al. The effects of relative timing of sirolimus and cyclosporine microemulsion formulation coadministration on the pharmacokinetics of each agent. Clin Pharmacol Ther 1998;63(1):48–53.

99. Huyghe E, Zairi A, Nohra J, et al. Gonadal impact of target of rapamycin inhibitors (sirolimus and everolimus) in male patients: an overview. Transpl Int 2007; 20(4):305–11.

100. Webster A, Pankhurst T, Rinaldi F, et al. Polyclonal and monoclonal antibodies for treating acute rejection episodes in kidney transplant recipients. Cochrane Database Syst Rev 2006;(2):CD004756.

101. Webster AC, Pankhurst T, Rinaldi F, et al. Monoclonal and polyclonal antibody therapy for treating acute rejection in kidney transplant recipients: a systematic review of randomized trial data. Transplantation 2006;81(7):953–65.

102. Sarahrudi K, Estenne M, Corris P, et al. International experience with conversion from cyclosporine to tacrolimus for acute and chronic lung allograft rejection. J Thorac Cardiovasc Surg 2004;127(4):1126–32.

103. Chan MC, Kwok BW, Shiba N, et al. Conversion of cyclosporine to tacrolimus for refractory or persistent myocardial rejection. Transplant Proc 2002;34(5): 1850–2.

104. Everly JJ, Walsh RC, Alloway RR, et al. Proteasome inhibition for antibody-mediated rejection. Curr Opin Organ Transplant 2009;14(6):662–6.

105. Stegall MD, Gloor JM. Deciphering antibody-mediated rejection: new insights into mechanisms and treatment. Curr Opin Organ Transplant 2009;15(1): 8–10.

106. Flynn JM, Byrd JC. Campath-1H monoclonal antibody therapy. Curr Opin Oncol 2000;12(6):574–81.

107. Ciancio G, Burke GW, Gaynor JJ, et al. A randomized trial of thymoglobulin vs. alemtuzumab (with lower dose maintenance immunosuppression) vs. daclizumab in renal transplantation at 24 months of follow-up. Clin Transplant 2008; 22(2):200–10.
108. Teuteberg JJ, Shullo MA, Zomak R, et al. Alemtuzumab induction prior to cardiac transplantation with lower intensity maintenance immunosuppression: one-year outcomes. Am J Transplant 2010;10(2):382–8.
109. McAdam AJ, Schweitzer AN, Sharpe AH. The role of B7 co-stimulation in activation and differentiation of CD4+ and CD8+ T cells. Immunol Rev 1998;165: 231–47.
110. Suntharalingam G, Perry MR, Ward S, et al. Cytokine storm in a phase 1 trial of the anti-CD28 monoclonal antibody TGN1412. N Engl J Med 2006;355(10): 1018–28.
111. Vincenti F. Costimulation blockade in autoimmunity and transplantation. J Allergy Clin Immunol 2008;121(2):299–306 [quiz: 7–8].
112. Vincenti F, Larsen C, Durrbach A, et al. Costimulation blockade with belatacept in renal transplantation. N Engl J Med 2005;353(8):770–81.
113. Vincenti F, Grinyo JM, Charpentier B, et al. Primary outcomes from a randomized, phase III study of belatacept vs cyclosporine in kidney transplant recipients (BENEFIT study). Boston: American Transplant Congress; 2009.

Prevention and Treatment of Infectious Complications After Solid Organ Transplantation in Children

Upton Allen, MBBS, MSc, FRCPC[a,b,c],*, Michael Green, MD, MPH[d,e]

KEYWORDS

• Transplantation • Pediatric • Infections • Posttransplant
• Prophylaxis

Organ transplantation is the most practical means of rehabilitating patients with a variety of forms of end organ dysfunction. This procedure is arguably the outstanding clinical biomedical accomplishment of the last 3 decades. Potent immunosuppressive drugs have dramatically reduced the incidence of rejection of transplanted organs, but have also increased the susceptibility of patients to opportunistic infections.[1] Thus, the success of organ transplantation is dependent in part on effective prevention, diagnosis, and treatment of infectious diseases after transplantation. To this end, emphasis is increasingly being placed on prevention. Most transplant patients will have evidence of microbial invasion in the first year after transplant. The effects of this microbial invasion are diverse, resulting in direct and indirect consequences. The direct consequences result in a variety of clinical

[a] Department of Paediatrics, University of Toronto, 555 University Avenue, Toronto, ON M5G 1X8, Canada
[b] Department of Health Policy Management & Evaluation, University of Toronto, 555 University Avenue, Toronto, ON M5G 1X8, Canada
[c] Division of Infectious Diseases, Hospital for Sick Children, 555 University Avenue, Toronto, ON M5G 1X8, Canada
[d] University of Pittsburgh School of Medicine, Pittsburgh, PA, USA
[e] Division of Infectious Diseases, Children's Hospital of Pittsburgh, 4401 Penn Avenue, Pittsburgh, PA 15224, USA
* Corresponding author. Department of Paediatrics, University of Toronto, 555 University Avenue, Toronto, ON M5G 1X8, Canada.
E-mail address: upton.allen@sickkids.ca

Pediatr Clin N Am 57 (2010) 459–479
doi:10.1016/j.pcl.2010.01.005
0031-3955/10/$ – see front matter © 2010 Elsevier Inc. All rights reserved.

infectious disease syndromes such as mononucleosis, pneumonia, gastroenteritis, hepatitis, among other entities. The indirect consequences are mediated through cytokines, chemokines, and growth factors elaborated by the transplant recipient in response to microbial replication and invasion, which contribute to the net state of immunosuppression, the pathogenesis of acute and chronic allograft injury, and in some cases, the development of lymphoproliferative or malignant disorders.

GENERAL PRINCIPLES AND RISK FACTORS FOR INFECTION

The risk of infection in the solid organ transplant patient is largely determined by the interaction of 3 factors: technical/anatomic factors that involve the transplant procedure itself, and the perioperative aspects of care such as the management of vascular access, drains, and the endotracheal tube; environmental exposures (**Box 1**); and the patient's net state of immunosuppression (**Box 2**). In the case of technical/anatomic mishaps, the best way to prevent infection is to correct the anatomic abnormality under coverage of appropriate antimicrobial therapy as antimicrobial treatment alone will not eliminate the risk of developing recurrent infections related to the uncorrected problem. As a consequence, the transplant recipient remains at high risk of subsequent infections with an increased risk of developing antimicrobial resistance until successful correction of the underlying abnormality.[1,2]

When one is considering therapy in the transplant patient, the concept of the therapeutic prescription package is useful. This package has 2 major components: an immunosuppressive component to prevent and treat rejection and an antimicrobial component to make it safe. Thus, the nature of the antimicrobial program being administered must be closely linked to the nature and intensity of the immunosuppressive program required and the resulting net state of immunosuppression.[1,2]

There are 3 modes in which antimicrobial agents can be administered to the transplant recipient: a therapeutic mode, in which antimicrobial agents are administered in the treatment of established clinical infection; a prophylactic mode, in which antimicrobial agents are administered to an entire population before an event to prevent the occurrence of an infection important enough to justify this intervention: and a preemptive mode, in which antimicrobial agents are administered to a subpopulation noted to be at particular risk of clinically important infection based on clinical, epidemiologic, or laboratory markers. This review focus on preventive strategies (prophylactic and preemptive) and on the diagnosis and management of established infection.

Infection in the posttransplant period has a stereotyped temporal pattern, a timetable. Although some clinical syndromes, such as pneumonia, can occur at any time point after transplant, the causes may be very different at different time points. **Fig. 1** delineates the timetable for the onset of infections after organ transplantation in the absence of effective preventative strategies. When preventative antimicrobial therapy fails to completely protect the patient, a common clinical effect is to extend the time period in which the infectious complication will likely appear. For example, in the case of cytomegalovirus (CMV) infection, in the absence of prophylaxis CMV-induced clinical disease is most common 1 to 3 months after transplantation. When prophylaxis is used, but fails, it is common for the disease to occur 4 to 8 months after transplantation (depending on the nature and duration of the prophylaxis and the immunosuppressive regimen).[2,3]

Like all patients, the transplant recipient is at risk of acquiring infections in the health care and community settings. Such infections are not necessarily transplant specific.

TIME LINE OF INFECTIONS AFTER TRANSPLANTATION

Fig. 1 is a graphical representation of the timing of infections during the posttransplant period.[2] In general, 3 time periods are recognized, each with differing forms of infection:[1–3]

First Month After Transplantation

In the first month, there are 3 major causes of infection: (1) infection that was present in the recipient before transplant, with its effects now increased as a result of surgery, anesthesia, and immunosuppressive therapy; (2) infection conveyed with a contaminated allograft; and (3) the same bacterial and candidal infections of the wound, lungs, drainage catheters, and vascular access devices that are seen in nonimmunosuppressed patients undergoing comparable surgery. Most (more than 95%) of the infections occurring in the first month after transplant fall into this last category; the main factor determining the incidence of such infections is the technical aspects of surgery as well as specific aspects of perioperative and postoperative care.

One to 6 Months After Transplantation

This second time period is when the effect of immune suppression is most notable on the risk of infection. During this period, 2 major classes of infection predominate. The first of these is attributable to a group of viral pathogens that are associated with latent and/or chronic infections. Examples include CMV, Epstein-Barr virus (EBV), human herpes virus 6 (HHV-6), and the hepatitis viruses (B and C); all of which may cause disease through acquisition of primary infection (typically from the donor) or secondary infection within the recipient under the pressure of immune suppression (secondary infection includes reactivation of latent pathogens and reinfection with a new strain). The second set of pathogens observed in this time period cause so-called opportunistic infections and include organisms such as *Listeria monocytogenes*, *Aspergillus fumigatus*, and *Pneumocystis jiroveci*. Development of infection with these opportunistic pathogens is attributable to the combination of sustained immunosuppression, which is often combined with the immunomodulating effects of viral infection creating a net state of immunosuppression great enough that these opportunistic infections can occur without an especially intensive environmental exposure.

More Than 6 Months After Transplantation

Information describing infections occurring in children more than 6 months after transplant is limited because transplant recipients commonly return to their homes, which are often far from their transplant centers. Accordingly, details regarding infectious complications occurring in this time period may be biased to include more significant infections resulting in hospitalization. Despite this limitation, experience supports dividing individuals with infections during this last time period into 2 main categories: (1) most patients with a good result from transplantation (maintenance immunosuppression, good allograft function) are at greatest risk from typical community-acquired infections (such as influenza, parainfluenza, and respiratory syncytial virus); (2) a smaller group of patients with poorer outcomes from transplantation (excessive acute and chronic immunosuppression, poor allograft function, and, often, chronic viral infection). These patients remain at high risk for recurrent infections related to uncorrected mechanical problems as well as opportunistic infections attributable to organisms like *Pneumocystis jiroveci*, *Listeria monocytogenes*, *Cryptococcus neoformans*, and *Nocardia asteroides*.

Box 1
Epidemiologic exposures of importance for the organ transplant recipient

A. In the community

1. *Mycobacterium tuberculosis*
2. Geographically restricted systemic mycoses

   Blastomycosis, coccidioidomycosis, histoplasmosis
3. *Strongyloides stercoralis*
4. Respiratory viruses

   Influenza

   Parainfluenza

   Respiratory syncytial virus

   Adenoviruses
5. Infections acquired by the ingestion of contaminated food/water

   Salmonella species

   Campylobacter jejuni

   Listeria monocytogenes

   Giardia lamblia
6. Environmental fungi (*Aspergillus* species and others)
7. Vector-borne (eg, West Nile virus)

B. In the hospital

1. From the contaminated air

   Aspergillus species

   Pseudomonas aeruginosa and other gram-negative bacilli
2. From contaminated potable water

   Legionella pneumophila

   Other *Legionella* species
3. Unwashed hands of medical personnel

   Candida species (including azole resistant)

   Methicillin-resistant *Staphylococcus aureus*

   Vancomycin-resistant enterococci

   Highly resistant gram-negative bacilli

C. Global travel (selected examples only)

1. Gastrointestinal bacterial and viral pathogens

   Salmonella, Shigella, Campylobacter, Vibrio

   Escherichia coli (multiple types)

   Viral gastroenteritis (eg, on cruise ships)
2. Parasitic infections

   Malaria

   Strongyloidiasis and other intestinal parasitic diseases

   Leishmaniasis

3. Respiratory infections

   SARS coronavirus

4. Viral hepatitis

   Hepatitis A, E or hepatitis B for long-term travel or residence

SUMMARY OF SPECIFIC INFECTIONS IN THE POSTTRANSPLANT PERIOD

The time line of infections after transplantation outlines the wide spectrum of infections that occur after transplantation. Among these infections, the major burden is represented by bacteria, *Candida* species, CMV, EBV, adenovirus, varicella zoster virus, and community-acquired respiratory viruses. In addition, certain infections represent challenges for specific organ groups (eg, BK virus infection in renal transplant recipients and toxoplasma infection in heart/heart-lung transplant recipients). Selected aspects of these infections are summarized later.

Bacterial Infections

As indicated earlier, bacterial infections are most commonly seen during the early posttransplant period. However, bacterial infections can occur at any time after transplantation. Risk factors include the presence of indwelling catheter devices, including endotracheal tubes, Foley catheters and central venous catheters. In this regard, hospital-acquired gram-negative organisms, coagulase-negative staphylococci and *Staphylococcus aureus* are often encountered. The nature of these infections and the specific pathogens involved vary according to the organ transplanted, sites of infection, the microbiologic flora of the institution, and the pretransplant status of the patient.

In general, the most common site of bacterial infection is at or near the site of transplantation. Urinary tract infection, notably pyelonephritis, has been recognized as the most common infectious complication among renal transplant recipients.[4] Among

---

Box 2
Factors contributing to the net state of immunosuppression in the organ transplant recipient

1. Dose, duration, and temporal sequence of immunosuppressive therapy
2. Neutropenia, lymphocytopenia
3. Metabolic abnormalities

   Protein-calorie malnutrition

   Uremia

   Hyperglycemia
4. Infection with immunomodulating viruses

   Cytomegalovirus

   Epstein-Barr virus

   Human herpes virus 6

   Hepatitis B virus

   Hepatitis C virus

   Human immunodeficiency virus

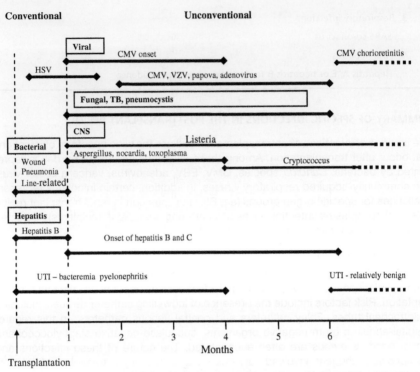

Fig. 1. Timetable of infection following organ transplantation. (*Adapted from* Rubin RH, Wolfson JS, Cosimi AB, et al. Infection in the renal transplant recipient. Am J Med 1981;70:405–11; with permission.)

liver transplant recipients, the most frequent site of bacterial infection is within the intraabdominal space, often accompanied by bacteremia.[5,6] Intraabdominal and wound infections are also commonly seen in intestinal transplant recipients. Bacteremia, which can be partly explained by disruption of the mucosal barrier associated with harvest injury or rejection, is commonly seen.[7,8] Infection of the lower respiratory tract (including pneumonia and lung abscess) is the most common site of infection reported in most, but not all, series of pediatric heart transplant recipients.[9–12] Mediastinitis is another important infection after thoracic transplantation, particularly if re-exploration of the chest is required. Pathogens associated with mediastinitis include *S aureus* and gram-negative enteric bacilli. Children undergoing lung transplantation because of cystic fibrosis experience a high rate of infectious complications as they often have preexisting colonization with resistant organisms, including *Pseudomonas* species, *Burkholderia* species and other bacterial pathogens.[13–16] Given the importance and difficulty in treating these often resistant organisms, transplant centers usually recommend a thorough microbiologic evaluation of heart-lung or lung transplant candidates before transplantation.

The transplant patient is also at risk of developing infection as a result of community-acquired bacterial pathogens, the most important of which is *Streptococcus pneumoniae* (pneumococcus). Transplant recipients are known to be at increased risk of pneumococcal sepsis.[17] Among these patients, heart recipients who have been transplanted at a young age seem to be at an increased risk compared with other pediatric organ recipients.[17]

Fungal Infections

The frequency of fungal infections varies according to the type of organ transplanted.[18–20] For example, invasive fungal infections are uncommon after renal transplantation. For these patients, the most frequently encountered entity is *Candida* urinary tract infection. Similarly for liver, heart, and intestinal transplant recipients, the major fungal infections are also caused by *Candida* species. For all of these patients, invasive aspergillosis and other mycoses occur uncommonly. The consequences of invasive aspergillosis and other noncandidal mycoses associated with invasive infections are frequently devastating. Lung transplant recipients are unique in that they experience proportionately more infections with *Aspergillus* species compared with other organ recipients. These infections are often seen in children undergoing transplantation as treatment of cystic fibrosis and reflect infection with *Aspergillus* that was present in the recipient before transplantation. However, *Aspergillus* is also frequently recovered from the lungs of transplant recipients with obliterative bronchiolitis (chronic rejection of the lung) regardless of the cause of their original lung disease leading to transplantation.[21]

CMV

CMV infection and disease remain important causes of mortality and morbidity among pediatric organ transplant recipients.[22] Data on the precise burden in pediatric organ transplant recipients are limited, however, by wide differences in data collection and reporting. In addition, nonuniform approaches to the laboratory diagnosis and definition of CMV disease applied in retrospective studies affects the ability to interpret available data. In 5 centers in the United States, 10% to 20% of liver transplant patients experienced CMV disease within 2 years after transplantation.[23] A review of first-time pediatric lung transplant patients indicated that among at-risk subjects, the incidence of CMV viremia was 29% to 32%, whereas the incidence of CMV pneumonitis was 20% during the first year after transplantation.[24,25]

CMV disease is often associated with fever and hematologic abnormalities, including leucopenia, atypical lymphocytosis, and thrombocytopenia. Visceral sites affected may include the gastrointestinal tract, lungs, and liver. Central nervous system involvement, including chorioretinitis, is rare in organ transplant recipients.

The diagnosis of CMV infection and disease in organ transplant recipients can be affected by the variable lack of sensitivity and/or specificity of different diagnostic tests. Serology has no role in the diagnosis of active CMV disease after transplantation as it does not differentiate between prior infection and active disease. The interpretation of serologic results is further confused by the potential presence of passive antibody from blood products provided during or after the transplant procedure. In addition, the altered immune responses after transplantation might impair the patient's ability to mount predictable humoral responses. Viral culture of blood for CMV has limited clinical usefulness for diagnosis of disease caused by poor sensitivity. There is no role for CMV urine culture in the diagnosis of disease caused by poor specificity.[26] A positive culture from bronchoalveolar lavage specimens may not correlate with disease.[27,28] The presence of a positive measurement of CMV load in the peripheral blood (measured by either nucleic acid amplification techniques (NAT) or pp65 antigenemia assay) in a patient with a compatible CMV clinical syndrome is strongly suggestive of CMV disease. However, the CMV load may be positive before the onset or in the absence of clinical disease and may be seen in the presence of disease from other causes. Further, the CMV load in the peripheral blood may be negative in some patients with tissue invasive disease, especially

CMV involving the gastrointestinal tract. Given the variable usefulness of these tests, histopathologic examination of involved organs is essential to confirm the presence of CMV when the diagnosis of invasive CMV disease is being considered.

Intravenous ganciclovir (10 mg/kg/d, given twice daily) remains the preferred drug for the treatment of CMV disease in pediatric transplant recipients. Reduction of immunosuppression is desirable unless concurrent evidence of rejection precludes this. Ganciclovir therapy is sometimes accompanied by CMV hyperimmune globulin therapy in some centers. Typically, a clinical response to treatments is expected in 5 to 7 days after treatment has been initiated. Foscarnet and cidofovir may be considered in the setting of ganciclovir resistance. The optimal length of treatment should be determined by monitoring viral loads weekly.[22] Treatment is typically continued until 2 consecutive negative samples are obtained. In cases of serious disease and in tissue invasive disease without viremia, longer treatment periods with clinical monitoring of the specific disease manifestation are recommended.

Data are emerging on the use of valganciclovir in the prevention and treatment of CMV infection/disease among adult transplant recipients.[29,30] Considerably less data are available for children.[31] A summary of the approach to prophylaxis is outlined in **Table 1**, including the roles of ganciclovir with or without immune globulin and suggestions on duration of their use, where indicated.

EBV

Although the most feared EBV-associated disease after transplantation is posttransplant lymphoproliferative disorder (PTLD), patients may experience a broad range of clinical symptoms that do not meet the definitions of PTLD. These might include the manifestations of infectious mononucleosis (fever, malaise, exudative pharyngitis, lymphadenopathy, hepatosplenomegaly, and atypical lymphocytosis), specific organ diseases such as hepatitis, pneumonitis, gastrointestinal symptoms, and hematological manifestations such as leucopenia, thrombocytopenia, hemolytic anemia, and haemophagocytosis.[32] EBV-associated leiomyosarcoma has also been described.[33] EBV disease is seen most frequently in patients experiencing primary EBV infections following transplantation. Rates of EBV disease and PTLD vary according to the organ transplanted with recipients of intestines and lungs being at the highest risk and those receiving liver, kidney, and heart at lower risk.

As for CMV disease, serology is not useful for diagnosis in the posttransplant period. The presence of increased EBV viral load in the peripheral blood as determined by quantitative polymerase chain reaction (PCR) is widely accepted as an assay to predict or indicate the likely presence of PTLD. However, these assays are limited in specificity and may remain persistently elevated in asymptomatic patients. The definitive diagnosis of EBV diseases, including PTLD requires histopathologic examination of biopsy material. The use of EBV-specific assays (eg, EBV encoded RNA [EBER] staining) enhances the sensitivity and specificity of histologic examination in these patients.

The approach to the treatment of EBV disease and PTLD remains somewhat controversial. Reduction of immune suppression is widely accepted as critical in the management of patients with these complications. The role of the antiviral agents acyclovir and ganciclovir are unproven, although many transplant clinicians use them in the treatment of EBV infection.[34,35] Treatment approaches are often modified from regimens used to treat CMV disease. Currently, when antiviral agents are used to treat EBV, the agent of choice is ganciclovir, as in vitro it is 10 times more active against EBV compared with acyclovir. The controversy on the use of these agents for EBV/PTLD arises because although these agents can suppress EBV lytic infection,

Table 1
Regimens and targets for prophylaxis in the posttransplant period

Infections	Target Groups	Prophylaxis Regimens/Comments	Suggested Duration of Prophylaxis
Bacterial infection (postoperative wound infection and sepsis)	All recipients	Perioperative antimicrobials regimens vary depending on organ, nature of surgery, and recipient factors (eg, selected regimens for cystic fibrosis)	48–72 h
Herpes simplex	Seropositive recipients	Acyclovir	3 months
CMV	Stratification of risk based on CMV donor/recipient serostatus	Intravenous ganciclovir (with/without intravenous immune globulin in some centers) Emerging data for valganciclovir in low- to intermediate-risk older children	Typically 3 months; some centers use prophylactics for shorter periods (2 weeks) or longer (6 months)
EBV	High-risk patients are D+R− patients	No established regimens; preemptive reduction in immune suppression in response to rising EBV load in peripheral blood in use by growing number of centers; ganciclovir with/without immune globulin used in some centers	Duration variable if antivirals with/without immune globulin used
Candida species	All recipients	Fluconazole selectively; lipid amphoterin B products selectively; nystatin often used	Up to 4 weeks depending on risk factors
Aspergillus	Lung/heart-lung recipients	Voriconazole; intraconazole; amphotericin B products	Duration variable; up to 4–6 months depending on risk
Pneumocystis jiroveci	All recipients	Trimethoprim-sulfamethoxazole	Typically 6–12 months; for lung and small bowel transplant recipients, as well as any transplant patient with a history of prior PCP infection or chronic CMV disease, lifelong prophylaxis may be indicated
Toxoplasma gondii	Heart/heart-lung recipients	Pyrimethamine/sulfa for D+R− patients Trimethoprim/sulfa of some value for R+ patients	6 months

they seem to be of limited value in treatment nonlytic EBV proliferation, which is believed to be the dominant component of EBV-related PTLD. Increasing evidence (albeit anecdotal) supports the use of the anti-CD20 monoclonal rituximab in the treatment of EBV disease and PTLD. However, the optimal timing and treatment strategy for this agent remain to be defined. Additional alternative strategies such as the use of chemotherapy require collaborative input from oncologists familiar with the management of EBV-related disease in organ transplant recipients.

The prevention of posttransplant EBV diseases, including PTLD remains controversial. Antiviral regimens have been modeled from the CMV scenario. To date, preemptive reduction in immunosuppression in the setting of increasing viral load may have the most supportive data and is increasingly being used (see **Table 1**).

Adenovirus

Adenovirus infection may be acquired by exogenous means or endogenously as a result of reactivation of latent infection. The clinical spectrum of infection and disease in pediatric transplant recipients is variable.[36] There are more than 51 serotypes that generally show some fidelity as this relates to the types of organs affected and the resultant syndromes.[37] Among liver transplant patients, disease manifestations include self-limited fever, gastroenteritis, cystitis, hepatitis, and pneumonitis. These manifestations may occur in other transplant recipients, depending on the level of immunosuppression. Adenovirus DNA can be detected in the peripheral blood using qualitative or quantitative PCR techniques. In the appropriate clinical setting, the presence of adenovirus DNA in the blood provides presumptive evidence of infection, with examination of tissue by histopathology providing more definitive evidence of infection. The management of adenovirus infection poses challenges because of limited effective treatment options. Cidofovir is currently accepted as the drug of choice. However, this conclusion is primarily based on a retrospective review of historical experience and the agent is not approved for this indication by the US Food and Drug Administration or similar agencies. Nonetheless, ongoing experience continues to support a role for the treatment of adenoviral infections with this agent. Before the advent of cidofovir, intravenous ribavirin was used with anecdotal reports of successes and failures.[38]

BK Virus

Although the major burden of BK virus infection is among adult renal transplant patients, the role of this virus in pediatric organ transplantation is becoming more clearly defined. Most infections are as a result of reactivation in adults. Primary infection may occur, notably among pediatric transplant recipients. The major clinical manifestation in the renal transplant recipient is tubulointerstitial nephritis. Renal biopsy is required for definitive diagnosis. Noninvasive testing modalities include screening of blood and urine for BK DNA using PCR.[39] There is no firm consensus on the preferred approach to the management of BK nephropathy. Early detection is a desired goal. To that end, quantitative PCR monitoring for BK DNA is performed in some centers. This often provides opportunities to modulate immunosuppression. In situations where antiviral therapy is used, the agent most often used is cidofovir, for which there are reports of success.[40] However, at present no consensus exists supporting the therapeutic efficacy of this agent.

Varicella Zoster Virus

Varicella zoster virus (VZV) is a major threat to pediatric transplant patients and many individuals enter transplantation without immunity to this virus.[41] Immunosuppressed individuals are at risk of severe outcomes from VZV infection. Visceral involvement may accompany severe infection and clinicians should be reminded that disseminated disease can rarely occur in the absence of typical cutaneous vesicles.[42] Pretransplant vaccination has been shown to provide sustained humoral immunity for at least 2 years after transplantation.[43] It is strongly recommended that transplant candidates be vaccinated before transplantation. Given that this is a live vaccine, the minimum interval between vaccination and transplantation is recommended to be 4 to 6 weeks. Although some centers have selectively considered the use of VZV vaccine in susceptible children after transplantation, this approach cannot be recommended at this time because of the lack of safety data, given the known risk of live vaccines in immunosuppressed individuals.

Families of transplant patients should be educated to be alert to potential exposures in settings such as schools and should report them promptly to health care providers to allow for postexposure prophylaxis. Varicella-susceptible transplant recipients should receive varicella zoster immune globulin within 96 hours after a varicella exposure.[44] If this window has passed or if varicella zoster immune globulin is not available, there is the option for the use of postexposure chemoprophylaxis with acyclovir (80 mg/kg/d, given 4 times daily for 7 days; maximum dose 800 mg, 4 times daily) starting at day 7 to 10 after exposure.[44] In the absence of profound immunosuppression, no prophylaxis is usually necessary for exposed organ recipients who are immune to VZV as a result of prior infection or vaccination before transplantation.

Treatment of the transplant patient with VZV infection is usually initiated with intravenous acyclovir until there is evidence of clinical improvement (fever abates, no new lesions, lesions starting to crust, no visceral disease). Outpatient treatment with oral acyclovir or valacyclovir has been used in children with mild infection, low levels of immunosuppression, and when there are no concerns regarding the adequacy of follow-up. Famciclovir and valacyclovir are approved for use in adults. Famciclovir is the prodrug of penciclovir, which has an extended half-life in infected cells. Valayclovir is the prodrug of acyclovir and produces fourfold greater serum levels than those produced by acyclovir. Pediatric formulations are current not available.

Community-acquired Respiratory Viruses

Most children who have undergone organ transplantation experience community-acquired viral infections and have no significant problems. However, it is well recognized that children who are significantly immunocompromised can have severe disease caused by these viruses, including respiratory syncytial virus infection, parainfluenza, and influenza viruses.[45,46] For pediatric transplant recipients, the likelihood of more severe outcomes is greater during the early months after transplantation or during periods of peak immunosuppression.

In 2009, the advent of a pandemic strain of influenza A (pandemic H1N1 2009) has been cause for concern.[47,48] In general, the principles that govern the prevention and treatment of pandemic H1N1 in pediatric transplant patients are similar to those for seasonal influenza. Transplant patients are among those who are known to be at increased risk of severe outcomes from pandemic H1N1. They are candidates for treatment with oseltamivir or zanamivir (where appropriate) if they have acute respiratory illness that is suspected or confirmed to be caused by H1N1.[49] Like other immunocompromised patients, they are at an increased risk of having prolonged shedding of virus and the harboring of drug-resistant strains of influenza A, including pandemic H1N1. Pediatric transplant patients are candidates for vaccination against this virus (as they are for seasonal influenza A) if they are greater than 6 months of age. Most experts currently delay vaccination until after the first months following organ transplantation.[49]

Selected Opportunistic Pathogens

Pneumocystis jiroveci pneumonia

Pneumocystis pneumonia (PCP) is a recognized threat in the posttransplant period.[50,51] The risk is greatest during the first 6 to 12 months after transplantation, with the time of onset being usually after the first month. Trimethoprim-sulfamethoxazole remains the prophylactic agent of choice.[52] This agent is also preferred for initiation of therapy in individuals who develop PCP. Although the optimal duration of PCP prophylaxis remains unclear, most experts provide PCP prophylaxis for a minimum of 6 to 12 months, with some recommending indefinite use, especially for solid organ transplant recipients requiring more prolonged periods of higher levels of immunosuppression.

Intravenous pentamidine is an alternative for treatment of PCP for patients who are intolerant of trimethoprim-sulfamethoxazole or whose disease has not responded to this agent after 5 to 7 days.[52] However, pentamidine is associated with a relatively high incidence of adverse events, including pancreatitis, renal dysfunction, hypoglycemia, and hyperglycemia. Atovaquone may be used to treat milder forms of PCP among adults; however, pediatric data are limited.

Alternatives to trimethoprim-sulfamethoxazole for prophylaxis include oral atovaquone or dapsone. Aerosolized pentamidine is recommended if children cannot tolerate these oral agents. Another alternative is intravenous pentamidine, albeit at the risk of greater toxicity.[52]

Toxoplasma gondii

Toxoplasma gondii infection is of greatest concern among heart transplant patients, but infection can occur in other categories of transplant recipients, including kidney and liver recipients.[53,54] Toxoplasma organisms can remain encysted within muscle tissue, such as cardiac muscle. Thus, infection is acquired as a result of the reactivation of cysts that remain dormant in the donor hearts of toxoplasma seronegative children. Clinical manifestations can occur as early as 2 weeks after transplantation. Manifestations include pneumonia, fever syndrome, myocarditis, chorioretinitis, and central nervous system disease. Current prophylaxis includes pyrimethamine/sulfadiazine for D+R− patients. Trimethoprim-sulfamethoxazole is typically used in R+ patients. However, some experts also recommend trimethoprim-sulfamethoxazole for D+R− patients. The duration of prophylaxis is usually 6 months.

Strongyloides stercoralis

Infection with this parasitic worm is of relevance to individuals who previously acquired infection following a period of residence in endemic regions.[55,56] Donor-associated transmission of Stronygloides has also occurred. Asymptomatic immunocompromised persons, including transplant recipients are at risk of strongyloides hyperinfection, which results from dissemination of larvae via the systemic circulation, resulting in abdominal pain, diffuse pulmonary infiltrates, and septicemia or meningitis from enteric gram-negative bacilli. Serologic screening is recommended for individuals from endemic regions (**Table 2**). Ivermectin treatment is indicated for screen-positive individuals.

Mycobacterium tuberculosis

Tuberculosis (TB) is always a concern for immunocompromised hosts.[57–60] Incidence rates are low in most transplant centers in the developed world, but outcomes of TB

Table 2
Screening tests for transplant candidates

Tests	Comments/Action Required for Abnormal Results
HIV-1 and 2	HIV-related management as indicated
HTLV-1 and 2	Counselling as indicated
Hepatitis A	IgG and IgM serology
Hepatitis B	Obtain full panel of hepatitis B serology, including surface antigen and anti-core antibody
Hepatitis C	
Hepatitis D	Obtain if hepatitis B seropositive
CMV	Obtain IgG; urine culture for seropositive infants <2 years
EBV	Viral capsid antigen and EBNA
Herpes simplex virus	
Varicella zoster virus	Vaccinate seronegative candidates at least 6 weeks before transplantation
Toxoplasma gondii	Obtain heart, heart-lung candidates
Measles	Immunize if ≥3 months before expected transplantation
Mumps	Immunize if ≥3 months before expected transplantation
Rubella	Immunize if ≥3 months before expected transplantation
Mycobacterium tuberculosis	Mantoux test; IGRA being evaluated; intervention for latent TB may be required
Strongyloides sterocoralis	Positive serology requires intervention; ivermectin
Respiratory tract pathogens	Sputum cultures on patients with cystic fibrosis and other heart-lung transplant candidates; Aspergillus colonization indication for suppressive therapy
Radiographic imaging	These tests are as clinically indicated

Abbreviations: EBNA, Epstein-Barr nuclear antigen; HTLV, human T-lymphotrophic virus; IGRA, interferon-gamma release assays.

can be devastating in organ transplant recipients. Before transplantation a careful history for TB exposure or infection, Mantoux test screening, and a chest radiograph can assists in establishing the diagnosis of latent tuberculosis infection. The interferon-gamma release assays are currently being evaluated to define their role in settings where the TB skin test has poor utility.[61,62] The use of antituberculous agents in transplant patients poses challenges because of the interaction between isoniazid and rifampin with immunosuppressive medications. However, this should not be seen as a contraindication to the use of antituberculous agents, which have to be used when warranted by the clinical situation.

STRATEGIES FOR PREVENTION OF POSTTRANSPLANT INFECTIONS
Pretransplant Evaluation

The pretransplant phase is arguably the most important phase of transplantation. A detailed history and physical examination are necessary to identify conditions that influence the risk or management of infections after transplantation. This assessment allows for the identification of preexisting conditions that require treatment or prophylaxis in the period before or after transplantation. **Table 2** summarizes screening tests that should be performed in the pretransplant period.

Immunizations

Immunizations represent an important strategy for preventing infections in the transplant patient.[63–72] Wherever possible, vaccines should be administered in the pretransplant period to improve the chances of optimal immunologic take. A guideline on vaccinations for the transplant candidate/patient has recently been published.[73] In some situations, accelerated vaccination schedules may be used for selected vaccines. Given differences in childhood vaccination schedules in different jurisdictions, clinicians should acquaint themselves with the appropriate schedules and the circumstances under which accelerated schedules could be used. When using vaccines after transplantation, one needs to be concerned about safety as well as efficacy. In general, all live virus vaccines should be avoided in the transplant recipient. The oral polio, yellow fever, and oral typhoid vaccines are live and are contraindicated in immunosuppressed patients. The live attenuated intranasal influenza vaccine is also contraindicated. Measles, mumps, and rubella vaccines are somewhat contraindicated and their use should be limited to outbreak scenarios. The varicella vaccine is also somewhat contraindicated and is not approved for use in transplant patents. Although limited published data support the potential use of this vaccine in transplant recipients,[72] most experts continue to advise against this practice. In the cases of the nonlive vaccines, the major concern is not safety, but efficacy. Thus, in general, it is advisable to give nonlive vaccines at times when the level of immunosuppression would allow for immunogenicity. **Table 3** summarizes the vaccines that are indicated and contraindicated in transplant recipients. Given the relative burden and importance of invasive pneumococcal disease in pediatric transplant recipients, the importance of pneumococcal vaccination should not be underestimated.[17,63,69]

Donor Organ Screening

The organ donor is a frequent source of exposure to pathogens in the organ transplant recipient. Accordingly, screening of the donor organ is a crucial aspect of the preventive strategies aimed at minimizing adverse outcomes from infections in the posttransplant period. Despite a long-standing recognition of the importance of donor-derived infections, increased concern about this problem has emerged because of recent donor-related transmission of human immunodeficiency virus (HIV). This case, as well as concerns about the lack of sensitivity of serologic testing and the relatively long time period until seroconversion against HIV, hepatitis B virus (HBV), and hepatitis C virus (HCV), have led to interest in the use of NAT-based testing for the pathogens HIV, HCV, and HBV. Although arguments exist for and against the use of NAT testing, a final international consensus addressing if and when to use these tests is only beginning to emerge.[74] Decisions relating to the use of such tests must consider not only the reliability of this technology but also the feasibility of universal implementation of these testing procedures for all procurement organizations. Recent cases of donor-associated transmission of lymphocytic choriomeningitis virus and West Nile virus have also raised questions on whether the panel of routine tests performed on potential donors should be expanded to include these and other potential donor-derived pathogens. To date, a consensus has not been reached on whether or not screening against these pathogens should be routinely included in donor testing panels. It is to be hoped that the implementation of working groups and committees focusing on the problem of donor-derived infections in North America and Europe will lead to improved data to better inform subsequent recommendations regarding donor testing. Current requirements for screening of nonliving donors are shown in **Table 4**. At present, no specific requirements have been implemented for screening

Table 3
Vaccines that are recommended and contraindicated in transplant recipients

Vaccine	Inactivated/Live Attentuated (I/LA)	Recommended Before Transplantation	Recommended After Transplantation
Influenza	I	Yes	Yes
	LA	No	No
Hepatitis B	I	Yes	Yes
Hepatitis A	I	Yes	Yes
Pertussis	I	Yes	Yes
Diphtheria	I	Yes	Yes
Tetanus	I	Yes	Yes
Inactivated polio vaccine	I	Yes	Yes
Haemophilus influenzae	I	Yes	Yes
Streptococcus pneumoniae (conjugate/ 23-valent polysaccharide)	I/I	Yes	Yes
Neisseria meningitidis (conjugate and polysaccharide)	I	Yes	Yes
Human papillomavirus	I	Yes	Yes
Rabies	I	Yes	Yes
Varicella	LA	Yes	No
Rotavirus	LA	Yes	No
Measles	LA	Yes	No
Mumps	LA	Yes	No
Rubella	LA	Yes	No
BCG[a]	LA	Yes	No
Smallpox	LA	No	No
Anthrax	I	No	No

[a] Where appropriate.

of live donors. In general, testing strategies that are in place for deceased donors are applied to the use of these organs. The importance of documenting the presence of potential donor-transmissible pathogens is imperative not only to inform decision making regarding the use of potential donor organs but also because results of donor testing can inform specific preventative strategies even when donor-associated exposure to pathogens is unavoidable.

Specific Preventive Strategies

Various prophylaxis regimens are used in the posttransplant period. Although there are common basic principles, the specific regimens vary across centers and by the type of organ transplanted. For most patients, the major targets of prophylaxis are

Table 4
Screening tests for donor organs

Tests	Comments/Action Required for Abnormal Results
HIV-1 and 2	Positive test contraindicates organ use
HTLV-1 and 2	Positive test contraindicates organ use[a]
Hepatitis A virus	Positive IgM contraindicates organ use
Hepatitis B virus	Obtain full panel of hepatitis B serology, including surface antigen and anti-core antibody; positive HBsAg contraindicates organ use
Hepatitis C virus	Some centers use positive organ only for positive candidates
CMV	Obtain IgG; urine culture for seropositive infants <2 years
EBV	Viral capsid antigen and EBNA
Toxoplasma gondii	Obtain on heart, heart-lung donor
Treponema pallidum	Positive confirmatory test contraindicates organ use

Abbreviation: HBsAg, hepatitis B surface antigen.
[a] This is currently being reexamined in some jurisdictions given lack of availability of testing platforms.

bacterial pathogens, herpes group viruses, and fungal pathogens, including pneumocystis. Perioperative antibiotics are typically used for 48 to 72 hours to provide prophylaxis against surgical contamination. The burden of CMV infection in transplant patients is such that it represents the major focus of prevention in the posttransplant period, when intravenous ganciclovir is usually used with or without CMV hyperimmune globulin in selected patient groups. **Table 1** summarizes various pathogens and the regimens that are often used for prevention of infection in the posttransplant period.

EVALUATION OF THE FEBRILE TRANSPLANT PATIENT

In the evaluation of the febrile transplant patient, clinicians should consider if the child's fever is related to common childhood infections or infections that are unique to the immunosuppressed transplant recipient. To this end, the timing of infections after transplantation (see **Fig. 1**) provides guidance regarding the most likely pathogens. For example, as discussed earlier, the most likely causes of infection within the first month after transplantation are often bacterial or candidal and are largely similar to what is seen in nonimmunosuppressed patients who have undergone comparable surgery. The nature of the evaluation will depend on the clinical status of the patient and whether or not a source of infection has been identified.

Examination abnormal, focus of infection defined. Admission to hospital may be indicated depending on the clinical status of the patient and the site of the infection. The diagnostic evaluation varies, but should include a minimum of a complete blood count and differential, blood, and urine cultures. Additional investigations depend on the clinical assessment and the timing of presentation after transplantation.

Examination normal, no focus of infection defined. Patients who are clinically unwell typically require admission for evaluation and treatment. The diagnostic evaluation should consider the likely differential diagnoses. Consultation with infectious diseases is recommended.

Patients who are well may not necessarily require admission. However, this depends on several factors, including the adequacy of follow-up, the degree of immune suppression and the suspected diagnoses. The diagnostic evaluation should include a minimum of a complete blood count and differential, blood, and urine cultures.

In all of these situations, clinicians need to be aware of the spectrum of viral infections that are associated with febrile syndromes without necessarily having a readily apparent organ focus of infection (eg, CMV virus).

REFERENCES

1. Fishman JA, Rubin RH. Infection in organ-transplant recipients. N Engl J Med 1998;338:1741–51.
2. Rubin RH, Wolfson JS, Cosimi AB, et al. Infection in the renal transplant patient. Am J Med 1981;70:405–11.
3. Rubin R, Ikonen T, Gummert J, et al. The therapeutic prescription for the organ transplant recipient: the linkage of immunosuppression and antimicrobial strategies. Transpl Infect Dis 1999;1(1):29–39.
4. Krieger JN, Brem AS, Kaplan MR. Urinary tract infection in pediatric renal transplantation. Urology 1980;15(4):362–9.
5. Zitelli BJ, Gartner JC, Malatack JJ, et al. Pediatric liver transplantation: patient evaluation and selection, infectious complications, and life-style after transplantation. Transplant Proc 1987;19(4):3309–16.
6. Colonna JO, Winston DJ, Brill JE, et al. Infectious complications in liver transplantation. Arch Surg 1988;123(3):360–4.
7. Sigurdsson L, Reyes J, Kocoshis SA, et al. Bacteremia after intestinal transplantation in children correlates temporally with rejection or gastrointestinal lymphoproliferative disease. Transplantation 2000;70(2):302–5.
8. Green M, Bueno J, Sigurdsson L, et al. Unique aspects of the infectious complications of intestinal transplantation. Curr Opin Organ Transplant 1999;4(4):361–7.
9. Green M, Wald ER, Fricker FJ, et al. Infections in pediatric orthotopic heart transplant recipients. Pediatr Infect Dis J 1989;8(2):87–93.
10. Baum D, Bernstein D, Starnes VA, et al. Pediatric heart transplantation at Stanford: results of a 15-year experience. Pediatrics 1991;88(2):203–14.
11. Bailey LL, Wood M, Razzouk A, et al. Heart transplantation during the first 12 years of life. Loma Linda University Pediatric Heart Transplant Group. Arch Surg 1989;124(10):1221–5.
12. Braunlin EA, Canter CE, Olivari MT, et al. Rejection and infection after pediatric cardiac transplantation. Ann Thorac Surg 1990;49(3):385–90.
13. Noyes BE, Michaels MG, Kurland G, et al. Pseudomonas cepacia empyema necessitatis after lung transplantation in two patients with cystic fibrosis. Chest 1994;105(6):1888–91.
14. De Soyza A, McDowell A, Archer L, et al. Burkholderia cepacia complex genomovars and pulmonary transplantation outcomes in patients with cystic fibrosis. Lancet 2001;358(9295):1780–1.
15. Aris RM, Routh JC, LiPuma JJ, et al. Lung transplantation for cystic fibrosis, patients with Burkholderia cepacia complex. Survival linked to genomovar type. Am J Respir Crit Care Med 2001;164(11):2102–6.
16. LiPuma JJ. Update on the Burkholderia cepacia complex. Curr Opin Pulm Med 2005;11(6):528–33.
17. Tran L, Hébert D, Dipchand A, et al. Invasive pneumococcal disease in pediatric organ transplant recipients: a high-risk population. Pediatr Transplant 2005;9(2):183–6.

18. Verma A, Wade JJ, Cheeseman P, et al. Risk factors for fungal infection in paediatric liver transplant recipients. Pediatr Transplant 2005;9(2):220–5.

19. Schaenman JM, Rosso F, Austin JM, et al. Trends in invasive disease due to *Candida* species following heart and lung transplantation. Transpl Infect Dis 2009;11(2):112–21.

20. van Hal SJ, Marriott DJ, Chen SC, et al. Australian Candidemia Study. Candidemia following solid organ transplantation in the era of antifungal prophylaxis: the Australian experience. Transpl Infect Dis 2009;11(2):122–7.

21. Weigt SS, Elashoff RM, Huang C, et al. Aspergillus colonization of the lung allograft is a risk factor for bronchiolitis obliterans syndrome. Am J Transplant 2009; 9(8):1903–11.

22. Kotton C, Kumar D, Caliendo A, et al. On behalf of The Transplantation Society International CMV Consensus Group. International consensus guidelines on the management of cytomegalovirus in solid organ transplantation. Am J Transplant 2010;10(1):18–25.

23. Green M, Michaels MG, Katz BZ, et al. CMV-IVIG for prevention of Epstein Barr virus disease and posttransplant lymphoproliferative disease in pediatric liver transplant recipients. Am J Transplant 2006;6(8):1906–12.

24. Danziger-Isakov LA, DelaMorena M, Hayashi RJ, et al. Cytomegalovirus viremia associated with death or retransplantation in pediatric lung-transplant recipients. Transplantation 2003;75(9):1538–43.

25. Danziger-Isakov LA, Worley S, Michaels MG, et al. The risk, prevention & outcome of cytomegalovirus after pediatric lung transplantation. Transplantation, in press.

26. Pillay D, Ali AA, Liu SF, et al. The prognostic significance of positive CMV cultures during surveillance of renal transplant recipients. Transplantation 1993;56(1): 103–8.

27. Storch GA, Ettinger NA, Ockner D, et al. Quantitative cultures of the cell fraction and supernatant of bronchoalveolar lavage fluid for the diagnosis of cytomegalovirus pneumonitis in lung transplant recipients. J Infect Dis 1993;168(6): 1502–6.

28. Buffone GJ, Frost A, Samo T, et al. The diagnosis of CMV pneumonitis in lung and heart/lung transplant patients by PCR compared with traditional laboratory criteria. Transplantation 1993;56(2):342–7.

29. Asberg A, Humar A, Jardine AG, et al. Long-term outcomes of CMV disease treatment with valganciclovir versus IV ganciclovir in solid organ transplant recipients. Am J Transplant 2009;9(5):1205–13.

30. Monforte V, Lopez C, Santos F, et al. A multicenter study of valganciclovir prophylaxis up to day 120 in CMV-seropositive lung transplant recipients. Am J Transplant 2009;9(5):1134–41.

31. Vaudry W, Ettenger R, Jara P, et al. Valganciclovir dosing according to body surface area and renal function in pediatric solid organ transplant recipients. Am J Transplant 2009;9(3):636–43.

32. American Academy of Pediatricas. Epstein-Barr virus infections. In: Pickering LK, Baker CJ, Kimberlin DW, et al, editors. Red Book. 2009 report of the Committee on infectious diseases. 28th edition. Elk Grove Village (IL): American Academy of Pediatrics; 2009. p. 289–92.

33. Nur S, Rosenblum WD, Katta UD, et al. Epstein-Barr virus-associated multifocal leiomyosarcomas arising in a cardiac transplant recipient: autopsy case report and review of the literature. J Heart Lung Transplant 2007;26(9): 944–52.

34. Green M. Management of Epstein-Barr virus-induced posttransplant lymphopro-liferative disease in recipients of solid organ transplantation. Am J Transplant 2001;1(2):103–8.

35. Preiksaitis JK. New developments in the diagnosis and management of post-transplantation lympholiferative disorders in solid organ transplant recipients. Clin Infect Dis 2004;39(7):1016–23.

36. de Mezerville MH, Tellier R, Richardson S, et al. Adenoviral infections in pediatric transplant recipients: a hospital-based study. Pediatr Infect Dis J 2006;25(9):815–8.

37. American Academy of Pediatricas. Adenovirus infections. In: Pickering LK, Baker CJ, Kimberlin DW, et al, editors. Red Book. 2009 report of the Committee on Infectious Diseases. 28th edition. Elk Grove Village (IL): American Academy of Pediatrics; 2009. p. 204–6.

38. Hoffman JA, Shah AJ, Ross LA, et al. Adenoviral infections and a prospective trial of cidofovir in pediatric hematopoietic stem cell transplantation. Biol Blood Marrow Transplant 2001;7(7):388–94.

39. Babel N, Fendt J, Karaivanov S, et al. Sustained BK viruria as an early marker for the development of BKV-associated nephropathy: analysis of 4128 urine and serum samples. Transplantation 2009;88(1):89–95.

40. Vats A, Shapiro R, Singh Randhawa P, et al. Quantitative viral load monitoring and cidofovir therapy for the management of BK virus-associated nephropathy in chil-dren and adults. Transplantation 2003;75(1):105–12.

41. Pandya A, Wasfy S, Hébert D, et al. Varicella Zoster infection in solid organ transplant recipients: a hospital-based retrospective study. Pediatr Transplant 2001;5(3):1–9.

42. Whitley RJ. Varicella zoster virus. In: Mandell GC, Bennett JE, Dolin R, editors. Principles and practice of infectious diseases. 5th edition. Philadelphia: Churchill Livingstone; 2000. p. 1580–5.

43. Barton M, Wasfy S, Melbourne T, et al. Sustainability of humoral responses to vari-cella vaccine in pediatric transplant recipients following a pre-transplantation immunization strategy. Pediatr Transplant 2008;13(8):1007–13.

44. American Academy of Pediatricas. Varicella-zoster infections. In: Pickering LK, Baker CJ, Kimberlin DW, et al, editors. Red Book. 2009 report of the Committee on Infectious Diseases. 28th edition. Elk Grove Village (IL): American Academy of Pediatrics; 2009. p. 714–27.

45. Pohl C, Green M, Wald ER, et al. Respiratory syncytial virus infections in pediatric liver transplant recipients. J Infect Dis 1992;165(1):166–9.

46. Apalsch AM, Green M, Ledesma-Medina J, et al. Parainfluenza and influenza virus infections in pediatric organ transplant recipients. Clin Infect Dis 1995;20(2):394–9.

47. Scalera NM, Mossad SB. The first pandemic of the 21st century: a review of the 2009 pandemic variant influenza A (H1N1) virus. Postgrad Med 2009;121(5):43–7.

48. Centers for Disease Control and Prevention. Outbreak of swine-origin influenza A (H1N1) virus infection – Mexico, March-April 2009. MMWR Morb Mortal Wkly Rep 2009;58:1–3.

49. Kumar D, Morris MI, Kotton CN, et al. Guidance on novel influenza A/H1N1 in solid organ transplant recipients. Am J Transplant 2010;10(1):18–25.

50. Schafers HJ, Cremer J, Wahlers T, et al. *Pneumocystis carinii* pneumonia following heart transplantation. Eur J Cardiothorac Surg 1987;1(1):49–52.

51. Gryzan S, Paradis IL, Zeevi A, et al. Unexpectedly high incidence of *Pneumocys-tis carinii* infection after lung-heart transplantation. Implications for lung defense and allograft survival. Am Rev Respir Dis 1988;137(6):1268–74.

52. American Academy of Pediatricas. *Pneumocystis jirovecii* infections. In: Pickering LK, Baker CJ, Kimberlin DW, et al, editors. Red Book. 2009 report of the Committee on Infectious Diseases. 28th edition. Elk Grove Village (IL): American Academy of Pediatrics; 2009. p. 536–40.
53. Luft BJ, Naot Y, Araujo FG, et al. Primary and reactivated toxoplasma infection in patients with cardiac transplants. Clinical spectrum and problems in diagnosis in a defined population. Ann Intern Med 1983;99(1):27–31.
54. Michaels MG, Wald ER, Fricker FJ, et al. Toxoplasmosis in pediatric recipients of heart transplants. Clin Infect Dis 1992;14(4):847–51.
55. Scoggin CH, Call NB. Acute respiratory failure due to disseminated strongyloidiasis in a renal transplant recipient. Ann Intern Med 1977;87(4):456–8.
56. Nolan TJ, Schad GA. Tacrolimus allows autoinfective development of the parasitic nematode *Strongyloides stercoralis*. Transplantation 1996;62(7):1038.
57. Sternecik M, Ferrell S, Asher N, et al. Mycobacterial infection after liver transplantation: a report of three cases and review of the literature. Clin Transplant 1992;6:55–61.
58. Higgins R, Kusne S, Reyes J, et al. *Mycobacterium tuberculosis* after liver transplantation: management and guidelines for prevention. Clin Transplant 1992;6: 81–90.
59. Singh N, Paterson DL. *Mycobacterium tuberculosis* infection in solid-organ transplant recipients: impact and implications for management. Clin Infect Dis 1998; 27(5):1266–77.
60. American Society of Transplantation Infectious Diseases Community of Practice. *Mycobacterium tuberculosis*. Am J Transplant 2004;10(Suppl 4):37–41.
61. Detjen AK, Keil T, Roll S, et al. Interferon-gamma release assays improve the diagnosis of tuberculosis and nontuberculous mycobacterial disease in children in a country with a low incidence of tuberculosis. Clin Infect Dis 2007;45(3):322–8.
62. Okada K, Mao TE, Mori T, et al. Performance of an interferon-gamma release assay for diagnosing latent tuberculosis infection in children. Epidemiol Infect 2008;136(9):1179–87.
63. Barton M, Wasfy S, Dipchand A, et al. Seven-valent pneumococcal conjugate vaccine in pediatric solid organ transplant recipients: a prospective study of safety and immunogenicity. Pediatr Infect Dis J 2009;28(8):688–92.
64. Madan RP, Tan M, Fernandez-Sesma A, et al. A prospective, comparative study of the immune response to inactivated influenza vaccine in pediatric liver transplant recipients and their healthy siblings. Clin Infect Dis 2008;46(5):712–8.
65. Arslan M, Wiesner RH, Sievers C, et al. Double-dose accelerated hepatitis B vaccine in patients with end-stage liver disease. Liver Transpl 2001;7(4):314–20.
66. Carey W, Pimentel R, Westveer MK, et al. Failure of hepatitis B immunization in liver transplant recipients: results of a prospective trial. Am J Gastroenterol 1990;85(12):1590–2.
67. Stark K, Gunther M, Neuhaus R, et al. Immunogenicity and safety of hepatitis A vaccine in liver and renal transplant recipients. J Infect Dis 1999;180(6):2014–7.
68. Balloni A, Assael BM, Ghio L, et al. Immunity to poliomyelitis, diphtheria and tetanus in pediatric patients before and after renal or liver transplantation. Vaccine 1999;17(20–21):2507–11.
69. Lin PL, Michaels MG, Green M, et al. Safety and immunogenicity of the American Academy of Pediatrics–recommended sequential pneumococcal conjugate and polysaccharide vaccine schedule in pediatric solid organ transplant recipients. Pediatrics 2005;116(1):160–7.
70. Centers for Disease Control and Prevention. Report from the Advisory Committee on Immunization Practices (ACIP): decision not to recommend routine

vaccination of all children aged 2–10 years with quadrivalent meningococcal conjugate vaccine (MCV4). MMWR Morb Mortal Wkly Rep 2008;57(17):462–5.

71. Olson AD, Shope TC, Flynn JT. Pretransplant varicella vaccination is cost-effective in pediatric renal transplantation. Pediatr Transplant 2001;5(1):44–50.

72. Danziger-Isakov L, Kumar D, AST Infectious Diseases Community of Practice. Guidelines for vaccination of solid organ transplant candidates and recipients. Am J Transplant 2009;9(Suppl 4):S258–62.

73. Weinberg A, Horslen SP, Kaufman SS, et al. Safety and immunogenicity of varicella-zoster virus vaccine in pediatric liver and intestine transplant recipients. Am J Transplant 2006;6(3):565–8.

74. Humar A, Morris M, Blumberg E, et al. Special report. Nucleic acid testing (NAT) of organ donors: is the "best" test the right test? Am J Transplant 2010. [Epub ahead of print].

Posttransplant Lymphoproliferative Diseases

Thomas G. Gross, MD, PhD[a], Barbara Savoldo, MD, PhD[b],
Angela Punnett, MD[c],*

KEYWORDS

- Posttransplant lymphoproliferative disease • Pediatric
- Solid organ transplantation

The risk of developing cancer after solid organ transplantation (SOT) is about 5- to 10-fold more than that of the general population. The cumulative risk of cancer rises to more than 50% at 20 years after transplant.[1] This risk increases with age, and so children receiving transplants are at high risk of developing a malignancy during their lifetime.[1,2] Posttransplant lymphoproliferative disease (PTLD) is the most common cancer observed in children following SOT, accounting for half of all such malignancies.[3] PTLD is a heterogeneous group of disorders with a wide spectrum of pathologic and clinical manifestations and is a major contributor to long-term morbidity and mortality in this population.[4] Among children, most cases are associated with Epstein-Barr virus (EBV) infection. This article reviews the pathology, immunobiology, epidemiology, and clinical aspects of PTLD, underscoring the need for ongoing systematic study of complex biologic and therapeutic questions.

PATHOLOGY

PTLD results from the uncontrolled proliferation of lymphocytes in the immunosuppressed transplant recipient. It encompasses a remarkable diversity of pathologic conditions, challenging the development of a standard classification of disease. The most commonly used pathologic classification scheme is the World Health Organization (WHO) categorization, outlined with diagnostic components in **Table 1**.[5] Pathologic evaluation requires assessment of tissue architecture and cytologic features;

[a] Division of Hematology/Oncology/BMT, Nationwide Children's Hospital, OSU School of Medicine, 700 Children's Drive, Columbus, OH 43205, USA
[b] Center for Cell and Gene Therapy, Baylor College of Medicine, The Methodist Hospital and Texas Children's Hospital, Houston, TX 77030, USA
[c] Division of Hematology/Oncology, SickKids Hospital, University of Toronto, 555 University Avenue, Toronto, ON M5G 1X8, Canada
* Corresponding author.
E-mail address: angela.punnett@sickkids.ca

Pediatr Clin N Am 57 (2010) 481–503
doi:10.1016/j.pcl.2010.01.011
0031-3955/10/$ – see front matter © 2010 Elsevier Inc. All rights reserved.
pediatric.theclinics.com

Table 1
WHO classification of PTLD

Pathology (Subtype)	Histopathology	Immunophenotype	EBV-ISH	Clonality	Other Genetics
Early lesions Reactive plasmacytic hyperplasia Infectious mononucleosis-like	No architectural effacement. Small lymphocytes, plasma cells, ± immunoblasts, ± hyperplastic follicles	Polyclonal B cells and admixed T cells	+ (often)	Polyclonal or small monoclonal population(s)	None
Polymorphic PTLD Polyclonal Monoclonal	Architectural effacement. Full spectrum of lymphoid maturation, ± atypical lymphoblasts	Polyclonal or monoclonal B cells and admixed T cells	+ (often)	Monoclonal B cells, nonclonal T cells	BCL6 somatic hypermutations may be seen
Monomorphic PTLD B-cell neoplasms DLBCL, diffuse large B-cell lymphoma Burkitt/Burkitt-like Plasma cell myeloma Plasmacytoma-like Other[a] T-cell neoplasms PTCL-NOS Hepatosplenic T cell Other	Architectural effacement usually seen. NHL or plasma cell neoplasm criteria	Dependent on neoplasm	Variable	Clonal B cells or T cells	Usually present
Classic HL-type PTLD	Architectural effacement. Classic HL criteria	Similar to classic HL	+	IgH not easily demonstrated	Unknown

[a] Indolent small B-cell lymphomas including follicular and mucosa-associated lymphoid tissue lymphomas are not included among PTLD.
Data from Swerdlow SH, Webber SA, Chadburn A, et al. Post-transplant lymphoproliferative disorders. In: Swerdlow SH, Campo E, Lee Harris N, et al, editors. WHO classification of tumors of haematopoietic and lymphoid tissues. Lyon (France): International Agency for Research on Cancer (IARC); 2008. p. 343, 348.

excisional biopsies are preferred and tissue samples should be submitted fresh rather than in formalin. EBV-associated disease is best determined by EBV-encoded RNA in situ hybridization (ISH) testing of diagnostic tissues. Cytogenetic studies assist with determination of clonality (immunoglobulin heavy [IgH] gene rearrangement; T-cell receptor gene rearrangement) and identify disease-associated chromosomal abnormalities.

There are 4 categories of PTLD in the WHO categorization. Early lesions refer to lymphoid proliferations with preservation of normal tissue architecture and occur more frequently in previously EBV-naive SOT recipients.[6] Polymorphic PTLD is the most commonly diagnosed PTLD among pediatric transplant recipients,[4] often following primary EBV infection. Morphology can be variable and include areas that seem more monomorphic, suggesting a continuum between polymorphic and mono-morphic disease.[5] Monomorphic disease is classified according to the B-cell or T/natural killer (NK)-cell neoplasms described in the immunocompetent host. Markers of oncogenes and tumor suppressor genes (eg, C-myc, N-ras, and p53) may be used to facilitate diagnosis in more complex cases.[7] Recurrent chromosomal abnormalities have been reported in some series of B-cell PTLD[8] and may portend a worse prognosis.[8,9] Reed-Sternberg-like cells may be seen in early, polymorphic, and some monomorphic PTLD. The diagnosis of true classic Hodgkin lymphoma (cHL)-type PTLD relies on morphologic and immunophenotypic features of the diagnostic sample.[10,11] The expression pattern of EBV proteins (EBV-latency pattern) may aid in the diagnosis of cHL.[12]

In contrast to the typical T/NK-cell disease spectrum among immunocompetent children, the most common T/NK-cell PTLD described is peripheral T-cell lymphoma (PTCL), followed by hepatosplenic T-cell lymphoma. T/NK-cell disease tends to occur later and is rare (approximately 15%), although it may be increasing.[13,14] The disease is more common in certain geographic regions possibly because of the greater prevalence of human T-lymphotropic virus 1 (HTLV-1) infection in these areas.[15] It more commonly presents late, is more likely to present at extranodal sites, and is more often EBV negative (two-thirds of cases).[16,17] T/NK-cell pathology seems to be rare in the pediatric SOT population.[18] The available literature suggests that T/NK-cell PTLD is clinically aggressive and associated with a poor prognosis,[17] although the natural history of the disease in children remains to be defined.[16]

IMMUNOBIOLOGY OF EBV

Most cases of PTLD following pediatric SOT are associated with EBV, a latent human lymphotropic virus discovered in 1964 by Epstein, Barr, and Achong.[19] More than 90% of the world's population is infected with EBV and infected individuals remain life-long carriers of the virus.[20] The life cycle of EBV is outlined in **Fig. 1**. Primary infection occurs through the oropharynx, where the virus infects resting B cells that become proliferating lymphoblasts with expression of EBV nuclear antigen 2 (EBNA2),[21] which activates the promoters necessary to produce all latent proteins (growth program or latency III) (**Table 2**). The virus gains access to the memory B-cell compartment following the steps required for a normal B cell to move along the pathway from naive to memory cell. After migration of the infected cells into the follicle, EBNA2 is turned off, together with the latent genes that drive proliferation. Infected cells acquire a germinal center phenotype and start the default program (latency II), which is accompanied by the expression of latent membrane protein 1 (LMP1) and LMP2,[21] which provide the necessary signals, T-cell help and B-cell receptor, respectively, that physiologically rescue latently infected germinal center cells into memory cells.

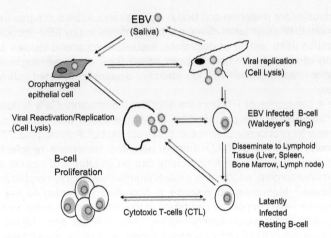

Fig. 1. EBV life cycle.

These infected B cells that have the surface phenotype of long-lived memory B cells and do not express any of the known latent proteins (latency O)[22] or only EBNA1 (latency I), mature and circulate in the peripheral blood. Release of the virus into the saliva occurs when circulating memory B cells transit the nasopharyngeal lymphoid tissue and differentiate into plasma cells.

Control of virus spread and of unrestrained infected B-cell proliferation is guaranteed by the development of a specific immune response that occurs in healthy immunocompetent individuals and consists of T cells specifically recognizing immunodominant latent EBV proteins presented in the context of major histocompatibility complex (MHC) molecules.[23] NK, CD8+, and CD4+ T cells generally control and contain the proliferation of EBV-infected B cells during primary infection. CD8+ cells, particularly those directed against lytic EBV antigens, expand dramatically during acute infection, and then contract at the resolution of the primary EBV infection.[24] During persistent EBV infection, lytic and latent EBV antigen-specific T cells are maintained at a frequency of 1% to 5% of peripheral blood T cells to immune survey and eliminate reactivating/proliferating infected B cells when they express the growth program.[25] CD4+ T cells directed against lytic and latent EBV antigens are also implicated in controlling EBV responses.[26]

Table 2			
EBV gene expression patterns			
B Cell Type	**Program**	**Gene Expressed**	**Function**
Naive	Growth (latency III)	EBNAs (1,2,3a,3b,3c) LP, LMP1, LMP2	Activation of B cells
Germinal center	Default (latency II)	EBNA1, LMP1, LMP2	Entry of B cells into memory pool
Memory, or dividing memory B cells	Latency, or EBNA1 only (latency 0 or I)	None or EBNA1	Persistence
Plasma cells	Lytic	Lytic antigens	Replication of the virus

In the immunocompetent host, T cell–mediated responses to the immunogenic proteins prevent outgrowth of EBV-infected B cells. In contrast, when T cell–mediated responses are impaired, as in immunocompromised individuals, including hematopoietic stem cell transplant (HSCT) recipients and SOT recipients, uncontrolled proliferation of EBV-infected B cells will lead to the development of EBV-associated lymphoproliferative diseases (PTLDs).

EPIDEMIOLOGY OF PTLD

It is difficult to precisely define the incidence and potential changes in the biologic characteristics of PTLD observed over time. First, there is a lack of large registry data with mandatory reporting of PTLD, established over the long periods of time required to appreciate changes in epidemiology of disease. Second, because of the heterogeneity of disease, a consensus for PTLD diagnosis has been lacking. Nonetheless, the incidence of PTLD seems to be related to several risk factors. The factor that has consistently been demonstrated to convey highest risk for PTLD is EBV seronegativity at time of transplant.[27,28] Similarly, younger age at transplant is a strong risk factor for PTLD, but likely reflects the proportion of recipients who are EBV naive.[29] The risk is highest following primary EBV infection,[27] which may occur via transmission from the allograft or the natural route via salivary secretion.

In general, it seems that risk of PTLD correlates with the intensity and cumulative exposure to immunosuppression.[1] It is difficult to assess the effect of individual immunosuppressive agents on PTLD risk for several reasons. There is no reliable and reproducible method to measure intensity of immunosuppression. A patient is typically on more than 1 immunosuppressive agent. There is often a learning curve with new agents, such that the incidence of PTLD is often higher when an agent is first introduced to clinical care.[28,30–32] To obtain sufficient numbers of patients to assess risk, large registries are required. Registry data are often limited by providing information only if an agent was used, not dosage or duration, or in combination with other agents.[31–34] Despite the lack of conclusive data, it can be surmised that the more T cell–specific the immunosuppression used, the higher the incidence of PTLD. Therefore, the use of anti-T-cell antibodies is usually associated with the highest risk of PTLD.[33,34] However, it seems that monoclonal antibodies convey a higher risk than polyclonal antibodies, and cytotoxic antibodies (ie, OKT3 and antithymocyte globulin) increase risk more than anti-interleukin 2 (anti-IL-2) antibodies.[34] The use of calcineurin inhibitors seems to confer the next highest risk.[28,30,32,33] Although early studies suggested the use of tacrolimus increases the risk of PTLD compared with cyclosporine, more recent studies suggest that if serum levels are monitored closely there is no difference in risk of PTLD.[28,30–32,35] It seems that the risk of PTLD is low with the use of mycophenolate mofetil or mammalian target of rapamycin inhibitors such as sirolimus.[31,36,37]

PTLD is an early event (ie, within the first 2 years after transplant) in most cases,[4,33] likely because of more intense immunosuppression used for induction therapy or the exposure of the EBV-naive host to the virus, often from EBV-infected passenger lymphocytes in the allograft. However, in children who receive allografts from EBV-negative donors, primary exposure to EBV is via the natural route of salivary secretion and may occur during adolescence.[4]

Most analyses suggest that the risk of PTLD is associated with the type of organ transplanted. Low-risk patients (eg, renal, heart, and liver recipients) are generally reported to have a risk of PTLD less than 5%, whereas high-risk patients (eg, those with lung, small bowel, and multiple organ grafts) have an incidence greater than

10%.[38] In pediatrics the variability in PTLD incidence between various allografts is less. The incidence seems to be 5% to 10% for most pediatric recipients regardless of allograft,[4,38] likely reflecting a stronger effect of EBV-naive status compared with type of allograft. The reasons for the observed differences in incidence of PTLD with various allografts are complex. There are recipient factors, such as age and EBV serostatus, but also allograft factors, such as the amount of immunosuppression required to prevent rejection and the differing risk of transmitting EBV-infected B cells (in associated lymphoid tissue) with intestine and lung transplants compared with liver, heart, and kidney transplants.[39,40]

It seems that the incidence of PTLD in pediatric renal transplant recipients may have been increasing since the 1990s,[28] whereas it may be decreasing in pediatric liver or intestinal transplant recipients.[30,41] The reasons for these observations are not clear.

CLINICAL PRESENTATION

Every visit by an SOT survivor to a primary care provider represents an opportunity for surveillance for malignancy/PTLD. The clinical presentation of PTLD is variable, depending on the underlying pathologic condition, the type of transplant, and the time since transplant. It is important to maintain a high index of suspicion because the onset of PTLD can be insidious and nonspecific. Frequently, patients present with relatively benign findings (episodic and unexplained fever, weight loss, fatigue) before developing more significant symptomatology. Patients considered high risk and managed as such may be diagnosed with PTLD before becoming symptomatic. Rarely, SOT recipients may present with so-called fulminant PTLD. This term refers to rapidly progressive, disseminated disease resulting in multiorgan failure and is more commonly seen following HSCT than in the SOT context.[42] Other EBV-associated diseases must be differentiated from PTLD, although the initial management is similar.[43]

Early-onset PTLD occurring within 1 to 2 years of transplantation is more common among pediatric SOT recipients because of their risk for primary EBV infection.[39] Early-onset disease is more likely to involve the allograft and present with declining allograft function, excepting heart allografts, in which direct involvement by PTLD is rare.[44] The major differential diagnostic considerations for early onset PTLD include allograft rejection and infection.[45] Later-onset disease is more likely to be EBV negative or include T/NK-cell disease[14,17,27,35,46] and to involve extranodal sites (especially gastrointestinal [GI] sites) or present with dissemination.[47]

Outside the allograft, common areas affected by PTLD include lymphoid tissues, GI tract, lung, and liver.[48] Patients may present with constitutional symptoms, lymphadenopathy, and organ dysfunction. Disease classified pathologically as early lesions often presents with adenotonsillar involvement with associated sore throat and obstructive symptoms (new onset snoring or mouth breathing).[49] Involvement of the GI tract may present with vomiting, diarrhea, bleeding, intussusception, or obstruction. Perforation may occur at presentation or immediately following initiation of therapy in the presence of transmural lesion necrosis. Chronic ulceration in intestinal transplant recipients should prompt a biopsy to rule out PTLD with samples from the ulcer edge and the intervening mucosa.[50] New-onset anemia or hypoalbuminemia may indicate GI involvement. Lung disease may result in respiratory insufficiency or asymptomatic nodules. Liver disease may present as diffuse hepatitis or nodular lesions. PTLD of the central nervous system (CNS), isolated or as part of multiorgan disease, has been described but is rare.[9,51] Patients may present with headache, seizures, or focal neurologic findings.

Initial assessment includes a full physical examination, screening blood tests, including a complete blood count with differential, chemistry panel to assess for tumor lysis syndrome, allograft function screening, and EBV viral-load studies. Variable disease presentation can make interpretation of imaging difficult.[52] Ultrasound seems to be effective for initial imaging in patients with suspected abdominal or soft-tissue PTLD.[53] Other imaging modalities should be pursued based on symptoms and initial screening results. The recommended diagnostic and staging procedures are similar to other non-Hodgkin lymphomas (NHLs) and are outlined in **Fig. 2**. Presentations according to selected patient series are outlined in **Table 3**.

The role of [^{18}F]2-fluoro-2-deoxyglucose (FDG)-positron emission tomography (PET) in the diagnosis of equivocal lesions, staging, and response assessment of PTLD is currently being defined.[54,55] Bakker and colleagues demonstrated additional extranodal sites on PET not appreciated on computed tomography (CT) in 50% of patients and concordance of PET response with outcome. However, false positives have been described when PET is used for disease monitoring in children[56] and for the evaluation of lung lesions.[57] An example of CT-PET imaging for the staging of PTLD is included in **Fig. 3**.

THERAPY

Although PTLD continues to be a significant cause of mortality in pediatric organ transplant recipients, there are data to suggest that the risk is decreasing.[33] It is unclear if this reflects monitoring of at-risk patients and earlier diagnosis, prevention (primary or secondary), or improved therapy.

PRIMARY PREVENTION

As the knowledge of the risk factors for PTLD increases, attention has turned to primary prevention of disease. Limiting as much as possible the total amount of immunosuppression by adjusting type, combination, and doses of drugs after transplant is key. For example, Opelz and Dohler[39] provided evidence in their analysis of the Collaborative Transplant Study data that the incidence of PTLD among cardiac transplant recipients decreased from 13.9% to 6.2% between 1985 to 1989 and 1995 to 2001, concomitant with reduced use of OKT3 in recent years. Avoiding EBV-positive donors in EBV-naive recipients to limit primary infection may prevent PTLD. However, such donors are in limited supply, with 1 survey study of donor EBV serologic status

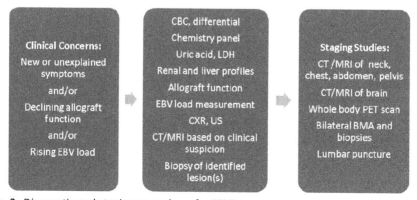

Fig. 2. Diagnostic and staging procedures for PTLD.

Table 3
Selected pediatric or mixed adult/pediatric SOT studies and PTLD

	Incidence	Mean Time to PTLD (Months)	Presenting Sites	Pathology	Survival
Pediatric Heart Transplant Study[A]	6% of patients surviving to 30 d after transplant	23.8 (3–91.1)	GI tract (39%) Respiratory system (25%) Cervical adenopathy (18%) CNS ds (3.6%)	p-PTLD 63% m-PTLD 32% Unknown 5% B cell 47/48 EBV + 39/45 (87%)	1 y: 75% 3 y: 68% 5 y: 67%
North American Pediatric Renal Transplant Cooperative Study[28,140]	2%–4% at 3–5 y	6.8	Lymph node (33%) Abdomen (29%) Kidney allograft (11%) CNS (11%)		
Charleston Liver Transplant Experience (including pediatric recipients)[141]	3.5% cumulative incidence (pediatric 7.5%, n = 5)	18	Extranodal (77%, one-third of whom had lesions in the allograft) Lymph nodes (23%)	p-PTLD 5/19 m-PTLD 13/19 EBV-positive 5/13 EBV-negative 8/13	
International Intestinal Transplant Registry (pediatric data only)[142]	Intestine only 13.5% Intestine + liver 15.4% Multivisceral 20.8% Cumulative incidence				As cause of death 19/270 versus rejection 33/270

Collaborative Transplant Study Report[39]	Relative risks: Kidney Age <10 y, 259.8; 10–20 y, 113.6; Heart Age <10 y, 1240.2; 10–20 y, 473.1; Liver Age <10 y, 565; 10–20, 368.6	Incidence highest in first year; most lymphomas diagnosed after first year; median time to occurrence 5 y	Preference to allograft (except heart) or region of allograft; GI tract; Disseminated disease		1-y mortality 40%–50%
Canadian PTLD Survey Group of Adult and Pediatric Transplant Centers[143]	90/4283 (2.1%) range 0%–14.6% with disproportionate representation of children	50% within first year after transplant	Lymph node as most common site (solitary and multiple lesions)	B cell 42%; T cell 15.6%; p-PTLD 18.9%; m-PTLD 31.1%	48.9% died, 25.6% CR, 8.9% PR

Abbreviations: CNS, central nervous system; CR, complete response; m-PTLD, monomorphic PTLD; p-PTLD, polymorphic PTLD; PR, partial response.

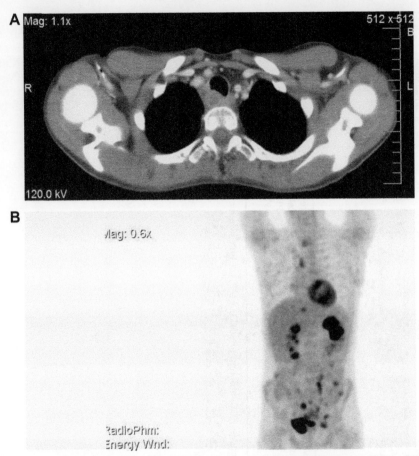

Fig. 3. A lung transplant recipient presented within 6 months of transplant with worsening pulmonary function tests and new onset of abdominal pain, weight loss, and diarrhea. Endoscopy was performed and biopsy specimens showed polymorphic EBV-associated PTLD. (*A*) Shown here on CT chest is 1 of 2 peripherally enhancing, centrally hypodense mass lesions posterior to and involving the membranous posterior wall of the trachea. (*B*) FDG-PET scanning showed 2 foci of marked uptake in the right paratracheal and pretracheal regions corresponding to the nodes seen on CT. Uptake in the liver, duodenal wall, scattered foci in the bowel, and lymph nodes in the left iliac chain inguinal areas were also noted and were consistent with disease.

documenting only 27 of 459 (6%) donors to be EBV negative.[58] An alternate approach is to immunize against EBV before immune suppression. Such vaccines are in development and early phase I/II trials are under way.[59]

The role for passive immunization with the use of anticytomegalovirus intravenous immune globulin (anti-CMV-IVIG) or the use of antiviral therapy for prophylaxis remains unclear. Green and colleagues[60] conducted a randomized, controlled trial of CMV-IVIG for the prevention of EBV disease and PTLD in EBV-seronegative SOT recipients. There was no difference from placebo at 2 years for either end point, although the study was underpowered and confounded by the clinical practice change of decreasing immunosuppression with the finding of rising EBV titres after the start of study recruitment. Another study by Humar and colleagues[61] was unable to demonstrate a benefit of the addition of CMV-IVIG to gancyclovir in EBV load or incidence of PTLD. Opelz and colleagues[62] conducted a large retrospective analysis of the effect of prophylactic anti-CMV-IVIG or antiviral therapy for renal allograft recipients on the incidence of PTLD. There was a statistically significant benefit to the use of CMV-IVIG in the first year after transplant, but not thereafter. This group was unable to detect a benefit to antiviral therapy as prophylaxis for PTLD, although other studies do suggest benefit.[63,64] Biologically, the role of antivirals in PTLD prevention has been questioned as they do not suppress EBV-driven B-cell proliferation. There may be a benefit to the EBV-naive recipient with an EBV-positive donor, with a reduction in the number of infected B cells.[65]

SECONDARY PREVENTION

Development of EBV-associated PTLD is usually preceded by an increase in the number of latently infected B cells, which can be revealed by increased levels of EBV DNA in peripheral blood or plasma.[66] Clinically, EBV DNA load is higher among SOT recipients subsequently diagnosed with PTLD than those who remain disease-free, with increasing risk with higher EBV loads.[67–69] EBV DNA loads seem to increase from 2 to 16 weeks before diagnosis of PTLD.[30,70] There is a trend towards higher EBV loads following primary infection compared with reactivation,[71] consistent with the clinical observation of higher risk of PTLD following primary infection.[27,48] Between 60% and 80% of EBV-negative children seroconvert within 3 months of transplant[72,73] and a small population maintain high viral loads after primary EBV infection or EBV-associated PTLD.[69,73,74] It is generally accepted practice to perform serial peripheral blood EBV polymerase chain reaction (EBV-PCR) monitoring or immune function monitoring with a planned decrease or change in specific drugs to decrease overall immunosuppression in the event of rising EBV load following SOT. Current guidelines suggest monthly to biweekly monitoring for the first 3 months following transplantation and then monthly EBV monitoring for 1 year in EBV-mismatched individuals.[66,75] Beyond the first year, monitoring at least every 3 months is recommended because of the risk of late-onset disease.

This practice assumes that EBV-PCR monitoring reliably detects those at high risk for PTLD. The first caution with this assumption relates to the significant variability between the different PCR techniques and laboratory tests.[66] Measurements of viral DNA are reproducibly obtained by amplifying short sequences of DNA currently using real-time PCR. Many studies have shown that most EBV genomes in the peripheral blood are cell-associated.[76,77] Although at lower quantities, cell-free, nonencapsulated EBV DNA can also be detected in the blood of patients with PTLD, indicating fragmented or naked DNA.[76] In many studies plasma or serum is used because they are readily obtained and handled, and have been proven capable of predicting the development of PTLD.[78,79] However, serum or plasma samples lack cell-associated virus and therefore plasma loads are not correlated with peripheral blood mononuclear cell (PBMC) values[77] and whole blood/PBMC might be better when screening for PTLD.[76,77,80] It remains challenging to identify which EBV load value should be used to identify high-risk patients, because different systems are used for different samples and patients so that quantitative values cannot be easily compared between laboratories.

The second caution relates to the absence of blinded, prospective trials to determine the predictive value of qPCR. EBV load seems to be sensitive for identifying patients at risk for, or presenting with, EBV-associated PTLD but lacks specificity for presence of disease.[76] Sensitivity (60%–100%) and specificity measures (4%–100%)

range depending on the threshold value of EBV DNA used,[66,81–83] differences in initial serologic status of recipients,[84] type of transplant, immunosuppressive regimen, and the blood compartment in which EBV is measured.[68] EBV DNA load alone cannot be used to make or exclude the diagnosis of PTLD.[85] Recent studies suggest that changes in viral-load kinetics better correlate with organ involvement compared with single viral-load measurements.[86]

Several laboratory findings have been proposed to increase the predictive value of EBV DNA load, including the concomitant use of gene-expression profiling of sentinel EBV genes,[74] cytokine polymorphisms,[87] and measurement of IL-6 and IL-10 levels.[88] Most promising is the development of monitoring techniques for T-cell reconstitution and function and particularly measures of anti-EBV T-cell immunity.[89] Low-quantity EBV cytotoxic T lymphocytes (EBV-CTL) in peripheral blood are a better predictor of patients who will develop PTLD or relapse after treatment for PTLD than is EBV viral load.[90,91] These laboratory techniques are not widely available.

The value of preemptive therapeutic strategies, including most commonly decreasing immunosuppression, in the presence of high or increasing EBV titres has been examined only compared with historical controls. The results in these small studies have been mostly positive, with the reported incidence of PTLD decreasing by 50% to 90%.[30,80,92,93] However, some groups report no difference in incidence of PTLD with this approach.[94] Ideally, clinicians would decrease and change immuno-suppression depending on the clinical context.[68] Rituximab is often given after HSCT, with the finding of increasing EBV load with variable success to control EBV-driven B-cell proliferation until EBV-CTL function develops to control proliferation.[95,96] Its use among SOT recipients for disease prevention is being studied further.[93,97]

THERAPY

The treatment of established PTLD presents a therapeutic challenge. These patients are susceptible to regimen-related toxicity (ie, infections and end-organ toxicity), as well as being at risk of rejecting the transplanted allograft. Therefore, ideal therapy for PTLD would be minimally toxic, while still being cytotoxic to the B-cell proliferation, preventing/treating allograft rejection, and minimizing the inhibition of immune responses required to control EBV-driven B-cell proliferation.

Numerous studies have attempted to identify prognostic factors. Because of heterogeneity of disease and treatment, there is not a consensus in the literature on prognostic factors. Some studies have suggested that monomorphic PTLD has a worse prognosis than polymorphic PTLD, but this has not been found in other series.[98–101] Some studies have demonstrated that clonality is a poor prognostic finding,[100] although other studies cannot confirm this.[99] A potential explanation for these apparent discrepancies is sampling bias. Single tumors may have areas of differing morphology and tumors at distinct sites may have different clonalities.[4,102] However, it is generally believed that monomorphic disease, clonal immunoglobulin gene rearrangement, and/or abnormal karyotype likely reflects a poorer prognosis.[4,9,98]

Extent of dissemination of disease has consistently been found to be prognostic. Local control with surgery or radiotherapy is effective in curing localized disease, but this represents only a small percentage of patients.[103] Even monomorphic, mono-clonal, or aggressive histology (ie, Burkitt histology) can be cured by local therapy alone if it is truly localized. Classic staging classifications for NHL have limited value in PTLD because of the high predilection for extranodal involvement.[100,104] Multiple (>2) sites of disease have consistently been found to confer poorer prognosis, and

CNS involvement portends a dismal outcome.[9,100,103–105] PTLD associated with primary EBV infection seems to have a superior prognosis,[4] whereas PTLD observed more than 1 year after transplant, non–B-cell phenotype, or tumor that is EBV negative has a poor prognosis.[100,106] The exception to this rule is posttransplant HL, which is often associated with EBV and responds well to standard therapy for HL.[107]

Reduction or withdrawal of immunosuppression is currently the cornerstone of PTLD treatment, but the reported success varies greatly, from 20% to 80%. This range of response is attributable to the differences in practice of reduction/withdrawal of immunosuppression and the wide spectrum of PTLD presentation, with localized or polymorphic disease more likely to respond.[4,98] Even for patients who have disease that is responsive to reduction of immunosuppression, there is an increased risk of rejection, which may threaten the viability of the allograft. This effect is most dramatically seen in cardiothoracic transplant recipients, in whom rejection and death are not infrequent.[4,108]

If disease is not amenable to local control and reduction/withdrawal of immunosuppression has failed, either because of progressive disease or development of allograft rejection, outcome has been poor. The outcome for such patients with refractory PTLD is again variable, with disease-free survival reported to be between 0% and 70%.[98,100,101,104,109–115] The efficacy of antiviral drugs in treating PTLD is controversial because they are seldom used without other interventions (eg, reduction of immunosuppression); in addition, if viral replication, which is lytic to the infected B cells, is suppressed, B-cell proliferation could theoretically be enhanced. A novel approach of using arginine butyrate, which upregulates expression of EBV thymidine kinase and stimulates viral replication, along with ganciclovir, which causes an abortive replicative cycle such that no virions are produced but cell death occurs, has been shown to be effective in highly refractory PTLD.[116]

The first report using anti-B-cell therapy used anti-CD21 and anti-CD23 antibodies and showed they were well tolerated, although only 35% of patients achieved long-term survival and only patients with monoclonal disease survived.[117] More recently, anti-CD20, or rituximab, has been used. All reports to date have had small numbers and results vary but it seems that about 50% of patients achieve complete remission with rituximab.[109,110,112,114,115] However, relapse has been reported in up to 25% of patients.[109,114] In addition, the significant effect of rituximab on normal B cells must be kept in mind and patients' immunoglobulin levels monitored closely.[118]

Chemotherapy has been used to treat resistant PTLD following SOT. Chemotherapy is attractive because it kills proliferating B cells and is immunosuppressive enough to treat or prevent graft-versus-host disease (GVHD) or organ rejection. However, at conventional doses used in the treatment of NHL, posttransplant patients have more end-organ toxicity and susceptibility to infection, with as many as 35% of patients dying of toxicity of the therapy,[110,111,119] although pediatric PTLD patients seem to tolerate standard-dose NHL regimens better.[98] One study demonstrated that overall outcome was improved when chemotherapy was reserved for patients who failed rituximab.[112] Therefore, a common practice at present is to treat with rituximab patients who have failed reduction of immunosuppression and reserve chemotherapy for patients who fail rituximab.[4,110,112] In attempts to avoid toxicity, regimens with lower-dose chemotherapy than used to treat B-cell NHL in children have been used. This approach has been shown to be effective in treating PTLD in children following organ transplant with little toxicity.[104] A report on a small series of children with PTLD, Burkitt lymphoma with c-myc translocation, and marrow involvement showed they could be successfully treated with reduced intensity chemotherapy.[113] These data suggest that most PTLD, even true lymphoma, may be more sensitive to chemotherapy than NHL that is seen in the general pediatric population. Studies are ongoing to determine if the addition of rituximab to these chemotherapy regimens improves outcome.

The role of EBV monitoring during treatment of PTLD as a measure of disease response remains unclear.[120,121] The relationship between clearance from PBMCs may not correlate with disease response as EBV-infected cells in peripheral blood are not found in the same compartment as the tumor cells.

Non-EBV-associated PTLD (B-cell, T-cell, Hodgkin, or plasmacytic myeloma) tends to occur late and rarely resolves with reduction of immunosuppression.[101,106] Despite the associated toxicity, standard-dosed chemotherapy regimens are usually required to achieve remissions; remissions are rare and recurrences are common. The possible exception is Hodgkin-PTLD; although there is more toxicity and inferior outcome compared with nontransplant patients, the use of standard Hodgkin regimens has produced a significant number of cures.[107]

ADOPTIVE IMMUNOTHERAPY WITH EBV-SPECIFIC T CELLS

The balance between EBV-infected proliferating B cells and frequency of functional EBV-specific T cells needs to be restored to ensure disease control and prevention. Therefore, T cell–based therapies capable of restoring EBV-specific immunity could be used to complement therapies directly aimed at destroying tumor cells and implement long-term control of EBV-infected B-cell proliferation.

Infusions of unmanipulated donor T lymphocytes containing a small proportion of EBV-reactive T cells can be effective for treating stem-cell recipients with established disease[122,123] but are limited by potentially fatal complications, including GVHD caused by contaminating alloreactive T cells, and by the time required for the EBV-CTL precursors in the infused population to expand in vivo to a number sufficient to contain the disease.

To overcome these obstacles strategies have been developed to expand donor-derived or patient-derived EBV-CTLs ex vivo.[124] These EBV-specific CTL lines expanded ex vivo are polyclonal, containing CD8+ and CD4+ EBV-CTLs to ensure recognition of multiple epitopes and minimize the risk of tumor escape mutants, as well as to promote long-term in vivo survival.[125] Donor-derived EBV-CTLs have been successfully used for prophylaxis and treatment of EBV-induced lymphoma in patients after HSCT.[95,125] In contrast, in solid-organ transplant recipients in whom tumor B cells are almost always of recipient origin, EBV-CTLs are generated from the recipients, either before transplantation[126] or from recipients receiving immuno-suppression following transplantation.[124] Infusions of EBV-CTLs in SOT patients are safe and do not cause graft rejection, have antiviral and antitumor effects, and increase in vivo EBV-specific cellular immune responses.[124,127] However, the infused EBV-CTLs in these patients persist only transiently and do not expand by several orders of magnitude, as opposed to results in HSCT recipients, likely because of the ongoing immunosuppression and the steady state of the patient's lymphocyte compartment, which limits CTL expansion rate.

Currently, efforts are being directed at reducing the time and labors required for CTL production[128,129] and at overcoming the difficulties encountered in generating CTLs from EBV-seronegative recipients.[130,131] A promising approach that bypasses the need to grow CTLs for individual patients is to develop a bank of allogeneic EBV-CTLs closely matched with human leukocyte antigen that could be available as an off-the-shelf product.[132,133] Recent studies have shown the safety, feasibility, and efficacy of this approach in patients with EBV lymphoma arising after HSCT or SOT.[134,135]

Obstacles to adoptive EBV-CTL therapy in HSCT and SOT remain, including cytokine dependency of CTLs, the role and direct immunosuppressive effects of the tumor environment, and the effect of immunosuppressive drugs. The combination of different strategies to overcome these limitations will help in designing the most successful approach.[136–139] In addition to these scientific developments, concomitant technical improvements in cell preparation that will simplify and accelerate the administration of these cells to patients with disease are critical to facilitate their application outside the current limited number of specialized centers.

SUMMARY

PTLD is a complex and heterogeneous disease requiring the collaborative efforts of the transplant, infectious diseases, and oncology teams for prevention, screening, and treatment. Ongoing clinical and translational studies are required to better understand the immunobiology and various pathologies of the disease for determination of risk factors and effective therapies. The heterogeneity of disease and patient populations and the differing approaches to immunosuppression, EBV detection methods, and therapeutic interventions are barriers to furthering our understanding of this disease process. The incidence of PTLD is expected to increase as greater numbers of children survive long-term after SOT.[39] There is an urgent need for multicenter trials to learn from larger numbers of patients and to determine best practice for this population.

REFERENCES

1. Buell JF, Gross TG, Woodle ES. Malignancy after transplantation. Transplantation 2005;80(Suppl 2):S254–64.
2. Bustami RT, Ojo AO, Wolfe RA, et al. Immunosuppression and the risk of post-transplant malignancy among cadaveric first kidney transplant recipients. Am J Transplant 2004;4(1):87–93.
3. Buell JF, Gross TG, Thomas MJ, et al. Malignancy in pediatric transplant recipients. Semin Pediatr Surg 2006;15(3):179–87.
4. Webber SA, Naftel DC, Fricker FJ, et al. Lymphoproliferative disorders after paediatric heart transplantation: a multi-institutional study. Lancet 2006; 367(9506):233–9.
5. Swerdlow SH, Webber SA, Chadburn A, et al. Post-transplant lymphoproliferative disorders. In: Swerdlow SH, Campo E, Lee Harris N, editors. WHO classification of tumours of haematopoietic and lymphoid tissues. Lyon (France): International Agency for Research on Cancer (IARC); 2008. p. 343–51.
6. Chadburn A, Chen JM, Hsu DT, et al. The morphologic and molecular genetic categories of posttransplantation lymphoproliferative disorders are clinically relevant. Cancer 1998;82(10):1978–87.
7. Chadburn A, Cesarman E, Knowles DM. Molecular pathology of posttransplantation lymphoproliferative disorders. Semin Diagn Pathol 1997;14(1):15–26.
8. Djokic M, Le Beau MM, Swinnen LJ, et al. Post-transplant lymphoproliferative disorder subtypes correlate with different recurring chromosomal abnormalities. Genes Chromosomes Cancer 2006;45(3):313–8.
9. Maecker B, Jack T, Zimmermann M, et al. CNS or bone marrow involvement as risk factors for poor survival in post-transplantation lymphoproliferative disorders in children after solid organ transplantation. J Clin Oncol 2007; 25(31):4902–8.

10. Pitman SD, Huang Q, Zuppan CW, et al. Hodgkin lymphoma-like posttransplant lymphoproliferative disorder (HL-like PTLD) simulates monomorphic B-cell PTLD both clinically and pathologically. Am J Surg Pathol 2006; 30(4):470–6.

11. Ranganathan S, Webber S, Ahuja S, et al. Hodgkin-like posttransplant lymphoproliferative disorder in children: does it differ from posttransplant Hodgkin lymphoma? Pediatr Dev Pathol 2004;7(4):348–60.

12. Rohr JC, Wagner HJ, Lauten M, et al. Differentiation of EBV-induced post-transplant Hodgkin lymphoma from Hodgkin-like post-transplant lymphoproliferative disease. Pediatr Transplant 2008;12(4):426–31.

13. Aucejo F, Rofaiel G, Miller C. Who is at risk for post-transplant lymphoproliferative disorders (PTLD) after liver transplantation? J Hepatol 2006;44(1): 19–23.

14. Leblond V, Davi F, Charlotte F, et al. Posttransplant lymphoproliferative disorders not associated with Epstein-Barr virus: a distinct entity? J Clin Oncol 1998;16(6): 2052–9.

15. Hoshida Y, Li T, Dong Z, et al. Lymphoproliferative disorders in renal transplant patients in Japan. Int J Cancer 2001;91(6):869–75.

16. Yang F, Li Y, Braylan R, et al. Pediatric T-cell post-transplant lymphoproliferative disorder after solid organ transplantation. Pediatr Blood Cancer 2008;50(2): 415–8.

17. Swerdlow SH. T-cell and NK-cell posttransplantation lymphoproliferative disorders. Am J Clin Pathol 2007;127(6):887–95.

18. Afify Z. T-cell post-transplantation lymphoproliferative disorder, a rare and challenging late complication of solid organ transplantation. Pediatr Transplant 2008;12(6):617–8.

19. Epstein MA, Achong BG, Barr YM. Virus particles in cultured lymphoblasts from Burkitt's lymphoma. Lancet 1964;1(7335):702–3.

20. Rickinson A, Kieff E. Epstein-Barr virus. In: Fields BN, Knipe DM, Howley PM, et al, editors. Fields virology. Philadelphia: Lippincott-Raven; 1996. p. 2397–446.

21. Thorley-Lawson DA. Epstein-Barr virus: exploiting the immune system. Nat Rev Immunol 2001;1(1):75–82.

22. Babcock GJ, Hochberg D, Thorley-Lawson AD. The expression pattern of Epstein-Barr virus latent genes in vivo is dependent upon the differentiation stage of the infected B cell. Immunity 2000;13(4):497–506.

23. Rickinson A, Kieff E. Epstein-Barr virus. In: Knipe DM, Howley PM, editors. Field's virology. Philadelphia: Lippincott, Williams and Wilkins; 2001. p. 2575–627.

24. Hislop AD, Gudgeon NH, Callan MF, et al. EBV-specific CD8+ T cell memory: relationships between epitope specificity, cell phenotype, and immediate effector function. J Immunol 2001;167(4):2019–29.

25. Steven NM, Leese AM, Annels NE, et al. Epitope focusing in the primary cytotoxic T cell response to Epstein-Barr virus and its relationship to T cell memory. J Exp Med 1996;184(5):1801–13.

26. Amyes E, Hatton C, Montamat-Sicotte D, et al. Characterization of the CD4+ T cell response to Epstein-Barr virus during primary and persistent infection. J Exp Med 2003;198(6):903–11.

27. Ho M, Jaffe R, Miller G, et al. The frequency of Epstein-Barr virus infection and associated lymphoproliferative syndrome after transplantation and its manifestations in children. Transplantation 1988;45(4):719–27.

28. Dharnidharka VR, Sullivan EK, Stablein DM, et al. Risk factors for posttransplant lymphoproliferative disorder (PTLD) in pediatric kidney transplantation: a report

of the North American Pediatric Renal Transplant Cooperative Study (NAPRTCS). Transplantation 2001;71(8):1065–8.

29. Newell KA, Alonso EM, Whitington PF, et al. Posttransplant lymphoproliferative disease in pediatric liver transplantation. Interplay between primary Epstein-Barr virus infection and immunosuppression. Transplantation 1996;62(3): 370–5.

30. McDiarmid SV, Jordan S, Kim GS, et al. Prevention and preemptive therapy of postransplant lymphoproliferative disease in pediatric liver recipients. Transplantation 1998;66(12):1604–11.

31. Dharnidharka VR, Ho PL, Stablein DM, et al. Mycophenolate, tacrolimus and post-transplant lymphoproliferative disorder: a report of the North American Pediatric Renal Transplant Cooperative Study. Pediatr Transplant 2002;6(5): 396–9.

32. Webster A, Woodroffe RC, Taylor RS, et al. Tacrolimus versus cyclosporin as primary immunosuppression for kidney transplant recipients. Cochrane Database Syst Rev 2005;(4):CD003961.

33. Faull RJ, Hollett P, McDonald SP. Lymphoproliferative disease after renal transplantation in Australia and New Zealand. Transplantation 2005;80(2): 193–7.

34. Opelz G, Naujokat C, Daniel V, et al. Disassociation between risk of graft loss and risk of non-Hodgkin lymphoma with induction agents in renal transplant recipients. Transplantation 2006;81(9):1227–33.

35. Guthery SL, Heubi JE, Bucuvalas JC, et al. Determination of risk factors for Epstein-Barr virus-associated posttransplant lymphoproliferative disorder in pediatric liver transplant recipients using objective case ascertainment. Transplantation 2003;75(7):987–93.

36. Kauffman HM, Cherikh WS, Cheng Y, et al. Maintenance immunosuppression with target-of-rapamycin inhibitors is associated with a reduced incidence of de novo malignancies. Transplantation 2005;80(7):883–9.

37. Birkeland SA, Hamilton-Dutoit S. Is posttransplant lymphoproliferative disorder (PTLD) caused by any specific immunosuppressive drug or by the transplantation per se? Transplantation 2003;76(6):984–8.

38. Dharnidharka VR, Tejani AH, Ho PL, et al. Post-transplant lymphoproliferative disorder in the United States: young Caucasian males are at highest risk. Am J Transplant 2002;2(10):993–8.

39. Opelz G, Dohler B. Lymphomas after solid organ transplantation: a collaborative transplant study report. Am J Transplant 2004;4(2):222–30.

40. Petit B, Le Meur Y, Jaccard A, et al. Influence of host-recipient origin on clinical aspects of posttransplantation lymphoproliferative disorders in kidney transplantation. Transplantation 2002;73(2):265–71.

41. Bond GJ, Mazariegos GV, Sindhi R, et al. Evolutionary experience with immunosuppression in pediatric intestinal transplantation. J Pediatr Surg 2005;40(1): 274–9 [discussion: 279–80].

42. Gross TG, Steinbuch M, DeFor T, et al. B cell lymphoproliferative disorders following hematopoietic stem cell transplantation: risk factors, treatment and outcome. Bone Marrow Transplant 1999;23(3):251–8.

43. Gross TG. Treatment for Epstein-Barr virus-associated PTLD. Herpes 2009; 15(3):64–7.

44. Bakker NA, van Imhoff GW, Verschuuren EA, et al. Early onset post-transplant lymphoproliferative disease is associated with allograft localization. Clin Transplant 2005;19(3):327–34.

45. Trpkov K, Marcussen N, Rayner D, et al. Kidney allograft with a lymphocytic infiltrate: acute rejection, posttransplantation lymphoproliferative disorder, neither, or both entities? Am J Kidney Dis 1997;30(3):449–54.

46. Nelson BP, Nalesnik MA, Bahler DW, et al. Epstein-Barr virus-negative posttransplant lymphoproliferative disorders: a distinct entity? Am J Surg Pathol 2000;24(3):375–85.

47. Verschuuren E, van der Bij W, de Boer W, et al. Quantitative Epstein-Barr virus (EBV) serology in lung transplant recipients with primary EBV infection and/or post-transplant lymphoproliferative disease. J Med Virol 2003;69(2):258–66.

48. Allen UD, Farkas G, Hebert D, et al. Risk factors for post-transplant lymphoproliferative disorder in pediatric patients: a case-control study. Pediatr Transplant 2005;9(4):450–5.

49. Herrmann BW, Sweet SC, Molter DW. Sinonasal posttransplant lymphoproliferative disorder in pediatric lung transplant patients. Otolaryngol Head Neck Surg 2005;133(1):38–41.

50. Selvaggi G, Sarkar S, Mittal N, et al. Etiology and management of alimentary tract ulcers in pediatric intestinal transplantation patients. Transplant Proc 2006;38(6):1768–9.

51. Castellano-Sanchez AA, Li S, Qian J, et al. Primary central nervous system posttransplant lymphoproliferative disorders. Am J Clin Pathol 2004;121(2):246–53.

52. Scarsbrook AF, Warakaulle DR, Dattani M, et al. Post-transplantation lymphoproliferative disorder: the spectrum of imaging appearances. Clin Radiol 2005;60(1):47–55.

53. Riebel T, Kebelmann-Betzing C, Scheer I. Ultrasound in abdominal and soft-tissue childhood PTLD (post-transplant lymphoproliferative disease). Ultraschall Med 2007;28(2):201–5.

54. Bakker NA, Pruim J, de Graaf W, et al. PTLD visualization by FDG-PET: improved detection of extranodal localizations. Am J Transplant 2006;6(8):1984–5.

55. von Falck C, Maecker B, Schirg E, et al. Post transplant lymphoproliferative disease in pediatric solid organ transplant patients: a possible role for [18F]-FDG-PET(/CT) in initial staging and therapy monitoring. Eur J Radiol 2007;63(3):427–35.

56. Rhodes MM, Delbeke D, Whitlock JA, et al. Utility of FDG-PET/CT in follow-up of children treated for Hodgkin and non-Hodgkin lymphoma. J Pediatr Hematol Oncol 2006;28(5):300–6.

57. McCormack L, Hany TI, Hubner M, et al. How useful is PET/CT imaging in the management of post-transplant lymphoproliferative disease after liver transplantation? Am J Transplant 2006;6(7):1731–6.

58. Lazda VA. Evaluation of Epstein-Barr virus (EBV) antibody screening of organ donors for allocation of organs to EBV serostatus matched recipients. Transplant Proc 2006;38(10):3404–5.

59. Shroff R, Rees L. The post-transplant lymphoproliferative disorder–a literature review. Pediatr Nephrol 2004;19(4):369–77.

60. Green M, Michaels MG, Katz BZ, et al. CMV-IVIG for prevention of Epstein Barr virus disease and posttransplant lymphoproliferative disease in pediatric liver transplant recipients. Am J Transplant 2006;6(8):1906–12.

61. Humar A, Hebert D, Davies HD, et al. A randomized trial of ganciclovir versus ganciclovir plus immune globulin for prophylaxis against Epstein-Barr virus related posttransplant lymphoproliferative disorder. Transplantation 2006;81(6):856–61.

62. Opelz G, Daniel V, Naujokat C, et al. Effect of cytomegalovirus prophylaxis with immunoglobulin or with antiviral drugs on post-transplant non-Hodgkin lymphoma: a multicentre retrospective analysis. Lancet Oncol 2007;8(3):212–8.
63. Funch DP, Walker AM, Schneider G, et al. Ganciclovir and acyclovir reduce the risk of post-transplant lymphoproliferative disorder in renal transplant recipients. Am J Transplant 2005;5(12):2894–900.
64. Green M, Kaufmann M, Wilson J, et al. Comparison of intravenous ganciclovir followed by oral acyclovir with intravenous ganciclovir alone for prevention of cytomegalovirus and Epstein-Barr virus disease after liver transplantation in children. Clin Infect Dis 1997;25(6):1344–9.
65. Green M, Michaels MG, Webber SA, et al. The management of Epstein-Barr virus associated post-transplant lymphoproliferative disorders in pediatric solid-organ transplant recipients. Pediatr Transplant 1999;3(4):271–81.
66. Rowe DT, Webber S, Schauer EM, et al. Epstein-Barr virus load monitoring: its role in the prevention and management of post-transplant lymphoproliferative disease. Transpl Infect Dis 2001;3(2):79–87.
67. Allen U, Hebert D, Petric M, et al. Utility of semiquantitative polymerase chain reaction for Epstein-Barr virus to measure virus load in pediatric organ transplant recipients with and without posttransplant lymphoproliferative disease. Clin Infect Dis 2001;33(2):145–50.
68. Schubert S, Renner C, Hammer M, et al. Relationship of immunosuppression to Epstein-Barr viral load and lymphoproliferative disease in pediatric heart transplant patients. J Heart Lung Transplant 2008;27(1):100–5.
69. Bingler MA, Feingold B, Miller SA, et al. Chronic high Epstein-Barr viral load state and risk for late-onset posttransplant lymphoproliferative disease/lymphoma in children. Am J Transplant 2008;8(2):442–5.
70. Webber SA. Post-transplant lymphoproliferative disorders: a preventable complication of solid organ transplantation? Pediatr Transplant 1999;3(2):95–9.
71. Kenagy DN, Schlesinger Y, Weck K, et al. Epstein-Barr virus DNA in peripheral blood leukocytes of patients with posttransplant lymphoproliferative disease. Transplantation 1995;60(6):547–54.
72. Smets F, Bodeus M, Goubau P, et al. Characteristics of Epstein-Barr virus primary infection in pediatric liver transplant recipients. J Hepatol 2000;32(1):100–4.
73. Green M, Webber SA. Persistent increased Epstein-Barr virus loads after solid organ transplantation: truth and consequences? Liver Transpl 2007;13(3):321–2.
74. Qu L, Green M, Webber S, et al. Epstein-Barr virus gene expression in the peripheral blood of transplant recipients with persistent circulating virus loads. J Infect Dis 2000;182(4):1013–21.
75. Humar A, Michaels M. American Society of Transplantation recommendations for screening, monitoring and reporting of infectious complications in immunosuppression trials in recipients of organ transplantation. Am J Transplant 2006;6(2):262–74.
76. Stevens SJ, Verschuuren EA, Pronk I, et al. Frequent monitoring of Epstein-Barr virus DNA load in unfractionated whole blood is essential for early detection of posttransplant lymphoproliferative disease in high-risk patients. Blood 2001;97(5):1165–71.
77. Wadowsky RM, Laus S, Green M, et al. Measurement of Epstein-Barr virus DNA loads in whole blood and plasma by TaqMan PCR and in peripheral blood lymphocytes by competitive PCR. J Clin Microbiol 2003;41(11):5245–9.

78. van Esser JW, Niesters HG, Thijsen SF, et al. Molecular quantification of viral load in plasma allows for fast and accurate prediction of response to therapy of Epstein-Barr virus-associated lymphoproliferative disease after allogeneic stem cell transplantation. Br J Haematol 2001;113(3):814–21.

79. Wagner HJ, Fischer L, Jabs WJ, et al. Longitudinal analysis of Epstein-Barr viral load in plasma and peripheral blood mononuclear cells of transplanted patients by real-time polymerase chain reaction. Transplantation 2002;74(5):656–64.

80. Bakker NA, Verschuuren EA, Veeger NJ, et al. Quantification of Epstein-Barr virus-DNA load in lung transplant recipients: a comparison of plasma versus whole blood. J Heart Lung Transplant 2008;27(1):7–10.

81. Wagner HJ, Cheng YC, Huls MH, et al. Prompt versus preemptive intervention for EBV lymphoproliferative disease. Blood 2004;103(10):3979–81.

82. Bakker NA, Verschuuren EA, Erasmus ME, et al. Epstein-Barr virus-DNA load monitoring late after lung transplantation: a surrogate marker of the degree of immunosuppression and a safe guide to reduce immunosuppression. Transplantation 2007;83(4):433–8.

83. Ahya VN, Douglas LP, Andreadis C, et al. Association between elevated whole blood Epstein-Barr virus (EBV)-encoded RNA EBV polymerase chain reaction and reduced incidence of acute lung allograft rejection. J Heart Lung Transplant 2007;26(8):839–44.

84. Wheless SA, Gulley ML, Raab-Traub N, et al. Post-transplantation lymphoproliferative disease: Epstein-Barr virus DNA levels, HLA-A3, and survival. Am J Respir Crit Care Med 2008;178(10):1060–5.

85. Henry DD, Hunger SP, Braylan RC, et al. Low viral load post-transplant lymphoproliferative disease localized within the tongue. Transpl Infect Dis 2008;10(6):426–30.

86. Funk GA, Gosert R, Hirsch HH. Viral dynamics in transplant patients: implications for disease. Lancet Infect Dis 2007;7(7):460–72.

87. Lee TC, Savoldo B, Barshes NR, et al. Use of cytokine polymorphisms and Epstein-Barr virus viral load to predict development of post-transplant lymphoproliferative disorder in paediatric liver transplant recipients. Clin Transplant 2006;20(3):389–93.

88. Baiocchi OC, Colleoni GW, Caballero OL, et al. Epstein-Barr viral load, interleukin-6 and interleukin-10 levels in post-transplant lymphoproliferative disease: a nested case-control study in a renal transplant cohort. Leuk Lymphoma 2005;46(4):533–9.

89. Lee TC, Goss JA, Rooney CM, et al. Quantification of a low cellular immune response to aid in identification of pediatric liver transplant recipients at high-risk for EBV infection. Clin Transplant 2006;20(6):689–94.

90. Smets F, Latinne D, Bazin H, et al. Ratio between Epstein-Barr viral load and anti-Epstein-Barr virus specific T-cell response as a predictive marker of post-transplant lymphoproliferative disease. Transplantation 2002;73(10):1603–10.

91. Savoldo B, Rooney CM, Quiros-Tejeira RE, et al. Cellular immunity to Epstein-Barr virus in liver transplant recipients treated with rituximab for post-transplant lymphoproliferative disease. Am J Transplant 2005;5(3):566–72.

92. Green M, Bueno J, Rowe D, et al. Predictive negative value of persistent low Epstein-Barr virus viral load after intestinal transplantation in children. Transplantation 2000;70(4):593–6.

93. Lee TC, Savoldo B, Rooney CM, et al. Quantitative EBV viral loads and immunosuppression alterations can decrease PTLD incidence in pediatric liver transplant recipients. Am J Transplant 2005;5(9):2222–8.

94. Benden C, Aurora P, Burch M, et al. Monitoring of Epstein-Barr viral load in pediatric heart and lung transplant recipients by real-time polymerase chain reaction. J Heart Lung Transplant 2005;24(12):2103–8.

95. Comoli P, Basso S, Zecca M, et al. Preemptive therapy of EBV-related lymphoproliferative disease after pediatric haploidentical stem cell transplantation. Am J Transplant 2007;7(6):1648–55.

96. Meerbach A, Wutzler P, Hafer R, et al. Monitoring of Epstein-Barr virus load after hematopoietic stem cell transplantation for early intervention in post-transplant lymphoproliferative disease. J Med Virol 2008;80(3):441–54.

97. Ghobrial IM, Habermann TM, Ristow KM, et al. Prognostic factors in patients with post-transplant lymphoproliferative disorders (PTLD) in the rituximab era. Leuk Lymphoma 2005;46(2):191–6.

98. Hayashi RJ, Kraus MD, Patel AL, et al. Posttransplant lymphoproliferative disease in children: correlation of histology to clinical behavior. J Pediatr Hematol Oncol 2001;23(1):14–8.

99. Dror Y, Greenberg M, Taylor G, et al. Lymphoproliferative disorders after organ transplantation in children. Transplantation 1999;67(7):990–8.

100. Leblond V, Dhedin N, Mamzer Bruneel MF, et al. Identification of prognostic factors in 61 patients with posttransplantation lymphoproliferative disorders. J Clin Oncol 2001;19(3):772–8.

101. Dotti G, Fiocchi R, Motta T, et al. Lymphomas occurring late after solid-organ transplantation: influence of treatment on the clinical outcome. Transplantation 2002;74(8):1095–102.

102. Chadburn A, Cesarman E, Liu YF, et al. Molecular genetic analysis demonstrates that multiple posttransplantation lymphoproliferative disorders occurring in one anatomic site in a single patient represent distinct primary lymphoid neoplasms. Cancer 1995;75(11):2747–56.

103. Trofe J, Buell JF, Beebe TM, et al. Analysis of factors that influence survival with post-transplant lymphoproliferative disorder in renal transplant recipients: the Israel Penn International Transplant Tumor Registry experience. Am J Transplant 2005;5(4 Pt 1):775–80.

104. Gross TG, Bucuvalas JC, Park JR, et al. Low-dose chemotherapy for Epstein-Barr virus-positive post-transplantation lymphoproliferative disease in children after solid organ transplantation. J Clin Oncol 2005;23(27):6481–8.

105. Buell JF, Gross TG, Hanaway MJ, et al. Posttransplant lymphoproliferative disorder: significance of central nervous system involvement. Transplant Proc 2005;37(2):954–5.

106. Hanson MN, Morrison VA, Peterson BA, et al. Posttransplant T-cell lymphoproliferative disorders–an aggressive, late complication of solid-organ transplantation. Blood 1996;88(9):3626–33.

107. Bierman PJ, Vose JM, Langnas AN, et al. Hodgkin's disease following solid organ transplantation. Ann Oncol 1996;7(3):265–70.

108. Aull MJ, Buell JF, Trofe J, et al. Experience with 274 cardiac transplant recipients with posttransplant lymphoproliferative disorder: a report from the Israel Penn International Transplant Tumor Registry. Transplantation 2004;78(11):1676–82.

109. Choquet S, Oertel S, LeBlond V, et al. Rituximab in the management of post-transplantation lymphoproliferative disorder after solid organ transplantation: proceed with caution. Ann Hematol 2007;86(8):599–607.

110. Elstrom RL, Andreadis C, Aqui NA, et al. Treatment of PTLD with rituximab or chemotherapy. Am J Transplant 2006;6(3):569–76.

111. Buell JF, Gross TG, Hanaway MJ, et al. Chemotherapy for posttransplant lymphoproliferative disorder: the Israel Penn International Transplant Tumor Registry experience. Transplant Proc 2005;37(2):956–7.
112. Trappe R, Riess H, Babel N, et al. Salvage chemotherapy for refractory and relapsed posttransplant lymphoproliferative disorders (PTLD) after treatment with single-agent rituximab. Transplantation 2007;83(7):912–8.
113. Windebank K, Walwyn T, Kirk R, et al. Post cardiac transplantation lymphoproliferative disorder presenting as t(8;14) Burkitt leukaemia/lymphoma treated with low intensity chemotherapy and rituximab. Pediatr Blood Cancer 2009; 53(3):392–6.
114. Choquet S, Leblond V, Herbrecht R, et al. Efficacy and safety of rituximab in B-cell post-transplantation lymphoproliferative disorders: results of a prospective multicenter phase 2 study. Blood 2006;107(8):3053–7.
115. Oertel SH, Verschuuren E, Reinke P, et al. Effect of anti-CD 20 antibody rituximab in patients with post-transplant lymphoproliferative disorder (PTLD). Am J Transplant 2005;5(12):2901–6.
116. Perrine SP, Hermine O, Small T, et al. A phase 1/2 trial of arginine butyrate and ganciclovir in patients with Epstein-Barr virus-associated lymphoid malignancies. Blood 2007;109(6):2571–8.
117. Benkerrou M, Jais JP, Leblond V, et al. Anti-B-cell monoclonal antibody treatment of severe posttransplant B-lymphoproliferative disorder: prognostic factors and long-term outcome. Blood 1998;92(9):3137–47.
118. Pescovitz MD. Rituximab, an anti-cd20 monoclonal antibody: history and mechanism of action. Am J Transplant 2006;6(5 Pt 1):859–66.
119. Choquet S, Trappe R, Leblond V, et al. CHOP-21 for the treatment of post-transplant lymphoproliferative disorders (PTLD) following solid organ transplantation. Haematologica 2007;92(2):273–4.
120. Machado AS, Apa AG, Magalhaes de Rezende LM, et al. Plasma Epstein-Barr viral load predicting response after chemotherapy for post-transplant lymphoproliferative disease. Clin Exp Med 2008;8(2):129–32.
121. Yang J, Tao Q, Flinn IW, et al. Characterization of Epstein-Barr virus-infected B cells in patients with posttransplantation lymphoproliferative disease: disappearance after rituximab therapy does not predict clinical response. Blood 2000;96(13):4055–63.
122. Papadopoulos EB, Ladanyi M, Emanuel D, et al. Infusions of donor leukocytes to treat Epstein-Barr virus-associated lymphoproliferative disorders after allogeneic bone marrow transplantation. N Engl J Med 1994;330(17):1185–91.
123. Heslop HE, Brenner MK, Rooney CM. Donor T cells to treat EBV-associated lymphoma. N Engl J Med 1994;331(10):679–80.
124. Savoldo B, Goss JA, Hammer MM, et al. Treatment of solid organ transplant recipients with autologous Epstein Barr virus-specific cytotoxic T lymphocytes (CTLs). Blood 2006;108(9):2942–9.
125. Rooney CM, Smith CA, Ng CY, et al. Infusion of cytotoxic T cells for the prevention and treatment of Epstein-Barr virus-induced lymphoma in allogeneic transplant recipients. Blood 1998;92(5):1549–55.
126. Haque T, Amlot PL, Helling N, et al. Reconstitution of EBV-specific T cell immunity in solid organ transplant recipients. J Immunol 1998;160(12):6204–9.
127. Sherritt MA, Bharadwaj M, Burrows JM, et al. Reconstitution of the latent T-lymphocyte response to Epstein-Barr virus is coincident with long-term recovery from posttransplant lymphoma after adoptive immunotherapy. Transplantation 2003;75(9):1556–60.

128. Gerdemann U, Christin AS, Vera JF, et al. Nucleofection of DCs to generate Multivirus-specific T cells for prevention or treatment of viral infections in the immunocompromised host. Mol Ther 2009;17(9):1616–25.
129. Vera JF, Brenner LJ, Gerdemann U, et al. Accelerated production of antigen-specific T-cells for pre-clinical and clinical applications using Gas-permeable Rapid Expansion cultureware (G-Rex). Mol Ther 2010, in press.
130. Savoldo B, Cubbage ML, Durett AG, et al. Generation of EBV-specific CD4+ cytotoxic T cells from virus naive individuals. J Immunol 2002;168(2):909–18.
131. Comoli P, Ginevri F, Maccario R, et al. Successful in vitro priming of EBV-specific CD8+ T cells endowed with strong cytotoxic function from T cells of EBV-seronegative children. Am J Transplant 2006;6(9):2169–76.
132. Sun Q, Burton R, Reddy V, et al. Safety of allogeneic Epstein-Barr virus (EBV)-specific cytotoxic T lymphocytes for patients with refractory EBV-related lymphoma. Br J Haematol 2002;118(3):799–808.
133. Haque T, Taylor C, Wilkie GM, et al. Complete regression of posttransplant lymphoproliferative disease using partially HLA-matched Epstein Barr virus-specific cytotoxic T cells. Transplantation 2001;72(8):1399–402.
134. Gandhi MK, Wilkie GM, Dua U, et al. Immunity, homing and efficacy of allogeneic adoptive immunotherapy for posttransplant lymphoproliferative disorders. Am J Transplant 2007;7(5):1293–9.
135. Haque T, Wilkie GM, Jones MM, et al. Allogeneic cytotoxic T-cell therapy for EBV-positive posttransplantation lymphoproliferative disease: results of a phase 2 multicenter clinical trial. Blood 2007;110(4):1123–31.
136. Quintarelli C, Vera JF, Savoldo B, et al. Co-expression of cytokine and suicide genes to enhance the activity and safety of tumor-specific cytotoxic T lymphocytes. Blood 2007;110(8):2793–802.
137. Dotti G, Savoldo B, Pule M, et al. Human cytotoxic T lymphocytes with reduced sensitivity to Fas-induced apoptosis. Blood 2005;105(12):4677–84.
138. De Angelis B, Dotti G, Quintarelli C, et al. Generation of Epstein-Barr-virus-specific cytotoxic T lymphocytes resistant to the immunosuppressive drug tacrolimus (FK506). Blood 2009;114(23):4784–91.
139. Brewin J, Mancao C, Straathof K, et al. Generation of EBV-specific cytotoxic T-cells that are resistant to calcineurin inhibitors for the treatment of posttransplantation lymphoproliferative disease. Blood 2009;114(23):4792–803.
140. Dharnidharka VR, Araya CE. Post-transplant lymphoproliferative disease. Pediatr Nephrol 2009;24(4):731–6.
141. Koch DG, Christiansen L, Lazarchick J, et al. Posttransplantation lymphoproliferative disorder–the great mimic in liver transplantation: appraisal of the clinicopathologic spectrum and the role of Epstein-Barr virus. Liver Transpl 2007;13(6):904–12.
142. International Transplant Registry. Pediatric data. Available at: http://www.intestinaltransplantregistry.org. Accessed October 30, 2009.
143. Allen U, Hebert D, Moore D, et al. Epstein-Barr virus-related post-transplant lymphoproliferative disease in solid organ transplant recipients, 1988-97: a Canadian multi-centre experience. Pediatr Transplant 2001;5(3):198–203.

Nonimmune Complications After Transplantation

Monique Choquette, MD[a], Jens W. Goebel, MD[b],
Kathleen M. Campbell, MD[c,d],*

KEYWORDS

- Pediatric transplantation • Long-term outcome
- Posttransplant renal dysfunction
- Immunosuppression complications

In the 1980s the introduction of the drug cyclosporine changed the face of solid organ transplantation, decreasing acute allograft rejection and early graft loss, and dramatically improving 1-year patient and graft survival. For the first time in history, organ transplantation became standard of care rather than an experimental procedure. However, as posttransplant longevity has increased, nonimmune complications related to the transplant and posttransplant course have emerged as important factors in defining long-term outcomes. The incidence of, and risk factors for these complications may vary by transplanted organ based on immunosuppressive protocols and preexisting risk factors. This article discusses the relevant nonimmune complications associated with posttransplant care, with a focus on risk factors and management strategies.

RENAL DYSFUNCTION

Renal dysfunction is one of the most common and well-described complications following solid organ transplantation. In their defining study on the topic, which included more than 69,000 predominantly adult nonrenal solid organ transplant recipients, Ojo and colleagues[1] found that the cumulative 5-year risk of chronic renal failure,

[a] Division of Gastroenterology, Hepatology and Nutrition, Cincinnati Children's Hospital Research Foundation, 3333 Burnet Avenue, Cincinnati, OH 45229, USA
[b] Division of Nephrology and Hypertension, Cincinnati Children's Hospital Medical Center, 3333 Burnet Avenue, Cincinnati, OH 45229, USA
[c] Pediatric Liver Transplant Program, Cincinnati Children's Hospital Medical Center, 3333 Burnet Avenue, Cincinnati, OH 45229, USA
[d] Division of Gastroenterology, Hepatology and Nutrition, Cincinnati Children's Hospital Medical Center, 3333 Burnet Avenue, Cincinnati, OH 45229, USA
* Corresponding author. Division of Gastroenterology, Hepatology and Nutrition, Cincinnati Children's Hospital Medical Center, 3333 Burnet Avenue, Cincinnati, OH 45229.
E-mail address: Kathleen.campbell@cchmc.org

Pediatr Clin N Am 57 (2010) 505–521
doi:10.1016/j.pcl.2010.01.008
0031-3955/10/$ – see front matter

defined as the need for either chronic dialysis or kidney transplantation, was 6.9% to 21.3% depending on type of organ transplanted. The onset of chronic renal failure was found to increase the risk of posttransplant death by more than 4-fold, and progression to end-stage renal disease (ESRD) dramatically increased posttransplant cost of care.[1] The relative morbidity and mortality of renal complications in pediatric solid organ recipients are potentially greater, as children have a longer life span following transplantation, with greater cumulative exposure to nephrotoxic medications and other renal insults.

Although the development of renal dysfunction following solid organ transplantation is a multifactorial process, the calcineurin inhibitors (CNI), cyclosporine and tacrolimus, constitute a major contributing factor. The nephrotoxic side effects of these medications have been well recognized since the introduction of cyclosporine in the 1980s. The CNI cause both acute and chronic nephrotoxicity. Acute nephrotoxicity involves afferent arteriolar vasoconstriction and reduced renal plasma flow, and is predictably associated with high trough levels. In contrast, chronic CNI-induced nephrotoxicity is not predicted by individual trough levels, and is characterized by potentially irreversible structural changes including arteriolopathy, tubulointerstitial fibrosis and, eventually, glomerulosclerosis.

Estimates of the incidence of posttransplant renal dysfunction in pediatric solid organ recipients have varied depending on the definition of renal dysfunction employed, the population examined, and the time frame post transplant (**Table 1**). Given that most published studies are single-center ones and do not allow for multivariate analysis, the identification of specific risk factors for posttransplant renal dysfunction has been difficult. However, based on the current data from a few large single-center or database studies, several risk factors have been suggested. In pediatric liver transplant patients, older age at transplant, decreased glomerular filtration rate (GFR) at 1 year post transplant, use of cyclosporine (vs tacrolimus), arterial hypertension, and primary disease with known renal involvement have all been associated with long-term posttransplant renal dysfunction.[1–3] In pediatric heart transplant recipients, higher CNI doses early post transplant, female sex, older age at transplant, early transplant era, pretransplant dialysis, longer duration of transplant listing, primary diagnosis of hypertrophic cardiomyopathy, African American race, renal dysfunction at 6 months post transplant, and previous transplant have emerged as risk factors.[4–6] In pediatric lung transplant patients, older age at transplant and the diagnosis of cystic fibrosis have been implicated, whereas in a mixed population of pediatric (66%) and adult (34%) intestinal transplant patients pretransplant renal impairment, pretransplant intensive care unit hospitalization, and high-dose tacrolimus therapy emerged as risk factors.[7,8] The drivers of posttransplant renal dysfunction in pediatric kidney graft recipients are more complicated and diverse. In this population, "chronic allograft nephropathy" may reflect chronic rejection, polyoma (BK virus) and other viral infections, and recurrent primary disease in addition to CNI nephrotoxicity.[9]

Additional, genetic susceptibility factors to CNI nephrotoxicity have been hypothesized for some time, and may be related to the pharmacokinetic pathway of CNI absorption and metabolism. The complex pharmacokinetics of these drugs are affected by the biologic activity of the p-glycoprotein cellular efflux pump (coded for by the gene ABCB1) and the cytochrome P450 enzyme system. The protein product of ABCB1, multidrug resistance protein 1 (MDR1), pumps a variety of compounds, including the CNI, from the cytoplasm to the cell exterior, while CYP3A4 is responsible for the oxidative metabolism of the drugs. The combined activity of these proteins in the intestinal epithelial cell creates an absorptive barrier, limiting CNI bioavailability

Table 1
Incidence of posttransplant renal dysfunction in nonrenal pediatric solid organ transplant recipients

Organ (Number of Patients)	Posttransplant Follow-Up Period	Definition of Renal Failure/Dysfunction	Incidence of Renal Dysfunction	References
Heart (2032)	Mean 7 y	Serum creatinine >2.5 mg/dL	11.8%	5
Heart (91)	Median 5 y	mGFR <90 mL/min/1.73 m^2	Cumulative incidence of 67% at 5 y, 8% with mGFR <30 mL/min/1.73 m^2 by 7 y post transplant	4
Heart (77)	Median 5.1 y	cGFR <90 mL/min/1.73 m^2	17% at 1 y, 38.7% at 5 y	6
Lung (125)	Mean 4.9 y	cGFR with National Kidney Foundation Chronic Kidney Disease staging	38% cGFR <60	8
Lung (19)	Mean 5.36 y	cGFR <80 mL/min/1.73 m^2	63%	76
Liver (352)	At 5-y visit	cGFR <90 mL/min/1.73 m^2	13%	53
Liver (117)	Mean 7.6 y	mGFR <70 mL/min/1.73 m^2	32%	3
Liver (101)	Median 6 y	mGFR <90 mL/min/1.73 m^2	28.7%	77
Intestinal (62 total, 45 pediatric)	Mean 30 mo	cGFR <75% of normal	16%	7

Abbreviations: cGFR, calculated glomerular filtration rate; mGFR, measured glomerular filtration rate.

and, thus, drug contact.[10,11] In addition, these proteins are present in the kidney (MDR1) and the liver (CYP3A4), thus both donor and recipient genetic variation may be relevant. Genetic polymorphisms, some of which influence the level of protein expression or activity, have been identified in both genes, and have been correlated with differing CNI dose requirements in adult renal and adult liver transplant recipients.[12,13] In addition, single reports have found associations between single nucleotide polymorphisms (SNPs) in ABCB1 and nephrotoxicity in adult liver and renal transplant recipients.[14,15]

In the complex pathway leading to CNI-induced nephrotoxicity, one of the final common mediators of the long-term structural kidney damage is the multifunctional, profibrogenic cytokine transforming growth factor (TGF)-β1. The CNI induce transcription of TGF-β1 in cultured renal tubular cells, rodent models, and human transplant recipients, and intrarenal levels of TGF-β1 RNA and protein correlate with the histologic findings of CNI-induced nephrotoxicity.[16,17] Reports in a predominantly adult population of cardiac transplant recipients have identified an SNP in codon 10 of the signal sequence of TGF-β1 that is associated with posttransplant renal dysfunction.[18] Polymorphisms of the renin-angiotensin system have also been implicated as genetic risk factors for posttransplant renal dysfunction in adult kidney transplant recipients.[19]

Strategies for management of posttransplant renal dysfunction have largely focused on CNI minimization, replacement, or avoidance. Delayed introduction of CNI post transplant via use of induction immunosuppression with either antithymocyte globulin or anti-CD25 monoclonal antibody has been postulated to preserve renal function (and protect kidney grafts from delayed graft function) by protecting the kidney from acute CNI-induced injury during the vulnerable immediate posttransplant period, when rapid fluid shifts, blood pressure instability, and multiple potentially nephrotoxic medications may impact renal function.[20,21]

Introduction of adjuvant immunosuppression with mycophenolate mofetil (MMF) in combination with decreased CNI dose is a widely employed method for preventing or managing renal dysfunction. CNI minimization with MMF has resulted in improvements in renal function (defined by either serum creatinine, calculated GFR, or measured GFR) in pediatric liver and heart transplant patients.[22,23] In addition, studies in pediatric renal transplant recipients have shown improved renal function with addition of MMF to a CNI-based regimen, with or without simultaneous decreases in CNI dosing.[24,25] This finding suggests that the benefit in these patients may be related to a combination of more effective immunosuppression and decreased CNI exposure.

Although less frequent, combination therapy with low-dose CNI and the non-nephrotoxic mTor inhibitor sirolimus has been associated with improved short-term renal function in pediatric heart transplant recipients.[26] However, this strategy may hold some risk. Although sirolimus alone is not nephrotoxic, there are concerns about its use in combination with CNI, in which instance potentiation of CNI nephrotoxicity has been reported.[27] There are also concerns regarding early posttransplant use of sirolimus associated with delayed graft function in renal transplant patients and hepatic artery thrombosis in liver transplant patients.[28] Although these associations have not been confirmed in large, multicenter studies these concerns, in addition to the delayed wound healing seen with sirolimus, have limited its use early post transplant. In contrast, late replacement of CNI with sirolimus may be a promising strategy, and has been associated with improvements in serum creatinine and calculated GFR in pediatric and adult solid organ recipients.[25,29]

The best combination of immunosuppressive agents for maintenance of excellent graft function while minimizing nephrotoxicity is unclear, and may need to be individualized based on patient- and organ-specific factors. In addition, the ideal timing of changes in immunosuppression is unknown. There are likely to be thresholds of renal function or time since transplant, beyond which changes in regimen are not effective at reversing renal disease. Identification of these thresholds is an area that requires further investigation.

The use of antihypertensive medications is another mechanism for renal protection. Calcium channel blockers and angiotensin-converting enzyme (ACE) inhibitors have both been associated with retained renal function post transplant; this is certainly related, in part, to the impact on blood pressure, chronic elevation of which can exacerbate kidney damage. However, these medications, particularly ACE inhibitors and angiotensin receptor blockers (ARBs), may have additional, direct beneficial effects on the pathway of CNI-induced nephrotoxicity, which involves activation of the renin-angiotensin system and downstream production of proinflammatory cytokines.

Attempts to minimize the impact of renal dysfunction on long-term posttransplant health and quality of life would be furthered by identification of easily available, noninvasive mechanisms for accurately assessing renal function, or biomarkers of early renal insufficiency. Formulas for estimating GFR based on serum creatinine are notoriously inaccurate in children following solid organ transplantation, routinely overestimating renal function. Estimation of GFR using cystatin-C–based equations may hold some promise in this area. In limited reports to date, cystatin C, a serum protein produced by all nucleated cells, independent of muscle mass, and freely filtered across the renal glomerular membrane, appears to be more accurate than serum creatinine at identifying mild and moderate degrees of renal dysfunction.[30,31]

Additional renal complications following solid organ transplantation include proteinuria and renal tubular dysfunction leading to hyperkalemia, hypomagnesemia, and metabolic acidosis. Proteinuria has been reported both in association with, and independent of decreased GFR, and is additionally a side effect of sirolimus.[32] In fact, proteinuria can be a limiting factor in the use of this otherwise renal sparing medication.[28,33] Proteinuria is a harbinger of later renal dysfunction in diabetic nephropathy, although its prognostic importance in the nondiabetic population is less clear.

Role of the Primary Care Provider

As in many aspects of chronic care, the primary care provider (PCP) is an essential member of the management team. In providing routine well-child care, management of acute illness, anticipatory guidance, and standard monitoring, the pediatrician often acts as the first line of defense against posttransplant complications. Detection and management of renal dysfunction is no exception. Heightened attention on the part of the PCP with regard to blood pressure monitoring is essential. Ensuring that a blood pressure is obtained with the appropriately sized cuff at each visit (acute care in addition to well child), and that abnormal blood pressures ($\geq$95% systolic or diastolic for age, sex, and height) is repeated expeditiously, is paramount. Close communication with the transplant center regarding the use of commonly prescribed antibiotics (which may impact CNI metabolism, leading to toxic levels and subsequent renal damage) and attention to the increased risk of dehydration in pediatric transplant patients, whose kidneys may already be compromised, are additional responsibilities.

CARDIOVASCULAR COMPLICATIONS

Several epidemiologic studies have shown that solid organ transplant recipients have an increased prevalence of risk factors for cardiovascular disease, often resulting from preexisting disease as well as the consequences of the transplant procedure and posttransplant regime.[34,35] Immunosuppressive agents are the primary culprits of cardiovascular toxicity, increasing the likelihood of hypertension, hyperlipidemia, hypercholesterolemia, and diabetes mellitus. For example, glucocorticoids and CNI are well-known precipitants of posttransplant hypertension, which has been documented in 62% to 75% of pediatric patients (**Table 2**).[36]

Although both tacrolimus and cyclosporine can cause significant hypertension, cyclosporine appears to have a more dramatic impact on blood pressure. A retrospective study of the North American Pediatric Renal Transplant Cooperative Study (NAPRTCS) database revealed that patients receiving tacrolimus/mycophenolate mofetil/steroids were less likely to require antihypertensive medications at 1 and 2 years post transplant compared with patients receiving cyclosporine/MMF/steroids.[37] A similar result was documented by Jain and colleagues[38] in pediatric liver transplant patients, in which there was a significant reduction in the incidence and severity of hypertension in patients treated with tacrolimus compared with those on cyclosporine.

The mechanism of drug-induced hypertension in solid organ transplant recipients likely involves renal and peripheral vasoconstriction via the renin-angiotensin system and the sympathetic nervous system, as well as release of various vasoconstrictors into the bloodstream. Glucocorticoid therapy is hypothesized to precipitate activation of the renin-angiotensin system, increase vasopressor responses to norepinephrine and angiotensin II, and reduce activity of vasodepressor systems such as the endothelial-derived vasodilator nitric oxide. The pathogenesis of CNI-dependent hypertension is comparatively complex. Acute administration of CNI induces sympathetic neural activity, and prolonged therapy often precipitates chronic sympathetic overactivity. Similar to treatment with glucocorticoids, CNI also stimulate the renin-angiotensin system while additionally up-regulating angiotensin II receptors in vascular smooth muscle.[34]

Although rare, hypertrophic cardiomyopathy is a serious complication associated with tacrolimus therapy. A study by Nakata and colleagues[39] found a relationship between high blood levels of tacrolimus and increased myocardial hypertrophy in a predominantly pediatric population. Specifically, the patients whose blood levels of tacrolimus were above 15 ng/mL had a higher percentage of left ventricular wall thickness than that of patients whose blood levels were less than 15 ng/mL. This life-threatening complication is specific to tacrolimus and mandates immediate discontinuation of that medication.

Treatment of vascular risk factors may reduce the incidence of cardiovascular disease in solid organ transplant recipients, further improving long-term survival.

Table 2
Incidence of hypertension in pediatric solid organ transplantation

Organ	Prevalence			References
	2 years	5 years	7 years	
Kidney	75%	70%		North American Pediatric Renal Transplant Cooperative Study
Liver	14.5%/15.7%			Studies in Pediatric Liver Transplantation
Heart			64.7%	International Society for Heart and Lung Transplantation
Lung		71.6%		

Data from Dharnidharka VR, Araya CE, Benfield MR. Organ toxicities. In: Fine RN, Webber S, Harmon WE, et al, editors. Pediatric solid organ transplantation. 2nd edition. Oxford (UK): Blackwell Publishing Ltd; 2007. p. 124–39.

Specific management protocols for risk reduction include therapeutic lifestyle changes, alteration of immunosuppressive regimen, or addition of specific medications to address each risk factor or complication.[34] As the mainstays of posttransplant immunosuppressive therapy, glucocorticoid and CNI-free protocols may be unrealistic. Adjustments of immunosuppressive regimens, however, may be feasible and more reasonable. Glucocorticoid withdrawal or reduction as well as choice of CNI may reduce the prevalence of cardiovascular risk factors and disease by decreasing rates of hypertension, dyslipidemia, or diabetes mellitus.[36] All classes of antihypertensive medications, including calcium-channel blockers, β-blockers, ACE inhibitors, ARBs, and diuretics, have been implemented effectively based on risk profile and therapeutic category. In addition to surveillance of tacrolimus levels and other parameters, long-term monitoring of cardiac function may also be warranted in high-risk populations.

Novel strategies for identification of high-risk populations include potential biomarkers such as B-type natriuretic peptide (BNP) or endothelin-1 (ET), which are elevated in pediatric liver transplant patients with early cardiac damage.[40] Because cardiovascular damage typically occurs decades before clinical outcomes become apparent, BNP and ET levels and trends may help identify patients to target for more intensive monitoring or novel interventions to reduce the risk of cardiovascular disease.

Role of the Primary Care Provider

Once again, the PCP plays a critical role in monitoring and identification of risk factors and disease. Aggressive blood pressure monitoring, determination of familial risk factors, and anticipatory guidance regarding lifestyle choices should be routine components of care, and can be reinforced between the transplant team and the PCP. In addition, the PCP may be presented with acute cardiac complications after transplant, including hypertensive crisis, vascular thromboses, and cardiomyopathy, all of which may present with vague symptoms not obviously related to the transplanted organ. Evaluation of the pediatric transplant recipient must include the potential for these complications, and prompt communication with the transplant team will help to ensure the best possible outcomes.

METABOLIC COMPLICATIONS

Posttransplant metabolic complications, including dyslipidemia, obesity, and glucose intolerance, are less common in pediatric than in adult solid organ transplant recipients, but still represent risks to the long-term health of the recipient and the graft. The incidence of diabetes mellitus (DM) after pediatric kidney transplantation, for example, had been estimated at 2% to 4% based on early registry studies.[36] However, a recent large-scale study using the United States Renal Data System found a 3-year incidence of diabetes of 7.1% in pediatric renal transplant patients. Risk factors for this complication included increased age at transplant, body mass index (calculated as the weight of the patient in kilograms divided by height in meters squared) of 30 kg/m^2 greater, use of tacrolimus (vs cyclosporine), and donor-positive/recipient-negative cytomegalovirus (CMV) status.[41] In contrast, the incidence of posttransplant DM in pediatric heart transplant recipients is much lower, affecting 1.8% to 2% of transplant recipients in median-term follow-up.[42] Tacrolimus and older age at transplant represent similar risk factors in this population. According to recent registry data from the Studies in Pediatric Liver Transplantation study group, the risk profile in pediatric liver recipients is somewhat different. While liver transplant recipients had a higher risk of DM overall (13%), only 3% had onset of DM more than 30 days post transplant, and the duration of DM was only 75 to 80 days.[43] Risk factors were similar to those seen in pediatric renal and heart recipients, namely older age at transplant, hospitalization at transplant, use of tacrolimus, early steroid use, and primary diagnosis other than biliary atresia.[43] Lung transplant recipients are at higher risk of posttransplant DM, with a cumulative incidence of 20% to 30% by 5 years post transplant, particularly when cystic fibrosis is the precipitant to end-stage lung disease and transplantation.[36]

Both CNI and corticosteroids predispose to DM: steroids by increasing resistance to peripheral and hepatic insulin, and CNI via a direct toxic effect on pancreatic β cells, decreasing insulin secretion.[44] Among the CNI, a meta-analysis of 16 prospective, randomized comparative studies in adults revealed a higher incidence of posttransplant new-onset DM in patients receiving tacrolimus versus cyclosporine (16.6% vs 9.8%).[45] In addition to type of immunosuppressive therapy, Greenspan and colleagues[46] identified 2 other significant risk factors for the development of posttransplant DM in pediatric renal transplant recipients, specifically a family history of type 2 DM and hyperglycemia in the peritransplant period. It remains unclear whether development of posttransplant DM is associated with poor outcomes, or associated with the development of classic DM later in life.

Although variable, the prevalence of dyslipidemia after pediatric solid organ transplantation is also noteworthy. According to registry data from the International Society for Heart and Lung Transplantation, the prevalence of hyperlipidemia 5 years after heart transplantation is approximately 21.4%, and 4.5% after lung transplantation.[36,47] Once again, the posttransplant immunosuppressive agents contribute to this trend. Among the CNI, Trompeter and colleagues[48] showed that cyclosporine is more often linked to hypercholesterolemia and hypertriglyceridemia after pediatric renal transplantation than tacrolimus. In fact, several studies in adult renal transplant patients have shown that conversion from cyclosporine to tacrolimus leads to an improvement in serum lipid levels, and may be an avenue of treatment in the setting of significant adverse effects.[49,50] Sirolimus is also strongly associated with dyslipidemia, causing hypercholesterolemia in nearly 44% of patients receiving the drug.[34] Obesity and genetic predisposition factor into the development of hyperlipidemia after transplant, of which the former may serve as a target for management.

Pediatric solid organ transplant recipients are not exempt from the epidemic of childhood obesity. The comorbid effects of obesity in this population extend beyond hypertension, DM, and dyslipidemia, and may include adverse effects on patient and allograft survival. In a study of the effect of obesity on pediatric renal transplant outcomes, Hanevold and colleagues[51] showed that obese patients aged 6 to 12 years had a higher risk of death than nonobese patients, and death was more likely secondary to cardiopulmonary disease (27% in obese vs 17% in nonobese children). Furthermore, obese children suffered a significant increase in graft loss as a result of vascular thrombosis in comparison with nonobese children.[51] In contrast, a study involving pediatric heart transplant patients showed that obesity at transplant or 1 year post transplant was not associated with decreased graft survival.[52] Nonetheless, weight gain after heart transplantation was a nearly universal phenomenon: at 1 year post transplant 17% of patients were overweight and only 4% of patients were underweight.[52] Although the data in pediatric liver transplant recipients is scarce, in one study of survivors 5 years or more post transplant, 12% had a body weight more than 95% for age.[53] While these rates of overweight/obesity may be similar to those of the entire North American pediatric population, the relative impact of obesity on pediatric transplant recipients may be greater. A complete discussion of growth following pediatric solid organ transplant is presented elsewhere in this issue in the article by Anthony and colleagues.

Drug regimens and total duration of therapy may be altered in the face of significant metabolic side effects. An early study by Curtis and colleagues[54] showed the benefit of equal total dose alternate-day steroid therapy over daily steroid therapy in lowering total cholesterol and triglyceride levels in a population of predominantly adult renal transplant patients. Later studies further demonstrated the benefit of early posttransplant corticosteroid withdrawal in adult renal transplant patients, who experienced reductions in total and low-density lipoprotein cholesterol levels as well as a decreased incidence of DM (from 30% to 8%) at 2 years post transplant.[55] In pediatric renal transplant recipients, steroid-free immunosuppression is associated with a decreased incidence of posttransplant DM (0.8% vs 9%), decreased need for antihypertensive agents, and decreased need for lipid-lowering agents as compared with patients on steroid-based therapy.[56]

Alteration of drug therapy may not be feasible in certain posttransplant regimens or metabolic parameters may become refractory to changes in immunosuppressive therapy. Lifestyle modification with diet and exercise remains the primary avenue to maintain adequate glycemic control and optimal lipid levels. Secondary measures with pharmacotherapy may nonetheless prove necessary. Management of posttransplant DM in pediatric patients may require insulin therapy, while implementation of HMG-CoA reductase inhibitors and fibrates may be beneficial in reducing total cholesterol and triglyceride levels, respectively.

Role of the Primary Care Provider

As members of the multidisciplinary care team, PCPs serve a pivotal role in ongoing monitoring for metabolic complications following transplantation. Identification of rapid weight gain, with counseling regarding nutrition and exercise, is a key role of the PCP, while pharmacologic therapy should be undertaken in concert with the transplant team and other subspecialists.

HEMATOLOGIC COMPLICATIONS

The major cell lines of the hematopoietic system are not exempt from the consequences of the transplant procedure or posttransplant regime. Hematologic adverse reactions occurring in renal, cardiac, and liver transplant recipients, respectively, include anemia (25.6%, 42.9%, 43%), leukopenia (23.2%, 30.4%, 45.8%), thrombocytopenia (10.1%, 23.5%, 38.3%), and leukocytosis (7.1%, 40.5%, 22.4%).[36] As the primary culprit of many end-organ toxicities, posttransplant immunosuppressive therapy can precipitate anemia, thrombocytopenia, or leukopenia. For example, several transplant medications, including MMF and its predecessor azathioprine, can induce bone marrow suppression, yielding anemia, thrombocytopenia, and leukopenia by direct nucleic acid synthesis inhibition. An alteration of cell counts, particularly anemia and leukopenia, appears to be more common with the use of MMF than with azathioprine. Khosroshahi and colleagues[57] compared the effects of MMF and azathioprine on the erythropoietic system of adult renal transplant recipients, and showed a lesser degree of bone marrow suppression by MMF, as demonstrated by a higher level of hemoglobin 6 months after transplantation. Although MMF has a more favorable effect on the erythropoietic system, it is a frequent cause of leukopenia. MMF leads to severe neutropenia (absolute neutrophil count <500/mm^3) in up to 2% of pediatric renal transplant patients, 2.8% of pediatric cardiac transplant patients, and 3.6% of pediatric liver transplant patients.[36]

The CNI, tacrolimus and cyclosporine, have both been implicated in the development of microangiopathic hemolytic anemia as well as hemolytic uremic syndrome, whereas only tacrolimus has been associated with the development of pure red cell aplasia.[58] As a newer immunosuppressive agent, sirolimus can induce leukopenia and thrombocytopenia. These risks appear to be directly related to trough concentrations of sirolimus greater than 15 ng/mL, highlighting the importance of therapeutic drug monitoring.[59]

Additional therapeutic agents of the posttransplant regime, including both antimicrobial and antihypertensive agents, can further serve as accomplices to immunosuppressive medications in perpetuating end-organ toxicity. Posttransplant antiviral drugs, including acyclovir and ganciclovir, can precipitate anemia by suppression of bone marrow. The combination of immunosuppression with MMF and anti-CMV prophylaxis with oral ganciclovir, for example, may further exacerbate the risk of blood dyscrasias. In a study of adult renal transplant recipients, significant changes in the blood profile did not resolve until discontinuation of both MMF and ganciclovir, implying a combined effect from both immunosuppressive and antiviral treatment.[60] In addition, the predicted incidences of neutropenia and leukopenia appear to be directly related to higher exposure to ganciclovir or valganciclovir.[60]

In addition to myelosuppression, other routine posttransplantation prophylactic or treatment agents may cause anemia by other means. For example, sulfur-containing drugs such trimethoprim-sulfamethoxazole and dapsone can lead to hemolytic anemia, whereas ACE inhibitors can cause pure red cell aplasia. Anemia may further be exacerbated by secondary erythropoietin deficiency from compromised kidney function as well as iron, vitamin B, or folic acid deficiencies from poor nutritional intake. More commonly, the causes of blood cell dyscrasias are multifactorial or unidentifiable, compounding the approach to management.

With the potential for significant toxicity to the hematopoietic system, routine monitoring of complete blood counts post transplant is imperative. Neutropenia most commonly occurs within 31 to 180 days after transplantation, particularly in association with MMF administration. Drug-induced alteration of cell counts may require adjustment of medication regimen or changes in drug dosage. For example, the MMF dosage is often reduced when the absolute neutrophil count (ANC) is less than 1500/mm^3, and the drug is typically discontinued at ANC less than 1000/mm^3. Similarly, prophylactic and therapeutic antiviral regimens, including ganciclovir and valganciclovir, should aim to control the risk of infection and disease while minimizing hematologic adverse effects. Minimization of anemia may further be achieved through adequate nutritional intake, therapeutic supplementation, and erythropoietin use. Similarly, neutropenia may be treated with granulocyte-colony stimulating factor. Although management of cytopenias after solid organ transplantation may be challenging, it is imperative to maintain a broad differential diagnosis in one's approach to the transplant patient, considering graft-versus-host disease, CMV infection, and acute viral infection as well as medication side effects in the differential diagnosis.[58]

Role of the Primary Care Provider

Hematologic complications following transplantation may be first identified in the primary care setting, where easy bruising, excessive bleeding, pallor, or fatigue may be presenting complaints. The PCP should be aware of the side effects associated with posttransplant medications, and should have a low threshold for blood work to assess hematologic parameters.

NEUROLOGIC AND CENTRAL NERVOUS SYSTEM COMPLICATIONS

A variety of central nervous system (CNS) complications are reported in pediatric solid organ transplant recipients. In general these are rather minor; headache and tremor are associated with the calcineurin inhibitors, while irritability and mood changes are well-known complications of high-dose corticosteroids. In pediatric liver transplant recipients, the incidence of CNS complications is 8% to 46%. Complications reported include seizures, posterior reversible encephalopathy syndrome (PRES), diffuse encephalopathy, psychiatric complaints, tremor, headache, and acute dystonic reaction.[61,62] Severe CNS complications have been reported in 19% of pediatric renal transplant recipients treated with CNI. These complications include seizures, hallucinations, visual disturbances, confusion, and drowsiness.[63]

PRES is the most severe CNS complication following solid organ transplant, and is believed to be a form of neurotoxicity associated with cyclosporine and tacrolimus. PRES may present with a variety of symptoms including headache, visual disturbances, altered behavior, or mentation or seizure. PRES is generally associated with hypertension, which is common in posttransplant patients, but 20% to 30% of reported patients are normotensive at presentation. Imaging by computed tomography or magnetic resonance imaging shows characteristic changes, including vasogenic edema in the occipital and parietal lobes (the "posterior" brain) and along the superior frontal sulcus, with variable involvement of the deep white matter, basal ganglia, and brainstem. The overall incidence of PRES following solid organ transplant is less than 1% and does not seem to vary based on organ; however, several striking organ-specific differences in presentation have been described in adult transplant populations. For example, after liver transplantation PRES is more likely to occur early (mean of 31 days) and in the setting of normal blood pressure, whereas kidney transplant recipients are more likely to be affected later post transplant (median of 53 months) and present with markedly elevated blood pressure. In addition, adult liver transplant patients present with more severe vasogenic edema than do other organ transplant recipients. In many cases, regardless of organ, development of PRES is associated with bacterial or viral infection, or with graft rejection, suggesting that the development of PRES is dependent on both drug exposure and a proinflammatory milieu.[64] Although believed to be related to CNI neurotoxicity, presentation with PRES is not necessarily accompanied by toxic drug levels. As the name would suggest, the CNS changes seen with PRES are often reversible with CNI withdrawal and aggressive medical support.

Although not as common as with the CNI, CNS side effects have also been noted with MMF. Both depression and progressive multifocal leukoencephalopathy (PML) have been reported in postmarketing data, although a causal association between MMF and these complications is not clear.[65,66] More subtle neurocognitive complications and side effects in pediatric solid organ transplant recipients are emerging as important components of posttransplant quality of life, and are discussed in detail elsewhere in this issue in the article by Anthony and colleagues.

Role of the Primary Care Provider

As with many of the complications described in this article, neurologic symptoms may first come to light in the PCP's office. A close partnership between the PCP and the transplant team is necessary to identify complications early, ensure appropriate workup and therapy, and help access support services for the patient and family.

BONE HEALTH

Decreased bone mineral density, fractures, avascular necrosis, and impaired linear growth are all potential complications following pediatric solid organ transplantation. Given the level of disability, growth failure, and malnutrition that many children face when suffering with end-stage renal, liver, heart, lung, and intestinal disease, it is amazing that these complications are not more prevalent post transplant. The afore-mentioned complications are most closely associated with corticosteroid use, and are frequently reported in populations who receive higher cumulative corticosteroid exposure.

Despite the osseous complications associated with long-standing renal disease (renal rickets), pediatric kidney transplant recipients experience relatively few frac-tures (2%), avascular necrosis (1%), and femoral deformities (4%) in the first 4 years following transplant, although bone mineral density more than 2 standard deviations below normal has been described in up to 26% of patients.[67,68] Pediatric liver recipients, who often enter transplant with significant cholestasis and associated vitamin D deficiency, have a fracture incidence of 5% to 18%, and more than half have a lumbar spine z-score of less than −1, although only 7.3% are reported to have a z-score of less than −2.[68,69] Osteopenia in pediatric liver transplant patients is directly associated with puberty and greater cumulative steroid exposure, and inversely associated with time since transplant.[69,70] In heart transplant patients, bone loss (z-score <−1) has recently been reported in almost 10% of recipients at a median of 3.4 years post transplant.[71] Although there are but few data on osseous complications following pediatric lung and intestinal transplant, similar trends are to be expected.

Prevention and management of osseous complications after transplant is similar to that employed in any chronic illness complicated by threats to bone health. Adequate vitamin D and calcium intake, minimization of corticosteroid exposure, and appropriate physical activity are the mainstays of treatment. In renal trans-plant patients with significant graft dysfunction, and nonrenal organ recipients with secondary renal dysfunction, monitoring for renal osteodystrophy and supplementation with 1,25-dihydroxyvitamin D_3 is warranted.[68] In patients with bone complications recalcitrant to these therapies, bisphosphonates are safe and effective at improving bone density and potentially reducing the risk of fractures.[71,72]

Role of the Primary Care Provider

The role of the PCP in monitoring for and preventing osseous complications post transplant includes routine counseling on diet (in particular on adequate calcium intake) and exercise, as well as maintaining a high level of suspicion for potential frac-tures, particularly in patients with any acute injury or unexplained focal pain.

OTHER COMPLICATIONS

Cosmetic side effects associated with cyclosporine (hirsutism and gingival hyper-plasia), prednisone (hirsutism, weight gain, Cushingoid features), and tacrolimus (hair loss), though not life-threatening, may have a serious impact on adherence, particularly in adolescent patients.[73,74] Birth defects and an increased rate of spon-taneous abortions have been reported in association with sirolimus and MMF; therefore, these medications should be avoided during pregnancy and adoles-cents, and young women of childbearing age should be educated about these risks.[75]

SUMMARY

Advances in transplant surgical techniques and in immunosuppressive medications have led to an age of unprecedented success in solid organ transplantation. As the number of long-term survivors of pediatric transplantation increases, this success is tempered by the potential for a large variety of posttransplant complications, the risk for many of which increases with increasing posttransplant longevity. Monitoring for and management of these complications, which range from minor cosmetic changes to life-threatening end-organ damage, requires vigilance and a multidisciplinary approach. Transplant professionals must partner with primary care physicians and with patients and families to identify and mitigate the impact of these nonimmune complications, and in so doing, to further improve the medical and psychosocial outcomes for pediatric transplant recipients.

REFERENCES

1. Ojo AO, Held PJ, Port FK, et al. Chronic renal failure after transplantation of a non-renal organ. N Engl J Med 2003;349:931.
2. Harambat J, Ranchin B, Dubourg L, et al. Renal function in pediatric liver transplantation: a long-term follow-up study. Transplantation 2008;86:1028.
3. Campbell KM, Yazigi N, Ryckman FC, et al. High prevalence of renal dysfunction in long-term survivors after pediatric liver transplantation. J Pediatr 2006;148:475.
4. Bharat W, Manlhiot C, McCrindle BW, et al. The profile of renal function over time in a cohort of pediatric heart transplant recipients. Pediatr Transplant 2009;13: 111.
5. Lee CK, Christensen LL, Magee JC, et al. Pre-transplant risk factors for chronic renal dysfunction after pediatric heart transplantation: a 10-year national cohort study. J Heart Lung Transplant 2007;26:458.
6. Sachdeva R, Blaszak RT, Ainley KA, et al. Determinants of renal function in pediatric heart transplant recipients: long-term follow-up study. J Heart Lung Transplant 2007;26:108.
7. Watson MJ, Venick RS, Kaldas F, et al. Renal function impacts outcomes after intestinal transplantation. Transplantation 2008;86:117.
8. Hmiel SP, Beck AM, de la Morena MT, et al. Progressive chronic kidney disease after pediatric lung transplantation. Am J Transplant 2005;5:1739.
9. Hocker B, Tonshoff B. Treatment strategies to minimize or prevent chronic allograft dysfunction in pediatric renal transplant recipients: an overview. Paediatr Drugs 2009;11:381.
10. Ishikawa T, Tsuji A, Inui K, et al. The genetic polymorphism of drug transporters: functional analysis approaches. Pharmacogenomics 2004;5:67.
11. Zhang Y, Benet LZ. The gut as a barrier to drug absorption: combined role of cytochrome P450 3A and P-glycoprotein. Clin Pharmacokinet 2001;40:159.
12. Roy JN, Barama A, Poirier C, et al. Cyp3A4, Cyp3A5, and MDR-1 genetic influences on tacrolimus pharmacokinetics in renal transplant recipients. Pharmacogenet Genomics 2006;16:659.
13. Wei-lin W, Jing J, Shu-sen Z, et al. Tacrolimus dose requirement in relation to donor and recipient ABCB1 and CYP3A5 gene polymorphisms in Chinese liver transplant patients. Liver Transpl 2006;12:775.
14. Hauser IA, Schaeffeler E, Gauer S, et al. ABCB1 genotype of the donor but not of the recipient is a major risk factor for cyclosporine-related nephrotoxicity after renal transplantation. J Am Soc Nephrol 2005;16:1501.

15. Hebert MF, Dowling AL, Gierwatowski C, et al. Association between ABCB1 (multidrug resistance transporter) genotype and post-liver transplantation renal dysfunction in patients receiving calcineurin inhibitors. Pharmacogenetics 2003;13:661.

16. Khanna AK, Cairns VR, Becker CG, et al. Transforming growth factor (TGF)-beta mimics and anti-TGF-beta antibody abrogates the in vivo effects of cyclosporine: demonstration of a direct role of TGF-beta in immunosuppression and nephrotoxicity of cyclosporine. Transplantation 1999;67:882.

17. Khanna AK, Hosenpud JS, Plummer MS, et al. Analysis of transforming growth factor-beta and profibrogenic molecules in a rat cardiac allograft model treated with cyclosporine. Transplantation 2002;73:1543.

18. van de Wetering J, Weimar CH, Balk AH, et al. The impact of transforming growth factor-beta1 gene polymorphism on end-stage renal failure after heart transplantation. Transplantation 2006;82:1744.

19. Siekierka-Harreis M, Kuhr N, Willers R, et al. Impact of genetic polymorphisms of the renin-angiotensin system and of non-genetic factors on kidney transplant function—a single-center experience. Clin Transplant 2009;23:606.

20. Neuberger JM, Mamelok RD, Neuhaus P, et al. Delayed introduction of reduced-dose tacrolimus, and renal function in liver transplantation: the 'ReSpECT' study. Am J Transplant 2009;9:327.

21. Wilson CH, Brook NR, Gok MA, et al. Randomized clinical trial of daclizumab induction and delayed introduction of tacrolimus for recipients of non-heart-beating kidney transplants. Br J Surg 2005;92:681.

22. Boyer O, Le Bidois J, Dechaux M, et al. Improvement of renal function in pediatric heart transplant recipients treated with low-dose calcineurin inhibitor and mycophenolate mofetil. Transplantation 2005;79:1405.

23. Evans HM, McKiernan PJ, Kelly DA. Mycophenolate mofetil for renal dysfunction after pediatric liver transplantation. Transplantation 2005;79:1575.

24. Henne T, Latta K, Strehlau J, et al. Mycophenolate mofetil-induced reversal of glomerular filtration loss in children with chronic allograft nephropathy. Transplantation 2003;76:1326.

25. Hocker B, Feneberg R, Kopf S, et al. SRL-based immunosuppression vs. CNI minimization in pediatric renal transplant recipients with chronic CNI nephrotoxicity. Pediatr Transplant 2006;10:593.

26. Balfour IC, Srun SW, Wood EG, et al. Early renal benefit of rapamycin combined with reduced calcineurin inhibitor dose in pediatric heart transplantation patients. J Heart Lung Transplant 2006;25:518.

27. Shihab FS, Bennett WM, Yi H, et al. Sirolimus increases transforming growth factor-beta1 expression and potentiates chronic cyclosporine nephrotoxicity. Kidney Int 2004;65:1262.

28. Pallet N, Thervet E, Legendre C, et al. Sirolimus early graft nephrotoxicity: clinical and experimental data. Curr Drug Saf 2006;1:179.

29. Tonshoff B, Hocker B. Treatment strategies in pediatric solid organ transplant recipients with calcineurin inhibitor-induced nephrotoxicity. Pediatr Transplant 2006;10:721.

30. Roos JF, Doust J, Tett SE, et al. Diagnostic accuracy of cystatin C compared to serum creatinine for the estimation of renal dysfunction in adults and children— a meta-analysis. Clin Biochem 2007;40:383.

31. Biancofiore G, Pucci L, Cerutti E, et al. Cystatin C as a marker of renal function immediately after liver transplantation. Liver Transpl 2006;12:285.

32. Dello Strologo L, Parisi F, Legato A, et al. Long-term renal function in heart transplant children on cyclosporine treatment. Pediatr Nephrol 2006;21:561.
33. Letavernier E, Legendre C. mToR inhibitors-induced proteinuria: mechanisms, significance, and management. Transplant Rev (Orlando) 2008;22:125.
34. Mells G, Neuberger J. Reducing the risks of cardiovascular disease in liver allograft recipients. Transplantation 2007;83:1141.
35. Petroski RA, Grady KL, Rodgers S, et al. Quality of life in adult survivors greater than 10 years after pediatric heart transplantation. J Heart Lung Transplant 2009; 28:661.
36. Dharnidharka VR, Araya CE, Benfield MR. Organ toxicities. In: Fine RN, Webber SA, Harmon WE, et al, editors. Pediatric solid organ transplantation. 2nd edition. Oxford (UK): Blackwell Publishing Ltd; 2007. p. 124–39.
37. Baluarte HJ, Gruskin AB, Ingelfinger JR, et al. Analysis of hypertension in children post renal transplantation—a report of the North American Pediatric Renal Transplant Cooperative Study (NAPRTCS). Pediatr Nephrol 1994;8:570.
38. Jain A, Mazariegos G, Kashyap R, et al. Comparative long-term evaluation of tacrolimus and cyclosporine in pediatric liver transplantation. Transplantation 2000; 70:617.
39. Nakata Y, Yoshibayashi M, Yonemura T, et al. Tacrolimus and myocardial hypertrophy. Transplantation 2000;69:1960.
40. Shalev A, Nir A, Granot E. Cardiac function in children post-orthotopic liver transplantation: echocardiographic parameters and biochemical markers of subclinical cardiovascular damage. Pediatr Transplant 2005;9:718.
41. Burroughs TE, Swindle JP, Salvalaggio PR, et al. Increasing incidence of new-onset diabetes after transplant among pediatric renal transplant patients. Transplantation 2009;88:367.
42. Simmonds J, Dewar C, Dawkins H, et al. Tacrolimus in pediatric heart transplantation: ameliorated side effects in the steroid-free, statin era. Clin Transplant 2009; 23:415.
43. Hathout E, Alonso E, Anand R, et al. Post-transplant diabetes mellitus in pediatric liver transplantation. Pediatr Transplant 2009;13:599.
44. Gomes MB, Cobas RA. Post-transplant diabetes mellitus. Diabetol Metab Syndr 2009;1:14.
45. Heisel O, Heisel R, Balshaw R, et al. New onset diabetes mellitus in patients receiving calcineurin inhibitors: a systematic review and meta-analysis. Am J Transplant 2004;4:583.
46. Greenspan LC, Gitelman SE, Leung MA, et al. Increased incidence in post-transplant diabetes mellitus in children: a case-control analysis. Pediatr Nephrol 2002; 17:1.
47. Singh TP, Naftel DC, Webber S, et al. Hyperlipidemia in children after heart transplantation. J Heart Lung Transplant 2006;25:1199.
48. Trompeter R, Filler G, Webb NJ, et al. Randomized trial of tacrolimus versus cyclosporin microemulsion in renal transplantation. Pediatr Nephrol 2002;17: 141.
49. Vincenti F, Jensik SC, Filo RS, et al. A long-term comparison of tacrolimus (FK506) and cyclosporine in kidney transplantation: evidence for improved allograft survival at five years. Transplantation 2002;73:775.
50. Ligtenberg G, Hene RJ, Blankestijn PJ, et al. Cardiovascular risk factors in renal transplant patients: cyclosporin A versus tacrolimus. J Am Soc Nephrol 2001;12: 368.

51. Hanevold CD, Ho PL, Talley L, et al. Obesity and renal transplant outcome: a report of the North American Pediatric Renal Transplant Cooperative Study. Pediatrics 2005;115:352.

52. Rossano JW, Grenier MA, Dreyer WJ, et al. Effect of body mass index on outcome in pediatric heart transplant patients. J Heart Lung Transplant 2007;26:718.

53. Ng VL, Fecteau A, Shepherd R, et al. Outcomes of 5-year survivors of pediatric liver transplantation: report on 461 children from a North American multicenter registry. Pediatrics 2008;122:e1128.

54. Curtis JJ, Galla JH, Woodford SY, et al. Effect of alternate-day prednisone on plasma lipids in renal transplant recipients. Kidney Int 1982;22:42.

55. Hricik DE, Knauss TC, Bodziak KA, et al. Withdrawal of steroid therapy in African American kidney transplant recipients receiving sirolimus and tacrolimus. Transplantation 2003;76:938.

56. Li L, Chang A, Naesens M, et al. Steroid-free immunosuppression since 1999: 129 pediatric renal transplants with sustained graft and patient benefits. Am J Transplant 2009;9:1362.

57. Khosroshahi HT, Asghari A, Estakhr R, et al. Effects of azathioprine and mycophenolate mofetil-immunosuppressive regimens on the erythropoietic system of renal transplant recipients. Transplant Proc 2006;38:2077.

58. Maheshwari A, Mishra R, Thuluvath PJ. Post-liver-transplant anemia: etiology and management. Liver Transpl 2004;10:165.

59. Gupta P, Kaufman S, Fishbein TM. Sirolimus for solid organ transplantation in children. Pediatr Transplant 2005;9:269.

60. Danziger-Isakov L, Mark Baillie G. Hematologic complications of anti-CMV therapy in solid organ transplant recipients. Clin Transplant 2009;23:295.

61. Erol I, Alehan F, Ozcay F, et al. Neurological complications of liver transplantation in pediatric patients: a single center experience. Pediatr Transplant 2007;11:152.

62. Cilio MR, Danhaive O, Gadisseux JF, et al. Unusual cyclosporin related neurological complications in recipients of liver transplants. Arch Dis Child 1993;68:405.

63. Bohlin AB, Berg U, Englund M, et al. Central nervous system complications in children treated with ciclosporin after renal transplantation. Child Nephrol Urol 1990;10:225.

64. Bartynski WS, Tan HP, Boardman JF, et al. Posterior reversible encephalopathy syndrome after solid organ transplantation. AJNR Am J Neuroradiol 2008;29:924.

65. Draper HM. Depressive disorder associated with mycophenolate mofetil. Pharmacotherapy 2008;28:136.

66. Neff RT, Hurst FP, Falta EM, et al. Progressive multifocal leukoencephalopathy and use of mycophenolate mofetil after kidney transplantation. Transplantation 2008;86:1474.

67. Goksen D, Darcan S, Kara P, et al. Bone mineral density in pediatric and adolescent renal transplant patients: how to evaluate. Pediatr Transplant 2005;9:464.

68. Saland JM. Osseous complications of pediatric transplantation. Pediatr Transplant 2004;8:400.

69. Valta H, Jalanko H, Holmberg C, et al. Impaired bone health in adolescents after liver transplantation. Am J Transplant 2008;8:150.

70. Guthery SL, Pohl JF, Bucuvalas JC, et al. Bone mineral density in long-term survivors following pediatric liver transplantation. Liver Transpl 2003;9:365.

71. Sachdeva R, Soora R, Bryant JC, et al. Bone mineral status in pediatric heart transplant recipients: a retrospective observational study of an "at risk" cohort. Pediatr Transplant 2009. [Epub ahead of print].

72. El-Husseini AA, El-Agroudy AE, El-Sayed MF, et al. Treatment of osteopenia and osteoporosis in renal transplant children and adolescents. Pediatr Transplant 2004;8:357.

73. Walker RG, Cottrell S, Sharp K, et al. Conversion of cyclosporine to tacrolimus in stable renal allograft recipients: quantification of effects on the severity of gingival enlargement and hirsutism and patient-reported outcomes. Nephrology (Carlton) 2007;12:607.

74. Shiboski CH, Krishnan S, Besten PD, et al. Gingival enlargement in pediatric organ transplant recipients in relation to tacrolimus-based immunosuppressive regimens. Pediatr Dent 2009;31:38.

75. Wielgos M, Pietrzak B, Bobrowska K, et al. Pregnancy after organ transplantation. Neuro Endocrinol Lett 2009;30:6.

76. Tsimaratos M, Viard L, Kreitmann B, et al. Kidney function in cyclosporine-treated paediatric pulmonary transplant recipients. Transplantation 2000;69:2055.

77. Herzog D, Martin S, Turpin S, et al. Normal glomerular filtration rate in long-term follow-up of children after orthotopic liver transplantation. Transplantation 2006; 81:672.

Tolerance: Is It Achievable in Pediatric Solid Organ Transplantation?

Vicki Seyfert-Margolis, PhD[a], Sandy Feng, MD, PhD[b],*

KEYWORDS

- Pediatric solid organ transplantation • Allo-immune response
- Tolerance • Immunosuppression withdrawal

In 1956, John Murray performed the first successful kidney transplant. A kidney from one identical twin was transplanted into the other.[1] Four years previously, the first attempt at pediatric kidney transplantation occurred in France.[2] In this case, a 16-year-old boy received a kidney from his mother after a nephrectomy of his right kidney and subsequent discovery that his left kidney was missing. Although the mother was ABO compatible, the outcome, rejection after 21 days and death of the boy, demonstrated the powerful effects of the immune system's allorecognition, a factor not at work in genetically identical transplants. At this point in history, the mechanisms underlying allorecognition were poorly understood, but 1 year later, in 1953, Peter Medawar performed the seminal experiment demonstrating the potential to overcome the alloimmune response and induce a state of immunologic tolerance.[3] Although much progress has been made in controlling alloimmunity through the use of ever-improving immunosuppressive therapies, the discoveries of Medawar still have yet to be translated such that tolerance can be successfully achieved routinely in the clinical transplant setting.

Therefore, in the clinical arena of transplantation, tolerance remains, for the most part, a concept rather than a reality. As delineated in many of the organ-specific articles in this issue, the current paradigm of lifelong immunosuppression leaves a lot to be desired, particularly for children who face a lifelong burden. Although modern immunosuppression regimens have effectively handled acute rejection, nearly all organs

No official support or endorsement of this article by the Food and Drug Administration is intended or should be inferred.

The views presented in this article do not necessarily reflect those of the Food and Drug Administration.

[a] Food and Drug Administration, 10903 New Hampshire Avenue, Silver Spring, MD 20903, USA

[b] University of California San Francisco, 505 Parnassus Avenue, Box 0780, San Francisco, CA 94143-0780, USA

* Corresponding author.

E-mail address: Sandy.feng@ucsfmedctr.org

Pediatr Clin N Am 57 (2010) 523–538

doi:10.1016/j.pcl.2010.01.015

0031-3955/10/$ – see front matter © 2010 Elsevier Inc. All rights reserved.

pediatric.theclinics.com

except the liver commonly suffer chronic immunologic damage that impairs organ function, threatening patient and allograft survival. In addition to the imperfect control of the donor-directed immune response, there are additional costs. First, there is the burden of mortality from infection and malignancy that can be directly attributed to a crippled immune system. Second, there are insidious effects on renal function, cardiovascular profile (hypertension, hyperglycemia, and dyslipidemia), bone health, growth, psychological and neurocognitive development, and overall quality of life. It is likely that the full consequences of lifelong immunosuppression on pediatric transplant recipients will not be fully appreciated until survival routinely extends beyond 1 or 2 decades after transplantation. Therefore, it can be argued that the holy grail of transplantation tolerance is of the utmost importance to children who undergo solid organ transplantation.[4,5]

THE ALLOIMMUNE RESPONSE

Responses to alloantigens are primarily mediated by host T cells. As naive alloreactive T cells must be activated to cause rejection, they require antigen to be presented on antigen-presenting cells (APCs). Antigen presentation can occur via direct or indirect antigen presentation. In direct antigen presentation, donor APCs leave the graft, migrate to regional lymph nodes, and activate host cells that recognize donor major histocompatibility complex (MHC). Indirect antigen presentation involves recipient APCs presenting peptides derived from donor MHC or other donor-specific proteins, and presenting them to host T cells. Direct allorecognition is believed to be largely responsible for mediating acute rejection. However, chronic rejection is more likely mediated via the indirect pathway, because self-APCs are resident and donor APCs eventually die out. Current strategies for suppressing the immune response to transplanted organs attempt to address both pathways of antigen presentation by suppressing the activation of T cells. However, it is not clear whether tolerance-induction strategies will adequately address both pathways, as protocols that affect direct presentation may not prevent slowly developing chronic rejection mediated by self-APCs continuing to present donor organ antigens.

DEFINITION OF TOLERANCE

Tolerance, a state of normal allograft function without histologic evidence of immunologic damage in the complete absence of immunosuppression, can be induced or occur spontaneously. Tolerance induction strategies refer to treatment regimens specifically designed to achieve the tolerant state that is typically delivered around the time of transplantation. In contrast, spontaneous or operational tolerance most often refers to achievement of the tolerant state without an induction regimen that is uncovered through successful withdrawal of immunosuppression. As such, biomarkers capable of identifying and/or monitoring the tolerant state are much needed to enhance the success and decrease the risk of discontinuation of immunosuppression.

MECHANISMS OF TOLERANCE

Immunologic tolerance is based on the fundamental premise of immunity, namely self-versus non-self discrimination. Because productive immune responses rely on the immune system's ability to recognize foreign antigens to protect the host, an elaborate process for ensuring proper recognition of foreign from self-antigens has evolved. To prevent one from responding to one's own cells and proteins, the immune system uses several mechanisms to induce self-tolerance. These mechanisms are mediated centrally and in the periphery, and are depicted in **Fig. 1**.

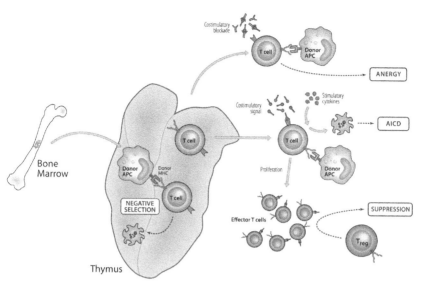

Fig. 1. The mechanisms of T cell tolerance. In central tolerance, T cells migrate from the bone marrow to the thymus where they are educated, such that those recognizing self-antigens are deleted. Peripheral mechanisms of tolerance for self-reactive T cells are also shown including activation-induced cell death (AICD), anergy, and suppression by regulatory T cells (T$_{reg}$ cells).

Central Tolerance

Central tolerance is the primary and most potent checkpoint to educate T and B cells during their development such that cells with high affinity receptors to self-antigens are deleted before they enter the periphery (see **Fig. 1**). For T cells, this process involves education in the thymus. Immature T lineage cells emerge from hematopoietic progenitors in the bone marrow and enter the thymus without expressing either the T cell receptor (TCR) or coreceptors, CD4 and CD8. On entry, these double-negative (DN) thymocytes (they lack CD4 and CD8) commit to 1 of 3 T-cell lineages by undergoing a succession of TCR gene rearrangements.[6,7] Murine studies indicate that different lineages populate in succession with γδ T cells comprising the first wave during embryogenesis followed by αβ T cells in a second wave.[8] The commitment to the γδ, αβ, or natural killer (NK) T-cell lineage is independent of peptide/MHC interactions.[6,7]

After lineage commitment, DN thymocytes undergo further development to express CD4 and CD8 receptors, thereby becoming double-positive (DP) thymocytes.[6,7] It is at this stage that a thymocyte's fate is determined by the nature of its interaction with self-peptides that are presented on the self-MHC of thymic stromal cells. The overall avidity of the thymocyte's TCR for self MHC/peptide complexes is based on the TCR structure and its density on the thymocyte cell surface. Thymocytes with TCRs that interact with self MHC/peptides are positively selected and evolve into mature T cells that express either the CD4 or CD8 receptor (single positive T cells). If a T cell then reacts too strongly with self-antigens presented on bone marrow–derived APCs, it is deleted in the thymus. This mechanism of self-tolerance is extraordinarily effective but clearly dependent on the expression of self-peptides by bone marrow–derived APCs in the thymus.[7,9]

Although it is not entirely clear how, many peripheral tissue-specific antigens are expressed and presented in the thymus to ensure central T-cell tolerance to antigens that will subsequently be encountered in the periphery. Insulin is a prime example. The expression of peripheral proteins in the thymus is driven in part by a gene called AIRE (autoimmune regulator). Mutations in the AIRE gene result in a disease known as autoimmune polyglandular syndrome type I. This condition emphasizes the importance of AIRE in ensuring that peripheral antigens are presented in the thymus to accomplish deletion of autoreactive T cells before their entry into the periphery.[10]

Similarly, B cells are tested for reactivity to self-antigens before they enter the periphery. Immature B cells developing in the bone marrow sample antigen through their antigen receptor, surface IgM (sIgM). If signaling through sIgM is sufficiently weak, immature B cells can be rendered permanently unresponsive or anergic. However, if immature B cells are strongly self-reactive, there are 2 possible scenarios to ensure central tolerance. The first is deletion of these self-reactive B cells. The second is receptor editing, a process by which a new receptor with altered specificity is generated through another sequence of B cell receptor gene rearrangements.[11,12]

Peripheral Tolerance

Although central tolerance is very effective at eliminating T and B cells with self-reactivity, not all peripheral self-antigens are expressed in the bone marrow and thymus. Moreover, some T or B cells with limited avidity to self-antigens may escape the deletion process. Therefore, peripheral tolerance mechanisms are in place to further ensure that immune responses to self are not initiated or are controlled. Peripheral tolerance either involves induction of activation-induced cell death (AICD), induction of anergy, or regulation of responses to self through regulatory lymphocytes (T or B cells). AICD is a mechanism used to delete T cells specific for self-antigen in the periphery (see **Fig. 1**). T cells that recognize self-antigens with high affinity in the periphery are initially activated and then die via apoptosis.[13] Similarly, mature B cells with a high affinity for self-antigen and thus, highly cross-linked receptors undergo clonal deletion in the periphery.[11]

Anergy is a state of functional inactivation of T or B cells in the periphery. T cell anergy can result from antigenic stimulation in the absence of costimulation. Activation signals generated by engagement of the TCR alone are insufficient to generate IL-2 production and therefore result in an abortive proliferative response. Engagement of CD28 by B7 molecules on APCs along with the TCR is required to induce the multiple pathways that ultimately activate IL-2 gene transcription leading to T cell activation and proliferation. It has been shown that IL-2 production and subsequent signaling through its receptor, IL-2R, is necessary for T cells to escape anergy, as blocking IL-2/IL-2R engagement even after stimulation through TCR and CD28 still results in induction of T cell anergy.[14]

Regulation of immune responses by regulatory T cells (T_{reg} cells) is a third mechanism of peripheral tolerance. T_{reg} cells are active in tolerance to self as well as in regulating adaptive immune responses to foreign antigens. In an adaptive immune response, T_{reg} cells control the type and magnitude of the immune response to foreign antigen to ensure that the host remains undamaged. T_{reg} cells also are integral to maintaining a lack of response to self-antigens or tolerance. There are 2 types of T_{reg} cells, natural and adaptive.[15]

Natural T_{reg} cells are committed to the regulatory lineage in the thymus and may express TCR reactive to peripheral self-antigens not encountered in the thymus. Natural T_{reg} cells are characterized by their expression of CD4 and high levels of

CD25 on their surface as well as intracellular expression of the transcription factor Foxp3. Foxp3 is the orchestrator of the cellular and molecular programs involved in mediating T_{reg} cell functions. It is a transcriptional regulatory factor that either directly or indirectly controls hundreds of genes, including signal transduction factors, cytokines, cell-surface receptors, enzymes for cell metabolism, and other proteins. Many of these genes are involved in activation and differentiation of T cells, such as the development of naive T cells into activated effectors. The importance of Foxp3 is underscored by the finding that mutations in this gene in humans causes the immune dysfunction, polyendocrinopathy, enteropathy, X-linked (IPEX) syndrome characterized by lethal autoimmunity.[15]

Adaptive T_{reg} cells are generated from naive T cells in the periphery as determined by the local cytokine milieu. In the presence of transforming growth factor-β (TGF-β), activation of naive T cells leads to expression of Foxp3 which represses the transcriptional apparatus for effector T cells, thereby converting the naive cells into T_{reg} cells. If naive T cells are stimulated by TGF-β in the presence of IL-6, they are converted to Th17 cells, effector T cells that secrete IL-17 and carry out immune tissue injury. However, the presence of retinoic acid, produced by a specialized set of dendritic cells, can block differentiation of naive CD4+ T cells into Th17 cells.[15,16] IL-2 also promotes T_{reg} cell development. Thus, there is tremendous plasticity in the peripheral development of adaptive T_{reg} cells from naive CD4+ T cells. A complex network of cytokines and developmental lineages has evolved to initiate and regulate proinflammatory responses in the T-cell compartment.

TOLERANCE IN SOLID ORGAN TRANSPLANTATION: INDUCED VERSUS SPONTANEOUS

In the clinical solid organ transplantation arena, it is useful to recognize that the tolerant state can be induced or occur spontaneously. Attempts to induce tolerance are discussed followed by experiences that have unmasked spontaneous tolerance. Induction strategies refer to treatment regimens typically delivered around the time of transplantation designed to achieve tolerance. Protocols exploiting 1 or more of the mechanisms of tolerance have been tried most often in the context of living donor kidney transplantation as candidates are not critically ill and the time of transplantation is known. No induction protocols have, as yet, included pediatric transplant candidates reflecting the preliminary nature of these efforts as well as the hesitation to expose children to highly experimental therapies. Nevertheless, it is instructive to consider the approaches that have been tried.

INDUCTION OF TOLERANCE: CENTRAL MECHANISMS

In transplantation, induction of central tolerance has been attempted through the induction of donor-recipient chimerism. In murine models, bone marrow chimeras, achieved by hematopoietic stem cell transplantation after host myelosuppression, are tolerant to skin grafts from the same donor. In these model systems, donor stem cells were shown to migrate to the thymus, leading to negative selection or elimination of newly emerging donor-specific T cells. These and other similar studies in nonhuman primates set the stage for recent clinical trials aimed at achieving chimerism as a tolerance induction strategy.[17]

There are several key components to regimens designed to induce donor-recipient chimerism. First the recipient must undergo some form of nonablative myelosuppression or conditioning to facilitate engraftment of donor hematopoietic cells while allowing ultimate survival of and repopulation by host hematopoietic cells. Total lymphoid irradiation and cyclophosphamide are 2 approaches that are actively being tested. Second, the immunosuppression regimen is designed to prevent rejection of the donor organ as well as graft-versus-host disease (GVHD), a risk of achieving chimerism particularly in the setting of HLA mismatch. T cell depletion, most commonly using a polyclonal preparation against T cells, has been the favored induction approach, followed by a period of standard immunosuppression before complete withdrawal. There are 1 or more infusions of donor bone marrow cells, either unsorted or enriched for hematopoietic stem cells.[17]

Currently, a few centers have used the chimerism approach to induce central tolerance in conjunction with adult kidney transplantation, with mixed success. The group from Stanford University has used total lymphoid irradiation with induction using rabbit antithymocyte globulin followed by maintenance immunosuppression with corticosteroids and cyclosporine. Of 4 HLA-mismatched, adult, living donor kidney transplant recipients treated, none achieved long-term chimerism or tolerance.[18] More recently, the same group reported on a single adult patient who underwent HLA-identical combined stem cell and kidney transplantation after total lymphoid irradiation followed by maintenance immunosuppression with cyclosporine and mycophenolate mofetil.[19] This patient showed persistent mixed chimerism, experienced neither allograft rejection nor GVHD, and was successfully withdrawn from all immunosuppression maintaining normal kidney function for 34 months after transplantation. However, 2 other patients achieved only transient chimerism such that immunosuppression has been maintained.[19] The protocol has been modified with intensification of the irradiation given for conditioning to enhance chimerism but results are, as yet, unpublished (clinicaltrials.gov identifier NCT00319657).

The best results to date have been achieved by the group at Massachusetts General Hospital. Initially, they reported on 6 adults undergoing combined bone marrow and kidney transplantation for multiple myeloma and end-stage renal disease (ESRD), again from HLA-identical donors.[17,20] All 6 patients developed evidence of mixed chimerism. Notably, the 2 patients who achieved full and durable donor chimerism developed GVHD that required treatment with maintenance immunosuppression. The other 4 showed only transient chimerism. When these 4 patients were weaned off immunosuppression, 1 experienced acute rejection that was treated with immunosuppression and the other 3 were tolerant to their kidney allografts, remaining off immunosuppression for 1.3 to 7 years after transplantation. Subsequently, the protocol was modified to accommodate ESRD candidates with single haplotype HLA-mismatched donors. All 5 adults enrolled in the protocol developed only transient mixed chimerism.[21] One of the 5 recipients suffered irreversible humoral rejection leading to graft loss. However, 4 have successfully withdrawn from immunosuppression, maintaining stable kidney function for 2.0 to 5.3 years after transplantation or 1.2 to 4.6 years after cessation of immunosuppression. All 4 tolerant recipients showed donor-specific hyporesponsiveness with high levels of Foxp3 transcripts in allograft tissue. Currently, a further modification of the protocol to accommodate complete HLA-mismatched donor-recipient combinations is undergoing testing (clinicaltrials. gov identifier NCT00801632).

Although the risks inherent in current chimerism approaches to induce central tolerance are substantial because of the requisite conditioning regimen and the risk of GVHD, this strategy may be especially promising for the pediatric population. Children have the advantage of a larger thymus which, in preclinical studies, correlates with better prospects to achieve a more robust state of tolerance. With aging, the thymus involutes leading to diminished capacity to educate T cells and thereby participate in central tolerance mechanisms.[5]

INDUCTION OF TOLERANCE: PERIPHERAL MECHANISMS

Even though commercial drug development programs do not aim to induce tolerance, recently developed therapies strongly reflect various approaches that may enhance mechanisms of peripheral tolerance. The strategy of T-cell depletion, most frequently using rabbit antithymocyte globulin has gained substantial popularity as induction immunosuppression for adult organ transplantation. Although the primary aim is to reduce the rate of acute rejection, depletion may indeed be pro-tolerogenic as T cell repopulation in the presence of the donor organ is believed to facilitate donor-specific hyporesponsiveness. A second attractive approach has been costimulatory blockade that leads to anergy of donor-specific T cells. LEA29Y, a humanized monoclonal antibody targeting the CD28-B7 costimulation pathway, is currently being tested in adult kidney and liver transplantation registration trials as a maintenance immuno-suppression agent to replace calcineurin inhibitors (clinicaltrials.gov identifiers NCT00455013, NCT00035555, NCT00256750, NCT00114777, and NCT00555321). Another costimulatory blockade agent, anti-CD154, that interferes with CD40/CD40L interaction, held substantial promise for tolerance induction until trials revealed an increased risk of thromboembolic events[22] and commercial development has ceased.

Another avenue of peripheral tolerance induction that is reflected in novel immuno-suppression strategies is the enhancement of T_{reg} cells. There is evidence for expansion of alloantigen cross-reactive natural T_{reg} cells and conversion of alloantigen-specific non-T_{reg} cells as part of the mechanisms that regulate antidonor responses.[23] Recent studies have pointed to the potential of certain immunosuppression regimens that seem to induce production of T_{reg} cells. In vitro, rapamycin has been shown selectively expand CD4+CD25+Foxp3+ T_{reg} cells.[24] The underlying target for rapamycin, mTOR or mammalian target of rapamycin, is a key player in signals generated via the TCR. Constitutive activation of the mTOR pathway antagonizes expression of FoxP3, thus inhibiting T_{reg} development. Conversely, blocking mTOR leads to de novo differentiation of naive CD4+ T cells into CD4+FoxP3+ regulatory T cells.[25] These findings have been confirmed in vivo; murine studies have shown that rapamycin promotes T_{reg} cell development, whereas calcineurin inhibitors inhibit their development.[26]

In the clinical setting, however, it is unclear whether the T_{reg} mechanism prevails in spontaneous or operational tolerance. One study by Yoshizawa and colleagues[27] reported donor alloantigen-specific T_{reg} cells as defined by CD4+CD25+ expression in 14 pediatric liver transplant recipients who had been successfully weaned off immu-nosuppression. However, functional studies did not suggest that T_{reg} cells were the primary means of anti-donor regulation. Even in the absence of CD4+CD25+ T_{reg} cells, effector (CD4+CD25−) T cells showed donor-specific hyporesponsiveness during in vitro mixed lymphocyte reactions. Moreover, several studies exploring biomarkers of operationally tolerant kidney and liver transplant recipients have not shown a definitive role for T_{reg} cells (see section on Markers of Tolerance in Solid Organ Transplantation).

SPONTANEOUS TOLERANCE IN SOLID ORGAN TRANSPLANTATION

In addition to the efforts to induce and/or exploit the tolerance mechanisms outlined earlier, there are reported examples of spontaneous tolerance after transplantation. Because spontaneous tolerance is only discovered through the successful cessation of immunosuppression, most transplant recipients were noncompliant with their prescribed regimens and, independent of their transplant physicians, discontinued their immunosuppression medications. The minority were obligatorily withdrawn from immunosuppression under physician direction as mandated by the emergence of a significant contraindication to ongoing immunosuppression. The most common contraindications, for both adults and children, have been posttransplant lymphoproliferative disorder, other malignancy, or life-threatening infection. Some recipients were electively withdrawn from immunosuppression *less than* physician direction, with no specific motivation other than to reduce the burden of immunosuppression. Currently, these reports are limited exclusively to kidney and liver transplant recipients. Normal or baseline allograft function has typically been evident solely from biochemical parameters without histologic confirmation. Although these cases are certainly notable, they are indeed rare, considering the total number of liver and kidney transplants performed.

Spontaneous Tolerance in Kidney Transplantation

In kidney transplantation, scattered reports of spontaneously tolerant recipients emerged in the 1970s. The first publication was in 1975 by Owens and colleagues[28] who identified 6 of 203 patients who had discontinued immunosuppression. Four of the 6, all recipients of living donor transplants, had maintained baseline renal function for 17, 23, 44, and 52 months although 1 patient was noted as taking 25 mg of azathioprine per day on a sporadic basis. Of the 2 recipients who developed rejection, 1 allograft was salvaged and the other was lost. These unusual and somewhat surprising cases led the investigators to survey 40 other renal transplant centers. Sixteen centers identified 24 patients who had discontinued immunosuppression for some period of time. Most of these recipients, 22 (92%), returned to immunosuppression; 8 recipients resumed treatment without experiencing rejection and 14 recipients resumed after experiencing rejection. Only 2 remained successfully off immunosuppression for 9 and 36 months at the time of publication. This report was extended 5 years later by Zoller and colleagues[29] who similarly conducted a survey of 165 renal transplant centers leading to the identification of 48 (16 deceased donor and 32 living donor recipients) who had discontinued immunosuppression for some period of time. Twenty-one of the 48 allografts (9 from deceased and 12 from living donors) failed wand 13 allografts maintained stable function for 1 year or more. The conclusions drawn by the investigators of these 2 experiences differed in tone. Owens and colleagues[28] highlighted the possibility of success, suggesting that immunosuppression should not be resumed unless rejection was to occur and that resumption of immunosuppression in response to rejection would likely salvage the allograft. However, in an accompanying editorial, Dr John Najarian, Chief of Transplantation at the University of Minnesota, strongly countered this perspective, calling it "dangerous" and "extremely controversial." Citing 6 cases of immunosuppression discontinuation at his transplant center that led to 5 episodes of severe rejection and, ultimately, 4 graft losses, he strongly advocated for reinstitution of immunosuppression for any recipient found to have discontinued treatment. Zoller and colleagues[29] echoed this cautious tone. These reports predate the modern era of immunosuppression. Therefore, the mere achievement of a stable state of good allograft function long after transplantation already provided evidence of an immunologically favorable situation.

There was then silence in the kidney transplant literature through much of the 1980s and 1990s with the exception of a single series from the University of Pittsburgh. Starzl and colleagues[30] reported on 5 long-standing (27–29 years) living donor kidney transplant recipients (1 or 0 haplotype-matched) with stable graft function without cover of immunosuppression. All 5 recipients had evidence of chimerism with detectible donor cells in the skin, lymph nodes, or blood. For the 4 whose donors were alive, all showed absent (n = 2) or depressed (n = 2) responses to donor lymphocytes but normal responses to third party lymphocytes. Moreover, donor cells failed to generate cytotoxic effector cells in vitro. This report is clearly unusual in its inclusion of mechanistic explorations to demonstrate a hypothesis of spontaneous tolerance.

More recently, however, there have been 2 important cohorts of spontaneously tolerant adult kidney transplant recipients, 1 from France and 1 from the United States. The French cohort comprised of 17 long-standing recipients of predominantly deceased donor, HLA-mismatched kidney transplants with stable long-term function (Cockcroft-Gault calculated creatinine clearance >60 mL/min/1.73 m^2 with absent or low-grade proteinuria <1.5 g/d) and a drug-free duration of at least 2 years but typically much longer.[31,32] Immunosuppression was discontinued in 15 secondary to noncompliance and in 2 secondary to medical necessity. The factors identified as favoring operational tolerance included long duration after transplantation, gradual drug discontinuation, and excellent graft quality from young donors. Notably, patients did not show general immune unresponsiveness in that the majority entered transplant with some evidence of sensitization after blood transfusions, they did not suffer opportunistic infections, and a subset had evidence of donor-specific antibodies against Class II MHC antigens. The American cohort has been presented at several national meetings but remains unpublished. It is comprised of 25 long-standing recipients of predominantly HLA-matched adult kidney transplants with stable long-term function (serum creatinine level within 25% of baseline) and a drug-free duration of at least 1 year. Both of these series have supported important mechanistic investigations with regard to biomarkers of tolerance (see section on Markers of Tolerance in Solid Organ Transplantation).

Spontaneous Tolerance in Liver Transplantation

In contrast to kidney transplantation, the setting of liver transplantation seems to have been more permissive of spontaneous operational tolerance. The transplant community generally perceives a higher likelihood of spontaneous tolerance and therefore, there are more withdrawal experiences and some that include children. The liver, a uniquely immunologic organ, has always been regarded as tolerogenic. This privilege is reflected by its anatomy and function.[33,34] The liver has 2 blood supplies, the portal venous and the hepatic arterial systems, which mix in the hepatic sinusoids, specialized blood channels lacking a discrete basement membrane but lined by fenestrated endothelial cells. This unique architectural arrangement facilitates the entry of circulating antigens and immune cells into these blood spaces. The sluggish sinusoidal flow patterns allow ample time and opportunity for antigens to interact with hepatocytes, endothelial, Kupffer, and other resident cells. This design is likely of integral importance to the liver's unique immunobiology. Compared with other organs and the peripheral blood compartment, the liver has a unique complement of lymphocytes. NK and NK-like T cells strikingly account for approximately 60% of resident lymphocytes compared with approximately 15% in the peripheral blood compartment. The liver is also enriched for CD8+ than for CD4+ T cells. When challenged by pathogens, the liver has the demonstrable capability to generate a protective immune response. However, because portal venous flow constitutively exposes the liver to nonpathogenic foreign antigens such as food derivatives, environmental toxins, and bacterial products, the liver must also possess potent mechanisms that suppress immune activation. Presentation of antigens via the portal venous system has long been recognized as more likely to result in a tolerizing response than presentation via the systemic venous system.

In the context of liver transplantation, multiple allogeneic models ranging from rodent to canine to swine have shown that minimal or even no immunosuppression has resulted in successful and durable graft function after transplantation.[35,36] This relative resistance against immunologic attack is also evident in many respects in the human setting. First, the recipient's sensitization status (the presence of preformed anti-HLA antibodies) seems to have no import. Crossmatching of the donor and recipient is unnecessary and hyperacute alloimmune responses are exceedingly rare. Second, acute rejection episodes, in general, do not compromise long-term allograft outcomes, presumably because regenerative processes enable full parenchymal recovery from injury. The liver is uniquely resistant to humoral and chronic rejection processes.

There have been multiple reports of spontaneously tolerant adult and pediatric liver transplant recipients.[37–54] Similar to the kidney transplant setting, most recipients were off immunosuppression secondary to noncompliance or mandatory withdrawal. However, reflective of the tolerogenic nature of the liver, some experiences reflect elective withdrawal rather than patient noncompliance or mandated withdrawal. **Table 1** summarizes the published experience for adults and children. Overall, among adults, the rate of spontaneous tolerance approximates 20% with low risk of graft loss, chronic rejection, and/or severe acute rejection. Favorable factors for success include increased time since transplantation, minimal maintenance immunosuppression such as a low dose of a single agent, transplantation for nonautoimmune diseases, and the presence of posttransplant lymphoproliferative disorder. There is some controversy as to the wisdom of weaning when hepatitis C (HCV) was the indication for transplantation. This population may face unique gains if fibrosis progression is retarded but unique risks if rejection occurs, particularly if treatment with corticosteroids or a depleting antibody is required.

Currently, in Europe and the United States, there are trials examining the safety and efficacy of immunosuppression withdrawal after liver transplantation. Two trials led by the Barcelona group target stable, long-term, adult liver transplant recipients. One trial, enrolling only recipients transplanted for nonimmune indications, Aims To Prospectively Validate A Signature Predictive Of Operational Tolerance (clinicaltrials. gov identifier NCT00647283; see section on Markers of Tolerance in Solid Organ Transplantation). The second trial, exclusive to adult HCV recipients, aims to assess the effect of withdrawal on HCV-induced allograft damage (clinicaltrials.gov identifier NCT00668369). The United States study is a large, randomized, multicenter trial enrolling adults undergoing transplantation for either hepatitis C or nonviral/nonimmune indications funded by the Immune Tolerance Network (ITN) and the National Institute of Allergy and Infectious Diseases (NIAID) (clinicaltrials.gov identifier NCT00135694). Qualified recipients are randomized during the second post-transplant year to withdrawing from immunosuppression or continuing immunosuppression according to standard of care. In addition to the safety and efficacy of withdrawal, this study aims to determine whether attempted withdrawal, even if unsuccessful, might result in renal, cardiovascular, metabolic, and malignancy benefit by reducing overall immunosuppression exposure. Concomitant to the clinical investigations are substantial mechanistic explorations based on peripheral blood and liver tissue samples to identify biomarkers predictive of successful withdrawal.

There are 2 significant experiences involving pediatric liver transplant recipients.[42,44,46,51,55] The University of Pittsburgh attempted withdrawal for 64 recipients of deceased donor grafts, succeeding in 22 (34%); Kyoto University attempted withdrawal for 191 recipients of living donor grafts, succeeding in 85 (45%). Acute rejection was fairly common, albeit readily reversed. A single patient between the 2 institutions developed chronic rejection that was successfully treated with triple immunosuppression. There were no graft losses or patient deaths related to withdrawal in either series.

Table 1
Summary of immunosuppression withdrawal experiences for adult and pediatric liver transplant recipients

Year	References	Center	No. of Patients	Adult or Children	Tolerant (%)	Rejection Acute	Rejection Chronic	Comments
1994	45	Mayo	12	Adult	0	6	3	2 deaths
1993, 1995, 1997, 2007	49,42,44,54	Pittsburgh	95	Adult + children	18 (19)	21	3	
1998, 2005	38,40	King's College	18	Adult	5 (17)	13[a]	1	1 retransplantation
2001, 2004, 2007	46,50,51	Kyoto	191	Children	81 (42)	?16	?1	
2003	53	Spain	9	Adult	3 (33)	6[a]	0	
2005	48	Miami	104	Adult	20 (19)	70[a]	2	1 retransplantation
2005	39	Ochsner	18	Adult	1 (6)	11	0	
2006, 2008	47,43	Tor Vergata	34	Adult	8 (23)	26	0	
2007	37	Ontario	26	Adult	2 (8)	15	0	
Total			677		138 (20)	178 (26)	10 (1)	

[a] Only a subset of the acute rejection episodes were biopsy-proven; 4 of 13 from King's College; 2 of 6 from Spain; and 30 of 70 from Miami.

These 2 series suggest that spontaneous tolerance occurs more frequently in children. There are many potential explanations. First, liver transplantation occurs predominantly in infants and toddlers, an age of immunologic immaturity that may favor the development of spontaneous tolerance. Second, diseases that necessitate pediatric liver transplantation typically do not recur. Third, management of immunosuppression is likely unique for children late after liver transplantation in that stable recipients with normal liver tests are typically maintained on monotherapy. Moreover, many transplant centers no longer adjust drug dosing to maintain target trough levels such that growth essentially accomplishes very gradual immunosuppression weaning.

Currently, there is a multicenter pilot trial of immunosuppression withdrawal for stable pediatric recipients of parental living donor grafts funded by the ITN/NIAID (clinicaltrials.gov identifier NCT00320606). Preliminarily, withdrawal has been safe and efficacious; 60% of all participants (12 of 20) attained the primary endpoint, defined as normal allograft function in the absence of immunosuppression for 1 year. Clinical follow-up of multiple parameters, including allograft histology, for up to 5 years after withdrawal is continuing. The inclusion of protocol liver biopsies spanning the 6-year study period is critical, in spite of their invasiveness, as a normal biochemical profile does not ensure normal allograft histology.[56,57] Mechanistic testing for biomarkers of spontaneous tolerance is just beginning.

MARKERS OF TOLERANCE IN SOLID ORGAN TRANSPLANTATION

The recently identified cohorts of spontaneously tolerant kidney and liver transplant recipients described earlier have supported fruitful efforts to identify biomarkers of tolerance. Two publications have shown distinct gene expression patterns characteristic of spontaneously tolerant kidney transplant recipients.[31,58] First, alterations in the repertoire of TCR variable region genes with a predominance of Vβ gene usage were associated with tolerance.[58] Second, a panel of several genes, including the B cell specific gene, CD20, was increased in spontaneously tolerant kidney transplant recipients.[31] In 2 unpublished studies of spontaneously tolerant kidney transplant recipients, increases in B cell specific genes were found in the peripheral blood of tolerant versus nontolerant kidney transplant recipients.

In the arena of liver transplantation, an early report showed that spontaneously tolerant adult liver transplant recipients showed a relative increase in plasmacytoid versus myeloid dendritic cells.[55] More recently, however, the Barcelona group studying adults[41,52] and the Kyoto group studying children[50,51] have both reported spontaneously tolerant liver transplant recipients, compared with those requiring maintenance immunosuppression and healthy non-transplant controls, had a relative increase in the proportion of $\gamma\delta$ T cells in the peripheral blood.[41,51] Moreover, the tolerant patients had an inverse ratio of $\delta1$ to $\delta2$ $\gamma\delta$ T cells with more $\delta1$ than $\delta2$ T cells. The Barcelona group has also investigated gene expression profiles of peripheral blood mononuclear cells in tolerant adult recipients and identified patterns correlated with the tolerant state.[41,52] Notably, the differentially expressed genes are attributable to NK or $\gamma\delta$ T cells. Currently, they have nearly completed a study aimed at prospective validation of their tolerance signature: the combination of a distinctive composition of circulating T-cell subsets and a distinctive pattern of peripheral blood gene expression (clinicaltrials.gov identifier NCT00647283). Overall, the putative signature suggests that the tolerance mechanism(s) operational in adult liver transplant recipients involve NK and/or $\gamma\delta$ T cells and therefore, may be specific to this organ. Again, the liver is uniquely an immunologic organ; it is a major site of $\gamma\delta$ T-cell development and a substantial reservoir for NK and $\gamma\delta$ T cells.[59]

OBSTACLES AND OPPORTUNITIES FOR TOLERANCE IN PEDIATRIC ORGAN TRANSPLANT RECIPIENTS

Intuition and evidence strongly suggest that pediatric organ transplant recipients face increased risk from the specter of lifelong conventional immunosuppression and therefore are at greatest need for innovation to achieve donor-specific tolerance. Moreover, it is thought that young children, in particular, may be particularly suitable, from an immunologic perspective, to become tolerant, either spontaneously or deliberately. However, thus far, children are under represented in the tolerance literature, most likely because clinical investigation in children must adhere to more rigorous ethical standards and a more favorable equipoise than in adults. In the case of attempted immunosuppression withdrawal to uncover operational tolerance, the risk of rejection endangering patient and/or graft survival, particularly in the setting of baseline graft function that is both normal and stable, is a dominant concern. In the case of tolerance-induction efforts, there is substantial reluctance to expose children to novel agents and/or treatments of unproven safety and/or efficacy.

From a scientific perspective, 1 of the primary obstacles to more rapid progress in tolerance after solid organ transplantation is the absence of validated biomarkers that predict or indicate the tolerant state. The availability of a fingerprint would substantially increase the safety of immunosuppression withdrawal to uncover either spontaneous or induced tolerance. Moreover, as the durability of spontaneous and operational tolerance remains unknown, an assay of immune status or function would be highly desirable as a monitoring tool. It is indeed exciting that gene expression signatures seem to be emerging for spontaneous tolerance after kidney and liver transplantation. However, enthusiasm is somewhat curbed by several considerations. First, these signatures have yet to be prospectively validated. Second, there is no information as to when after transplantation and under what circumstances the tolerance biomarker might emerge. Third, the currently available data from liver and kidney recipients suggest that the tolerance fingerprint may be unique to each transplanted organ, and therefore would need to be individually derived. Fourth, as the tolerance fingerprint likely reflects specific mechanism(s) of tolerance, the fingerprint of spontaneous tolerance may differ from that of induced tolerance. Gene expression profiles have been derived, thus far, from adult cohorts, and they may well be irrelevant for the pediatric population who may have alternative avenues to achieve tolerance.

Therefore, what are the true prospects for tolerance after solid organ transplantation for children? In spite of the obstacles outlined earlier, the authors believe that the critical groundwork has been laid for steady and stepwise progress toward the holy grail. In our opinion, for children, spontaneous tolerance after liver transplantation is the least treacherous terrain that should be traversed first. Establishing the safety and efficacy of immunosuppression withdrawal and deriving a robust signature of tolerance should be the first goals. Dissecting the signature to elucidate the operational mechanism(s) underlying spontaneous tolerance after liver transplantation will undoubtedly guide subsequent trials that will, gradually and safely, expand the benefits of tolerance to an increasing number of pediatric organ transplant recipients.

REFERENCES

1. Guild WR, Harrison JH, Merrill JP, et al. Successful homotransplantation of the kidney in an identical twin. Trans Am Clin Climatol Assoc 1955;67:167–73.
2. Michon L, Hamburger J, Oeconomos N, et al. [An attempted kidney transplantation in man: medical and biological aspects]. Presse Med 1953;61(70):1419–23.

3. Billingham RE, Brent L, Medawar PB. Actively acquired tolerance of foreign cells. Nature 1953;172(4379):603–6.
4. Bartosh SM, Ryckman FC, Shaddy R, et al. A national conference to determine research priorities in pediatric solid organ transplantation. Pediatr Transplant 2008;12(2):153–66.
5. Traum AZ, Kawai T, Vacanti JP, et al. The need for tolerance in pediatric organ transplantation. Pediatrics 2008;121(6):1258–60.
6. von Boehmer H. The developmental biology of T lymphocytes. Annu Rev Immunol 1988;6:309–26.
7. Murphy K, Travers P, Walport M, editors. Janeway's immunobiology. 7th edition. New York, London: Garland Science; 2007.
8. Dunon D, Courtois D, Vainio O, et al. Ontogeny of the immune system: gamma/delta and alpha/beta T cells migrate from thymus to the periphery in alternating waves. J Exp Med 1997;186(7):977–88.
9. Melchers F, ten Boekel E, Seidl T, et al. Repertoire selection by pre-B-cell receptors and B-cell receptors, and genetic control of B-cell development from immature to mature B cells. Immunol Rev 2000;175:33–46.
10. Peterson P, Org T, Rebane A. Transcriptional regulation by AIRE: molecular mechanisms of central tolerance. Nat Rev Immunol 2008;8(12):948–57.
11. Goodnow CC, Crosbie J, Jorgensen H, et al. Induction of self-tolerance in mature peripheral B lymphocytes. Nature 1989;342(6248):385–91.
12. Russell DM, Dembic Z, Morahan G, et al. Peripheral deletion of self-reactive B cells. Nature 1991;354(6351):308–11.
13. Tinckam KJ, Sayegh MH. Transplantation tolerance in pediatric recipients: lessons and challenges. Pediatr Transplant 2005;9(1):17–27.
14. Wells AD. New insights into the molecular basis of T cell anergy: anergy factors, avoidance sensors, and epigenetic imprinting. J Immunol 2009;182(12):7331–41.
15. Sakaguchi S, Yamaguchi T, Nomura T, et al. Regulatory T cells and immune tolerance. Cell 2008;133(5):775–87.
16. Feng G, Chan T, Wood KJ, et al. Donor reactive regulatory T cells. Curr Opin Organ Transplant 2009;14(4):432–8.
17. Fehr T, Sykes M. Clinical experience with mixed chimerism to induce transplantation tolerance. Transpl Int 2008;21(12):1118–35.
18. Millan MT, Shizuru JA, Hoffmann P, et al. Mixed chimerism and immunosuppressive drug withdrawal after HLA-mismatched kidney and hematopoietic progenitor transplantation. Transplantation 2002;73(9):1386–91.
19. Scandling JD, Busque S, Dejbakhsh-Jones S, et al. Tolerance and chimerism after renal and hematopoietic-cell transplantation. N Engl J Med 2008;358(4):362–8.
20. Fudaba Y, Spitzer TR, Shaffer J, et al. Myeloma responses and tolerance following combined kidney and nonmyeloablative marrow transplantation: in vivo and in vitro analyses. Am J Transplant 2006;6(9):2121–33.
21. Kawai T, Cosimi AB, Spitzer TR, et al. HLA-mismatched renal transplantation without maintenance immunosuppression. N Engl J Med 2008;358(4):353–61.
22. Buhler L, Alwayn IP, Appel JZ 3rd, et al. Anti-CD154 monoclonal antibody and thromboembolism. Transplantation 2001;71(3):491.
23. Nagahama K, Fehervari Z, Oida T, et al. Differential control of allo-antigen-specific regulatory T cells and effector T cells by anti-CD4 and other agents in establishing transplantation tolerance. Int Immunol 2009;21(4):379–91.
24. Battaglia M, Stabilini A, Roncarolo MG. Rapamycin selectively expands CD4+CD25+FoxP3+ regulatory T cells. Blood 2005;105(12):4743–8.

25. Haxhinasto S, Mathis D, Benoist C. The AKT-mTOR axis regulates de novo differentiation of CD4+Foxp3+ cells. J Exp Med 2008;205(3):565–74.
26. Gao W, Lu Y, El Essawy B, et al. Contrasting effects of cyclosporine and rapamycin in de novo generation of alloantigen-specific regulatory T cells. Am J Transplant 2007;7(7):1722–32.
27. Yoshizawa A, Ito A, Li Y, et al. The roles of CD25+CD4+ regulatory T cells in operational tolerance after living donor liver transplantation. Transplant Proc 2005; 37(1):37–9.
28. Owens ML, Maxwell JG, Goodnight J, et al. Discontinuance of immunosuppression in renal transplant patients. Arch Surg 1975;110(12):1450–1.
29. Zoller KM, Cho SI, Cohen JJ, et al. Cessation of immunosuppressive therapy after successful transplantation: a national survey. Kidney Int 1980;18(1): 110–4.
30. Starzl TE, Demetris AJ, Trucco M, et al. Chimerism and donor-specific nonreactivity 27 to 29 years after kidney allotransplantation. Transplantation 1993;55(6): 1272–7.
31. Brouard S, Mansfield E, Braud C, et al. Identification of a peripheral blood transcriptional biomarker panel associated with operational renal allograft tolerance. Proc Natl Acad Sci U S A 2007;104(39):15448–53.
32. Roussey-Kesler G, Giral M, Moreau A, et al. Clinical operational tolerance after kidney transplantation. Am J Transplant 2006;6(4):736–46.
33. Bertolino P, McCaughan GW, Bowen DG. Role of primary intrahepatic T-cell activation in the 'liver tolerance effect'. Immunol Cell Biol 2002;80(1):84–92.
34. Crispe IN. Hepatic T cells and liver tolerance. Nat Rev Immunol 2003;3(1):51–62.
35. Calne RY, Sells RA, Pena JR, et al. Induction of immunological tolerance by porcine liver allografts. Nature 1969;223(205):472–6.
36. Kamada N, Davies HS, Roser B. Reversal of transplantation immunity by liver grafting. Nature 1981;292(5826):840–2.
37. Assy N, Adams PC, Myers P, et al. Randomized controlled trial of total immunosuppression withdrawal in liver transplant recipients: role of ursodeoxycholic acid. Transplantation 2007;83(12):1571–6.
38. Devlin J, Doherty D, Thomson L, et al. Defining the outcome of immunosuppression withdrawal after liver transplantation. Hepatology 1998;27(4):926–33.
39. Eason JD, Cohen AJ, Nair S, et al. Tolerance: is it worth the risk? Transplantation 2005;79(9):1157–9.
40. Girlanda R, Rela M, Williams R, et al. Long-term outcome of immunosuppression withdrawal after liver transplantation. Transplant Proc 2005;37(4):1708–9.
41. Martinez-Llordella M, Puig-Pey I, Orlando G, et al. Multiparameter immune profiling of operational tolerance in liver transplantation. Am J Transplant 2007; 7(2):309–19.
42. Mazariegos GV, Reyes J, Marino IR, et al. Weaning of immunosuppression in liver transplant recipients. Transplantation 1997;63(2):243–9.
43. Orlando G, Manzia T, Baiocchi L, et al. The Tor Vergata weaning off immunosuppression protocol in stable HCV liver transplant patients: the updated follow up at 78 months. Transpl Immunol 2008;20(1–2):43–7.
44. Ramos HC, Reyes J, Abu-Elmagd K, et al. Weaning of immunosuppression in long-term liver transplant recipients. Transplantation 1995;59(2):212–7.
45. Sandborn WJ, Hay JE, Porayko MK, et al. Cyclosporine withdrawal for nephrotoxicity in liver transplant recipients does not result in sustained improvement in kidney function and causes cellular and ductopenic rejection. Hepatology 1994;19(4):925–32.

46. Takatsuki M, Uemoto S, Inomata Y, et al. Weaning of immunosuppression in living donor liver transplant recipients. Transplantation 2001;72(3):449–54.

47. Tisone G, Orlando G, Cardillo A, et al. Complete weaning off immunosuppression in HCV liver transplant recipients is feasible and favourably impacts on the progression of disease recurrence. J Hepatol 2006;44(4):702–9.

48. Tryphonopoulos P, Tzakis AG, Weppler D, et al. The role of donor bone marrow infusions in withdrawal of immunosuppression in adult liver allotransplantation. Am J Transplant 2005;5(3):608–13.

49. Starzl TE, Demetris AJ, Trucco M, et al. Cell migration and chimerism after whole-organ transplantation: the basis of graft acceptance. Hepatology 1993;17(6): 1127–52.

50. Li Y, Koshiba T, Yoshizawa A, et al. Analyses of peripheral blood mononuclear cells in operational tolerance after pediatric living donor liver transplantation. Am J Transplant 2004;4(12):2118–25.

51. Koshiba T, Li Y, Takemura M, et al. Clinical, immunological, and pathological aspects of operational tolerance after pediatric living-donor liver transplantation. Transpl Immunol 2007;17(2):94–7.

52. Martinez-Llordella M, Lozano JJ, Puig-Pey I, et al. Using transcriptional profiling to develop a diagnostic test of operational tolerance in liver transplant recipients. J Clin Invest 2008;118(8):2845–57.

53. Pons JA, Yelamos J, Ramirez P, et al. Endothelial cell chimerism does not influence allograft tolerance in liver transplant patients after withdrawal of immunosuppression. Transplantation 2003;75(7):1045–7.

54. Mazariegos GV, Sindhi R, Thomson AW, et al. Clinical tolerance following liver transplantation: long term results and future prospects. Transpl Immunol 2007; 17(2):114–9.

55. Mazariegos GV. Withdrawal of immunosuppression in liver transplantation: lessons learned from PTLD. Pediatr Transplant 2004;8(3):210–3.

56. Demetris AJ, Lunz JG 3rd, Randhawa P, et al. Monitoring of human liver and kidney allograft tolerance: a tissue/histopathology perspective. Transpl Int 2009;22(1):120–41.

57. Evans HM, Kelly DA, McKiernan PJ, et al. Progressive histological damage in liver allografts following pediatric liver transplantation. Hepatology 2006;43(5): 1109–17.

58. Brouard S, Dupont A, Giral M, et al. Operationally tolerant and minimally immuno-suppressed kidney recipients display strongly altered blood T-cell clonal regulation. Am J Transplant 2005;5(2):330–40.

59. Seyfert-Margolis V, Turka LA. Marking a path to transplant tolerance. J Clin Invest 2008;118(8):2684–6.

Approach to Optimizing Growth, Rehabilitation, and Neurodevelopmental Outcomes in Children After Solid-organ Transplantation

Saeed Mohammad, MD*, Estella M. Alonso, MD

KEYWORDS

- Growth • Cognitive function • Quality of life
- Liver transplantation • Kidney transplantation
- Heart transplantation • Intestinal transplantation

One of the most critical differences between the posttransplant care of children and adults is the essential requirement in children to maintain a state of health that supports normal physical and psychological growth and development. Most children with organ failure have some degree of growth failure and developmental delay, which is not quickly reversed after successful transplantation. Thus, the challenge for clinicians caring for these children is to use strategies that minimize these deficits before transplantation and provide maximal opportunity for recovery of normal developmental processes during posttransplant rehabilitation. The effect of chronic organ failure, frequently complicated by malnutrition, on growth potential and cognitive development is poorly understood. Likewise, although immunosuppressive medications including corticosteroids and calcineurin inhibitors have known side effects that negatively affect growth and neurologic function the dose-response relationships of these medications and time course of their toxicities are still an area of active investigation. This review presents a summary of what is known regarding risk factors for suboptimal growth and development following solid-organ transplant and describes possible strategies to improve these outcomes.

Department of Pediatrics, Northwestern University Feinberg School of Medicine, Siragusa Transplant Center, Children's Memorial Hospital, 2300 Children's Plaza, Box 65, Chicago, IL 60614, USA
* Corresponding author.
E-mail address: smohammad@childrensmemorial.org

Pediatr Clin N Am 57 (2010) 539–557
doi:10.1016/j.pcl.2010.01.014
0031-3955/10/$ – see front matter © 2010 Elsevier Inc. All rights reserved.

pediatric.theclinics.com

GROWTH

Measurements of physical growth include height, weight, and lean muscle mass. Few studies of pediatric solid-organ transplantation recipients have included measurements of muscle mass, making it difficult to comment on this element of growth. Weight gain is a parameter that has been carefully studied and it seems to be an aspect of growth that recovers fully in patients with adequate graft function, despite a history of previous malnutrition. Therefore, this review focuses on optimizing linear growth following transplantation in recipients of kidney, liver, cardiac, lung, and intestinal transplantation.

Kidney Recipients

There are multiple factors that impair linear growth in children with chronic kidney disease, including inadequate nutritional intake, chronic acidosis, renal osteodystrophy, and growth hormone resistance. Improvements in the care of children with end-stage renal disease (ESRD) targeting these clinical problems have reduced the severity of growth retardation in children approaching renal transplantation. Data collected through the North American Pediatric Renal Trials Collaborative (NAPRTCS) show the improvement in linear growth in children with ESRD in the past 20 years.[1] The mean height standard deviation score (SDS or z score) at the time of initial transplant has improved from a −2.4 in 1987 to −1.3 in the 2007 cohort (**Fig. 1**). Catch-up growth has been demonstrated in the youngest recipients, with a mean increase in height SDS of 0.55 for those aged 2 to 5 years and 0.66 for those aged 0 to 1 year by 2 years after transplant.[1] However, children older than 6 years at the time of transplant exhibit almost no increase in SDS for height in the early posttransplant period (**Fig. 2**).

Several factors have been identified that adversely affect catch-up linear growth following kidney transplant. A recent review by Fine[2] details early age at transplant,

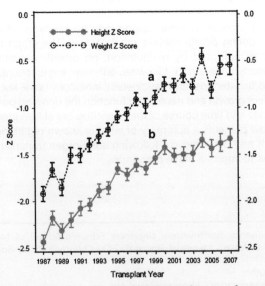

Fig. 1. Standardized *z* scores at time of kidney transplant by year of transplant. (a) Improvement in weight *z* scores at time of kidney transplant from −1.91 to −0.54. (b) Improvement in height *z* scores from −2.43 to −1.33. (*Courtesy of* NAPRTCS [North American Pediatric Renal Trials and Collaborative Studies]. https://web.emmes.com/study/ped/; with permission.)

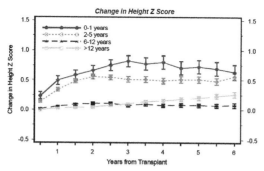

Fig. 2. Change in baseline height z scores by age at kidney transplant. The greatest change in scores occurs in the 0- to 1-year age group with rapid growth in the first 2 years after kidney transplant. Patients aged 6 to 12 years and greater than 12 years have stable linear growth. (*Courtesy of* NAPRTCS [North American Pediatric Renal Trials and Collaborative Studies]. https://web.emmes.com/study/ped/; with permission.)

maintenance of normal graft function, and early withdrawal of corticosteroids as measures that improve final height. However, patients who are transplanted later in childhood are less likely to achieve their predicted adult height despite these strategies.

Steroid-sparing strategies have been shown to be safe and effective in pediatric kidney recipients with a 5-year graft survival of 88%, which is comparable with current NAPRTCS data.[3] Steroid-sparing regimens improve catch-up growth at 1 year after transplant for patients aged 0 to 15 years with continued improvement up to 2 years in a subset of patients aged 0 to 5 years. Children less than 5 years of age also show an increase in height percentiles at 6 and 12 months when compared with patients on steroid-based therapy.[4] The effectiveness of recombinant human growth hormone (rhGH) therapy to promote growth in growth-stunted children is reasonably well established.[5–8] Serum insulinlike growth factor 1 (IGF-1) levels are increased in response to rhGH therapy; however, in many patients there seems to be a dose-dependent IGF-1 insensitivity resulting from prolonged corticosteroid exposure.[9] Studies with rhGH have demonstrated an improvement in final height without an increased risk of kidney dysfunction.[9,10] A significant increase in lipoprotein(a) levels, a risk factor for cardiovascular disease, has also been noted, but without corresponding increases in serum cholesterol and triglyceride levels.[10–12]

Of all clinical interventions, transplantation in children before age 6 years has the greatest beneficial effect on subsequent statural growth.[13–17] There is speculation that timing transplantation to ensure an optimal pubertal growth spurt is key. As detailed earlier, ensuring adequate nutrition, minimizing steroid exposure, and administering rhGH to the most growth-retarded recipients are also important strategies to maximize linear growth.[5,6,13,18,19] However, despite these interventions up to 25% of children do not reach their predicted adult height based on midparental height values.[2]

Liver Recipients

Linear growth failure in children with cirrhosis seems to be mediated in part by growth hormone resistance.[20] Malnutrition caused by fat malabsorption, abnormal nitrogen metabolism, and increased energy expenditure, which are all well-established features of end-stage liver disease in children, are also important determinants of growth failure in these patients. Following successful liver transplantation, GH, and IGF-I levels return to normal and the rate of linear growth improves.[21] However, it seems that many children do not achieve their height potential even years after transplantation.

Similar to kidney transplant recipients there does seem to have been an improvement in mean height z scores at the time of transplant and in catch-up growth for children with end-stage liver disease (**Fig. 3**). When examining height z scores in cohorts including children transplanted in the 1990s the mean height z score at transplant is approximately −1.5.[22–24] Separating patients by era of transplant reveals that with more recent experience, the mean height z scores are similar at transplant, but catch-up growth is more accelerated and prolonged. Catch-up growth is usually not observed until the second 12 months following liver transplantation.[22,23] Catch-up proceeds through intermediate follow-up after transplant (2–3 years) and then stalls, leaving up to 25% of these patients with heights that are less than the 5% for age in long-term follow-up. A recent multivariate analysis of patients included in the Studies of Pediatric Liver Transplant (SPLIT) registry revealed that linear growth impairment was more likely in patients with metabolic disease (odds ratio [OR] 4.4) and greater than 18 months of steroids exposure (OR 3.02). Higher percentiles for weight (OR 0.80) and height (OR 0.62) at liver transplantation were protective. Less linear catch-up growth was observed in patients with metabolic diseases, cholestatic diseases other than biliary atresia, and lower weight and higher height percentiles before liver transplantation. Prolonged steroid exposure and increased calculated glomerular filtration rate were also associated with less catch-up growth. However, the strongest predictors of catch-up growth following liver transplantation seem to be weight and height z scores at transplant. Patients with lower weight percentiles exhibit less growth acceleration, suggesting that complications of malnutrition must be reversed before catch-up growth is achievable. Conversely, patients with lower height percentiles at transplant exhibit more linear growth acceleration in early follow-up. Previous reports examining the relationships between pre- and posttransplant growth have been inconclusive, with some investigators reporting pretransplant

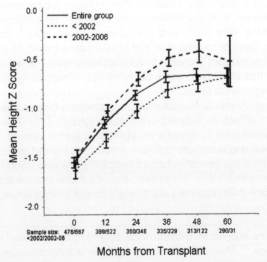

Fig. 3. Mean height z scores at liver transplant for 5 years after transplant. There is an increase in velocity of growth in the first 3 years after liver transplant, which is more accelerated and prolonged in the more recent cohort of liver transplant recipients. (*Courtesy of* SPLIT; with permission.)

growth failure to have a positive effect[23,25] and others reporting a negative effect.[26] Experience from the SPLIT registry suggests both observations may be valid. Children with more severe growth arrest before transplant have the most to recover, and without other limitations, the acceleration of their posttransplant linear growth may be more pronounced than that of patients with growth patterns closer to normal before transplant. However, even with an above-average degree of catch-up growth following transplant, patients with the lowest height percentiles at transplant would be less likely to achieve normal percentiles after transplant. Thus, catch-up growth occurs, but is incomplete.

Improvements in growth have been achieved with steroid withdrawal or discontinuation and by supplemental use of rhGH therapy.[27–30] rhGH treatment response has been sustained in the second and third treatment years without advancing the bone age beyond chronologic age, suggesting that prolonged rhGH therapy does not have a negative effect on duration of linear growth and adult height potential.[31] As in the kidney transplant population, concerns that rhGH may contribute to development of late allograft rejection have not been validated. However, these measures may not be enough to improve final height because up to 50% of recipients have a final adult height that is 1.3 SD lower than their genetic potential.[32] Studies examining the effect of transplant during or just before accelerated pubertal growth are forthcoming. However, in liver transplantation, which still includes a significant risk of early postoperative mortality, it is not clear that early transplantation to avoid adult short stature would be reasonable. Yet, preferential allocation of organs to patients at highest risk of posttransplant growth failure who also meet the standard indications for transplantation could have a significant positive effect.

Heart Recipients

Growth outcomes in pediatric heart transplantation have been encouraging and some reports have suggested that delayed linear growth may be less of a problem for heart recipients than liver or kidney recipients.[33–37] This phenomenon may be related to the practice of eliminating chronic steroid treatment in most patients and the dichotomy of ages at which children receive heart transplants, with very young children undergoing early transplantation to correct congenital disease and older children with acutely acquired cardiac disease undergoing transplantation before they develop chronic growth impairment. Both groups of heart transplant patients thus avoid the growth-retarding effects of disease during their most critical developmental years.[38–41]

Peterson[42] studied 46 heart transplant recipients less than 11 years of age and found that mean z scores for height were fairly static during the first 2 years after cardiac transplantation with a mean of -0.7 at transplant and -1.3 at 2 years' follow-up (**Fig. 4**). This analysis identified prolonged steroid exposure as a negative predictor and age at transplant as a positive predictor for height z score, with older patients showing more catch-up growth. Another report by Cohen and colleagues[43] examined bone age in patients transplanted before and after age 7 years and did not find a difference in height z scores based on age at transplant; however, these investigators did report worsening delay of bone age at 4 years after transplant in patients transplanted before age 7 years. For those who are growth delayed, rhGH may be used to improve growth velocity.[44]

Lung Recipients

As most older patients requiring lung transplantation are children with cystic fibrosis, it is not surprising that they also have suboptimal growth at the time of transplant. The indications for lung transplant in infants and toddlers are commonly alveolar

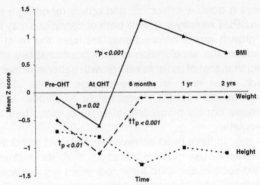

Fig. 4. Growth parameter trends from before orthotopic heart transplant (OHT) to 2 years after OHT. There was no significant change in mean height z score with time. Significant changes in mean weight and body mass index (BMI) z score are denoted by P values along the slopes between time points. *, mean BMI z score at pre-OHT versus at OHT; **, mean BMI z score at OHT versus 6 months after OHT; †, mean weight z score at pre-OHT versus at OHT; ††, mean weight z score at OHT versus 6 months after OHT. (*From* Peterson RE, Perens GS, Alejos JC, et al. Growth and weight gain of prepubertal children after cardiac transplantation. Pediatr Transplant 2008;12(4):438; with permission.)

proteinosis and interstitial diseases of infancy. A recent single-center study reported worsening of height z scores from −1.89 at time of transplant to −2.14 at 5 years after transplant.[45] This study focused on infants and toddlers and did not report data for older children who underwent lung transplantation. An older study from the same center reported growth at 64% of predicted values.[46] rhGH cannot be used in this group because of concern about bronchiolitis obliterans, which is the leading cause of retransplantation and death in children more than 3 years of age following lung transplantation.[45]

Intestine Recipients

Despite improvement in graft and patient survival, growth of the intestinal transplant recipient remains poor. This situation may be related to their primary disease which is commonly short bowel syndrome or because many are born prematurely. A positive trend in z scores for height/length was observed in only 26% of intestinal transplantation survivors in 1 study,[47] although another reported normal growth in 50% and catch-up growth in 15%.[48] There are no data on strategies to further improve growth, and prospective long-term data such as are collected with NAPRTCS and SPLIT are unavailable.

Summary of Growth

Further studies are needed to establish the optimal window for steroid withdrawal, and determine which long-term drug regimens preserve function of the transplanted organ and allow normal statural growth of the recipient. The observation that catch-up growth slows after the first few years following transplantation and that a large percentage of kidney and liver transplant recipients do not reach their predicted target adult height also warrants further investigation. Immunosuppression strategies that include limited steroid exposure seem to be safe in most forms of solid-organ transplantation and may significantly improve a patient's catch-up growth potential. The long-term effect of calcineurin inhibitors on linear growth is not known because there has been minimal opportunity to compare growth between children who have and have not received this therapy following transplantation. Treatment with rhGH should be considered for patients with slow catch-up growth who seem to be at risk for final adult height that is less than the fifth percentile. The timing of transplantation is critically important for children with ESRD and may also improve posttransplant growth in children with chronic liver disease and advancing signs of malnutrition.

Primary care providers play a critical role in monitoring growth of the pediatric solid-organ transplant recipient and ensuring that these patients achieve maximal nutritional rehabilitation. Setting expectations for linear growth and assisting the transplant team in recognizing suboptimal growth are important contributions to the overall care of these patients. The same programs that these providers implement to educate the families of healthy children regarding nutritional goals can be valuable for transplant recipients as well. Primary care providers should assist in monitoring for the long-term side effects of chronic steroid exposure, including decreased bone density, short stature, obesity, and metabolic syndrome. Their knowledge of community resources and their long-term relationship with the other family members are an invaluable resource in patient management of growth-related issues.

COGNITIVE FUNCTION

Developmental outcomes can be measured in several ways dependent on the age at testing. Measures of infant development focus on motor function, social and environmental interaction, and language development, whereas older children can be tested for intelligence, academic achievement, behavior, and adaptation skills. Abnormalities that are observed later in childhood are more predictive of static deficits that will persist into adulthood. Many forms of chronic disease in childhood can have a negative effect on cognitive development. Children who experience solid-organ failure during infancy may be at particular risk for cognitive delay because they experience the onset of their illness during a period of rapid neurologic maturation.

Kidney

Chronic renal failure is believed to have a negative effect on neurocognitive development, which may be alleviated by renal transplantation. Intelligence levels in children following kidney transplant are usually in the normal to low-normal range, with 1 study reporting a mean full scale intelligence quotient (FSIQ) of 87[49] (normative mean 100, SD 15) and a more recent study reporting 19 of 27 patients with normal IQ and 6 of 27 patients with an IQ only 1 SD less than normal.[50] It has been suggested that renal transplant recipients have lower verbal compared with nonverbal performance, shorter attention spans, and difficulty with memory, especially those who have had renal disease since birth.[49] In children who were older at the time of transplant significant deficits have been observed in performance IQ, which measures intellectual ability that is less dependent on one's fund of knowledge, vocabulary, and basic knowledge and more dependent on fluid mental abilities.[50] Early onset of renal disease, longer duration on dialysis, pretransplant morbidity (eg, seizures)[49] and lower socioeconomic status are believed to have a negative effect on developmental outcome.[51–53] Early transplant may mitigate some of these deficits and has been shown to improve head circumference from an SDS of -1.4 to -0.9 ($P = .02$) and significantly improve gross motor, social, and language development quotients ($P = .02–0.0006$) in infants 1 year after transplant.[54]

Following renal transplantation, approximately 70% of patients receive routine classroom instruction,[49,51] whereas the remainder require some special educational support[51] or have a history of serious neurologic morbidity such as stroke.[49] Several long-term studies have reported final education levels that are lower than national averages,[55,56] whereas others[57] have revealed education levels that were similar to the general population and their sibling controls.

Liver

Onset of chronic liver disease in infancy is believed to increase the risk of neurocognitive delay, which may persist even after successful liver transplantation. Children who have survived transplantation are more likely to have intelligence that is significantly lower than healthy children.[58-62] Infants, while awaiting transplant, have mental and motor developmental scores that are within the low average range,[63] which then drop even further in the posttransplant period and recover to pretransplant levels only at 12 months after the procedure. This observation suggests that infant recipients do not exhibit developmental catch-up until after the first posttransplant year. This study also demonstrated that infants with longer hospitalizations and those with growth impairment at transplant had more significant delays.[63] In long-term follow-up after transplantation, multiple small, single-center studies have demonstrated that patients have IQ scores in the low normal range, with 10% to 15% having IQ scores that indicate significant mental disability (IQ <70) (**Table 1**). Krull and colleagues[60] compared a group who received liver transplantation during early childhood with those with cystic fibrosis and found age at transplant to be a significant risk factor for delayed language skills. Patients also had lower verbal IQ and FSIQ scores than patients with cystic fibrosis. Kaller and colleagues[59] performed intelligence testing in a group of children who underwent transplant at a mean age of 32 months and reported mean intelligence scores that were not statistically significant from a normal population. These findings suggested that patients who receive liver transplantation in the current era may not be at the same risk for developmental delay as those transplanted 10 to 15 years ago. However, a recent article focusing on children with infantile onset of chronic liver disease[66] who were transplanted before age 6 months revealed even higher rates of developmental delay than that observed in many older studies, with only 46% having normal intelligence. These investigators also found that older children had lower composite FSIQ that was also associated with growth failure and increased days of high-trough calcineurin inhibitors levels. The Functional Outcomes Group (FOG) is an ancillary study conducted through a multicenter SPLIT registry focusing on the measurement of health-related quality of life (HRQOL) and cognitive outcomes in pediatric liver transplant recipients. It is the first multicenter study addressing these outcomes in any pediatric solid-organ transplant cohort. Through the SPLIT/FOG collaborative, longitudinal developmental testing has been performed on a group of 140 patients who received liver transplantation at the age 5 years or younger. Preliminary results from the first 92 patients tested confirm that mean FSIQ is significantly lower than population norms, but within the low normal range (93.8±14.5). Within

Table 1
Percentage of pediatric liver transplant recipients with serious developmental delay

References	Publication Year	Number of Patients (% Biliary Atresia)	IQ <70 (%)
Kennard et al[64]	1999	50 (50)	18
Gritti et al[65]	2001	18 (67)	0
Adeback et al[58]	2003	21 (38)	14
Krull et al[60]	2003	15 (87)	13

this group, 28% had evidence of mild to moderate delay (IQ ≤85) and 5% had evidence of serious delay (IQ ≤70) compared with the expected prevalence in the general population of 14% and 2%, respectively.

Analyses of risk factors for developmental delay in the more contemporary transplant experience included in the FOG study are under way. Previous studies suggest that younger children (those <6 months of age) with a shorter duration of illness, less evidence of malnourishment before transplant, and those with shorter hospital stays have a better prognosis regarding their cognitive functioning.[59,67]

Heart Recipients

Studies performed in children with cyanotic heart disease consistently show that chronic cyanosis is associated with progressive cognitive impairment and that earlier correction of cyanotic heart disease leads to more favorable cognitive outcomes.[68–70] Other factors including circulatory arrest, cardiopulmonary bypass, and embolic events have also been associated with lower than expected developmental outcomes.[71–74] Data are just now emerging regarding the developmental progress of these patients, primarily infants, following cardiac transplantation, which is discussed in a recent review.[75] In general, reports describing developmental outcomes in children who have received cardiac transplantation suggest these patients have intelligence in the low to normal range which is comparable with other children with surgically corrected congenital heart disease.[75] However, up to 10% may have significant neurologic injury, which could preclude testing. Freier and colleagues[76] in 2004 reported the longitudinal neurodevelopmental assessment, using the Bayley scales, of 39 patients transplanted as young infants (median age at transplant 53 days). Patients were tested 4 to 6 weeks after transplant and then every 6 to 12 months thereafter. The mean Mental Developmental Index (MDI) of the group was within normal limits and the mean Psychomotor Developmental Index (PDI) was in the mildly delayed range. Wray and Radley-Smith[77] in 2006 reported a longitudinal assessment of 34 patients who received heart and lung transplants spanning a wide age range from 1.3 to 15.3 years. Cognitive function and academic achievement were tested at 12 and 36 months after transplant. Mean scores of intelligence and academic achievement were within the normal range and appeared stable during the testing period, with the exception of a decrease in arithmetical scores for younger children. Several studies have examined risk factors for lower cognitive outcomes, finding that circulatory arrest, birth head circumference, prolonged hospital stay, cardiopulmonary bypass, embolic events, waiting time to transplant, and pretransplant diagnosis are all potentially associated with variability in developmental outcomes in this patient group.[71–75,77] Studies that have examined the effect of primary diagnosis suggest that patients transplanted for cardiomyopathy typically have higher scores than those with a history of cyanotic congenital heart disease.

Despite the encouraging results of studies examining intelligence in this patient group, the school performance of cardiac transplant recipients seems to be lower than healthy children and the prevalence of behavior problems may increase with time after transplantation.[78] Ikle and colleagues[79] studied 26 children who had received cardiac transplantation for hypoplastic left heart syndrome using the Vineland scales. The analysis found that many scored greater than 1 SD less than the mean for measures of daily living skills (39%), socialization (29%), communication skills (48%), and adaptive behavior (52%). These findings suggest that interventions that target improvement in these skill areas might improve functional outcomes, including school function in this population.

Lung Recipients

Lung transplant recipients have not been studied so extensively as cardiac recipients. As mentioned earlier, Wray and Radley-Smith[77] have reported means scores for intelligence and academic achievement in the normal range. Another study that focused on a cohort of infants and toddlers who underwent lung transplantation found that 50% to 60% of infants and 70% to 80% of the toddlers had developmental levels that ranged from normal to mild delay.[45]

Intestine

Intestinal transplant patients are at high risk for cognitive delay[80–82] and patients may display worsening developmental delay in the first 2 months[80] after transplant, similar to what has been reported in liver transplant recipients. Multivisceral transplant recipients are also more delayed than infants receiving liver-only transplantation.[81] These patients generally recover more slowly and have undergone a more extensive surgical procedure than patients receiving liver, heart, or kidney transplantation. Some patients may have an ostomy that necessitates repeat surgery for closure. Many continue to require parenteral nutrition while the transplanted intestine adapts to its new environment. Thus, intestinal recipients have a larger burden of chronic disease than other solid-organ recipients, which may contribute to the slower developmental rehabilitation. Common risk factors experienced by infants with end-stage liver disease compounded by chronic malnutrition and prolonged hospitalization and prematurity likely play an important role.

Summary of Cognitive Function

The existing body of literature examining neurodevelopmental outcomes in pediatric solid-organ transplant recipients is growing. The need to use different scales to measure cognitive ability in different age groups coupled with the small sample sizes available to study make it difficult to reach comprehensive conclusions. Children who receive heart transplantation may have better cognitive outcomes than expected considering the results of older studies of children with cyanotic congenital heart disease. The cognitive outcomes of liver and kidney transplant recipients may also be improving, but many still require special educational resources. Infants requiring intestine or liver and intestine transplant are probably at the highest risk for cognitive delay, but longitudinal studies that affirm that these delays are not recoverable are lacking. In all cases neurologic comorbidities increase the risk of delay. Despite recent advances, a significant proportion of liver and heart recipients have serious developmental delay or neurologic injury. Risk factors for developmental delay are still being examined, but strategies that limit the duration of unsupported organ failure and chronic malnutrition, especially during infancy, are likely to have a positive effect.

Solid-organ transplant recipients display a wide range of developmental outcomes, which include patients with normal development and those with significant delays. Although the exact mechanisms that contribute to these delays are not fully elucidated factors such as long-term hospitalization, chronic malnutrition in the pretransplant period, and a history of surgical complications likely all play a role. The primary care physician is an important partner in assisting in the early diagnosis of developmental delay and in facilitating appropriate evaluation and intervention within the patient's community. Early intervention with physical and occupational therapy can curtail physical disabilities. Prompt recognition of cognitive delay and abnormal school function can aid in securing special educational resources early in their academic experience. Again, setting expectations for the family and school system regarding cognitive outcomes is an important aspect of their anticipatory health care.

REHABILITATION AND QUALITY OF LIFE

Organ transplantation saves lives and reverses terminal illness, but the posttransplant condition is not equal to that of healthy children, and these patients struggle in a chronic health condition that can include physical and developmental deficits. Many patients who were transplanted as children are now surviving into young adulthood, gaining independence and joining the workforce. Functional outcomes include specific measures of everyday living, such as social and school functioning, which are components of generic HRQOL. Functional outcomes can also include results of direct patient testing of physical skills and cognitive status. All of these constructs are essential components of rehabilitation following transplant and it is important to examine functional outcomes of this growing population not only in intermediate follow-up during childhood but also in long-term follow-up as these children mature to adulthood.

Kidney

Several reports of pediatric patients with ESRD confirm that kidney transplant recipients experience a higher level of HRQOL than patients who continue hemodialysis or peritoneal dialysis with moderate effect sizes.[83–86]

Some, but not all, studies comparing kidney transplant recipients with healthy controls reveal lower levels of HRQOL.[83,84,87,88] Patients report distress regarding their physical appearance and physical symptoms, difficulty with peer and family interactions, and school disruption as significant concerns.[89] Primary caregivers report a significant negative effect on their emotional state and limitations on family activities because of their child's health.[88,89] Significant discordance exists between child and parental reports of HRQOL, with parents tending to report lower physical and psychosocial function.[84,88] Although most pediatric kidney transplant recipients who have transitioned into adulthood seem to be satisfied with their quality of life and report successful interpersonal relationships[90,91] up to 83% report they suffer from anxiety, depression, or both.[57] They are more likely to be unemployed and less likely to live independently when compared with the general population.[55–57] A correlation has also been noted between final adult height and measures of functional outcomes, including educational level, paid activity, marital life, and independent housing.[55]

Liver

Initial studies reporting HRQOL in children following liver transplantation suggested good quality of life.[92–94] However, when pediatric liver transplant recipients are tested with validated instruments their reported levels of HRQOL are significantly lower than control populations.[22,95,96] SPLIT/FOG recently conducted a large cross-sectional analysis of generic HRQOL in 873 (363 self-report) pediatric liver transplant recipients between the ages of 2 and 18 years using the PedsQL (Mapi Research Institute, Lyon, France) generic core scales. The mean age of the patients included in the sample was 8.2 ± 4.4 years and 55% were female. The median interval from transplant to survey was 3.1 years. Outcomes were compared with a sample of healthy children randomly matched by age group, gender, and race/ethnicity (**Fig. 5**). The physical and psychosocial function of the liver transplant recipients compared favorably with children with other chronic pediatric illnesses, but were not equal to the healthy sample. The total scale score and subscales of the PedsQL 4.0 Generic Core Scales were all significantly lower than those of healthy children ($P<.001$), with effect sizes ranging from 0.25, for self-reported emotional functioning, to 0.68 for self-reported school functioning.[22] Effect sizes greater than 0.5 are considered moderate, with those approaching 0.8 considered large. The altered school function that is observed in this group

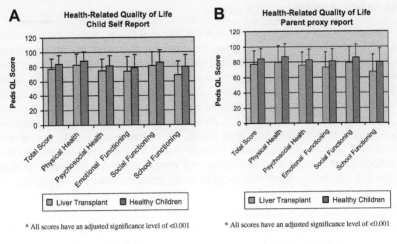

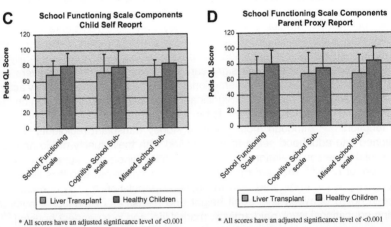

Fig. 5. Using the PedsQL generic core scales to assess quality of life in liver transplant recipients compared with a healthy sample matched for gender, race, and age. (*A*) Patient self-report (n = 363); patients report significantly lower scores when compared with healthy controls. (*B*) Parent proxy report (n = 869); parents report lower scores compared with healthy controls. (*C*) School functioning scale by patient self-report (n = 361); parents of liver transplant recipients report significantly lower scores than parents of healthy children with an effect size of 0.68. (*D*) School functioning scale parent proxy report (n = 746); parents of liver transplant recipients report significantly lower scores than parents of healthy children. (*Data from* Alonso EM, Limbers CA, Neighbors K, et al. Cross-sectional analysis of health-related quality of life in pediatric liver transplant recipients. J Pediatr 2009;156:270–6; with permission.)

may be secondary to an increased prevalence of developmental delay or learning disabilities. One study of long-term recipients aged 3 to 9 years revealed that almost 20% had an IQ of less than 70.[64] A recent survey of school outcomes conducted by the SPLIT network revealed that 40% have required some type of special educational services, with 8% having been classified as learning disabled and 5% having a reported IQ of less than 70. Missed school days may also contribute to compromised function. Data from the SPLIT network suggest that 30% to 40% of patients in long-term follow-up miss more than 10 days of school per year, with teenagers having the highest rate of absences.

Demographic as well as medical variables may predict levels of HRQOL in this population.[96–98] The effect of age on HRQOL in pediatric liver transplant recipients has been considered in several studies. In a small, multicenter report, younger survivors (< age 5 years) had physical and psychosocial health that was comparable with age-matched controls and higher than what was reported for older children in the same study. The SPLIT/FOG cross-sectional data set was analyzed to examine the effect of age at testing on parent report of HRQOL. Results suggest that age at testing may indeed have an important effect on HRQOL, with younger children having the highest scores (**Table 2**). The effect of age at testing seems to be more significant than interval from transplant. Initial results from multivariant analysis examining the effect of various factors on parent reported HRQOL in the SPLIT/FOG study identified single-parent household, length of initial hospitalization after transplant, older age, history of seizures, lower height z score at transplant, and days hospitalized in recent follow-up as negative predictors. The relationship between the patient's HRQOL and family dynamics bears further consideration. Studies that have included assessment of the effect of the child's health state on the parents have shown a considerable negative influence on parental emotional state and family life.[58,88,99] However, when formally measured, family function was found to be equal to that reported by a reference population.[99] These preliminary results suggest that services that support the parent's ability to cope with their child's health condition would likely improve the child's HRQOL. This strategy is especially important because the patient's level of HRQOL has been linked to adherence behaviors and possibly maintenance of graft function.[100]

Heart

Although it is reported that most patients adjust well after transplant, HRQOL has not been systematically studied. A recent study[101] of 23 adult patients who received heart transplants as children reported physical and mental health scores using the SF-36 (QualityMetric, Lincoln, RI, USA) that were similar to the general US population. Seventy percent lived with a parent or family member and had private medical insurance and all had completed high school.

Lung

Among lung transplant recipients there seems to be a significant percentage who have behavior problems at home, and decreased social competence with their peers, most commonly in male patients. The prevalence of depression has been explored, with reported rates of 23% at 1 year and 13% at the 3-year follow-up.[77,102]

Table 2
PedsQL 4.0 generic core scale scores by age at testing

Scale Score		<2 Years (n = 259)	2–4 Years (n = 254)	5–7 Years (n = 244)	≥8 Years (n = 169)
		Median (Interquartile Range)			
Total score	(P<.0001)	85.7 (73.8–94.4)	79.4 (63.0–90.2)	73.9 (59.8–84.2)	76.1 (59.8–88.0)
Physical health	(P<.0001)	93.8 (78.1–100.0)	87.5 (68.8–96.9)	83.3 (62.5–93.8)	81.3 (62.5–93.8)
Psychosocial health	(P<.0001)	82.7 (70.0–92.3)	76.7 (61.7–88.3)	69.2 (56.7–81.7)	73.3 (56.7–90.0)

Intestine

There is a dearth of literature on the assessment of quality of life after intestinal transplant. Scores for quality of life often deteriorate with time in patients on parenteral nutrition as complications, particularly liver disease, emerge. Conversely, after intestine transplantation, quality of life is reported to improve with time.[103] After the initial postoperative course, assessed quality of life was similar between patients dependent on parenteral nutrition and intestinal transplantation patients. In longitudinal follow-up, intestinal transplantation patients reported significant improvement in anxiety, sleep, and impulsiveness and control, which reflected a progressive adjustment to post-transplant status.[103] Parents of intestinal transplantation recipients have reported significant limitations in the physical and psychosocial well-being of their children, although the patients themselves reported little effect in most domains compared with other normal schoolchildren.[104] These investigators concluded that despite differences in life relative to their peers, these children do not find that these differences affect their functioning.

Summary of Rehabilitation and Quality of Life

The HRQOL and functional outcomes of children who have received solid-organ transplantation are lower than a normative population and seem to be most comparable with those of children with other chronic diseases. Parents of pediatric solid-organ transplant recipients experience stress related to their child's illness and tend to report functional outcomes that are lower than that reported by the children themselves. Age at the time of testing may have an influence on reporting of HRQOL, with parents of younger children reporting better functional outcomes. It seems that demographic factors have a significant effect on HRQOL and interventions that provide support and education for families caring for organ transplant recipients may improve outcomes for these children.

HRQOL is a global measure of how well patients feel, how they see themselves in relationship to others, and how they function within their environment. Despite good long-term patient and graft survival in solid-organ transplantation many recipients struggle with diminished HRQOL and suboptimal or incomplete rehabilitation. Data regarding long-term HRQOL in these pediatric groups are lacking and these children would be best served by a multicenter study design. The primary care provider, through their relationship with the family and other siblings, is well poised to assist families in determining needs for rehabilitation and social support. By facilitating evaluation and laboratory monitoring in the community, the primary provider may help to reduce the need for school absences and interruption of family activities. The primary provider can also help the family place their concerns within the context of those of parents of children with other chronic diseases and share intervention strategies that have improved functional outcomes for children with other more common diseases, such as asthma or diabetes.

REFERENCES

1. North American Pediatric Renal Trials and Collaborative Studies. Annual report 2008. Available at: https://web.emmes.com/study/ped/annlrept/annlrept.html. Accessed November 1, 2009.
2. Fine RN. Management of growth retardation in pediatric recipients of renal allografts. Nat Clin Pract Nephrol 2007;3(6):318–24.

3. Pedersen EB, El-Faramawi M, Foged N, et al. Avoiding steroids in pediatric renal transplantation: long-term experience from a single centre. Pediatr Transplant 2007;11(7):730–5.
4. Sarwal MM, Vidhun JR, Alexander SR, et al. Continued superior outcomes with modification and lengthened follow-up of a steroid-avoidance pilot with extended daclizumab induction in pediatric renal transplantation. Transplantation 2003;76(9):1331–9.
5. Ulinski T, Cochat P. Longitudinal growth in children following kidney transplantation: from conservative to pharmacological strategies. Pediatr Nephrol 2006; 21(7):903–9.
6. Haffner D, Schaefer F. Does recombinant growth hormone improve adult height in children with chronic renal failure? Semin Nephrol 2001;21(5):490–7.
7. Hokken-Koelega AC, Stijnen T, de Jong RC, et al. A placebo-controlled, double-blind trial of growth hormone treatment in prepubertal children after renal transplant. Kidney Int Suppl 1996;53:S128–34.
8. Maxwell H, Rees L. Randomised controlled trial of recombinant human growth hormone in prepubertal and pubertal renal transplant recipients. British Association for Pediatric Nephrology. Arch Dis Child 1998;79(6):481–7.
9. Clot JP, Crosnier H, Guest G, et al. Effects of growth hormone on growth factors after renal transplantation. Pediatr Nephrol 2001;16(5):397–403.
10. Motoyama O, Hasegawa A, Kawamura T, et al. Adult height of three renal transplant patients after growth hormone therapy. Clin Exp Nephrol 2007;11(4): 332–5.
11. Ghio L, Damiani B, Garavaglia R, et al. Lipid profile during rhGH therapy in pediatric renal transplant patients. Pediatr Transplant 2002;6(2):127–31.
12. Fine RN, Stablein D, Cohen AH, et al. Recombinant human growth hormone post-renal transplantation in children: a randomized controlled study of the NAPRTCS. Kidney Int 2002;62(2):688–96.
13. Melter M, Briscoe DM. Challenges after pediatric transplantation. Semin Nephrol 2000;20(2):199–208.
14. Ingelfinger JR, Grupe WE, Harmon WE, et al. Growth acceleration following renal transplantation in children less than 7 years of age. Pediatrics 1981; 68(2):255–9.
15. Tejani A, Fine R, Alexander S, et al. Factors predictive of sustained growth in children after renal transplantation. The North American Pediatric Renal Transplant Cooperative Study. J Pediatr 1993;122(3):397–402.
16. Tejani A, Sullivan K. Long-term follow-up of growth in children post-transplantation. Kidney Int Suppl 1993;43:S56–8.
17. Englund MS, Tyden G, Wikstad I, et al. Growth impairment at renal transplantation–a determinant of growth and final height. Pediatr Transplant 2003;7(3): 192–9.
18. Fine RN. Growth following solid-organ transplantation. Pediatr Transplant 2002; 6(1):47–52.
19. Harambat J, Cochat P. Growth after renal transplantation. Pediatr Nephrol 2009; 24(7):1297–306.
20. Maes M, Sokal E, Otte JB. Growth factors in children with end-stage liver disease before and after liver transplantation: a review. Pediatr Transplant 1997;1(2):171–5.
21. Sarna S, Laine J, Sipila I, et al. Differences in linear growth and cortisol production between liver and renal transplant recipients on similar immunosuppression. Transplantation 1995;60(7):656–61.

22. Alonso EM, Limbers CA, Neighbors K, et al. Cross-sectional analysis of health-related quality of life in pediatric liver transplant recipients. J Pediatr 2010; 156(2):270–6.
23. McDiarmid SV, Gornbein JA, DeSilva PJ, et al. Factors affecting growth after pediatric liver transplantation. Transplantation 1999;67(3):404–11.
24. Saito T, Mizuta K, Hishikawa S, et al. Growth curves of pediatric patients with biliary atresia following living donor liver transplantation: factors that influence post-transplantation growth. Pediatr Transplant 2007;11(7):764–70.
25. Bartosh SM, Thomas SE, Sutton MM, et al. Linear growth after pediatric liver transplantation. J Pediatr 1999;135(5):624–31.
26. Viner RM, Forton JT, Cole TJ, et al. Growth of long-term survivors of liver transplantation. Arch Dis Child 1999;80(3):235–40.
27. Balistreri WF, Bucuvalas JC, Ryckman FC. The effect of immunosuppression on growth and development. Liver Transpl Surg 1995;1(5 Suppl 1):64–73.
28. Kelly DA. Posttransplant growth failure in children. Liver Transpl Surg 1997; 3(5 Suppl 1):S32–9.
29. Reding R. Steroid withdrawal in liver transplantation: benefits, risks, and unanswered questions. Transplantation 2000;70(3):405–10.
30. Sarna S, Sipila I, Ronnholm K, et al. Recombinant human growth hormone improves growth in children receiving glucocorticoid treatment after liver transplantation. J Clin Endocrinol Metab 1996;81(4):1476–82.
31. Puustinen L, Jalanko H, Holmberg C, et al. Recombinant human growth hormone treatment after liver transplantation in childhood: the 5-year outcome. Transplantation 2005;79(9):1241–6.
32. Scheenstra R, Gerver WJ, Odink RJ, et al. Growth and final height after liver transplantation during childhood. J Pediatr Gastroenterol Nutr 2008;47(2): 165–71.
33. de Broux E, Huot CH, Chartrand S, et al. Growth after pediatric heart transplantation. Transplant Proc 2001;33(1–2):1735–7.
34. de Broux E, Huot CH, Chartrand S, et al. Growth and pubertal development following pediatric heart transplantation: a 15-year experience at Ste-Justine Hospital. J Heart Lung Transplant 2000;19(9):825–33.
35. Fortuna RS, Chinnock RE, Bailey LL. Heart transplantation among 233 infants during the first 6 months of life: the Loma Linda experience. Loma Linda Pediatric Heart Transplant Group. Clin Transpl 1999;263–72.
36. Hosenpud JD, Bennett LE, Keck BM, et al. The Registry of the International Society for Heart and Lung Transplantation: seventeenth official report-2000. J Heart Lung Transplant 2000;19(10):909–31.
37. Bauer J, Thul J, Kramer U, et al. Heart transplantation in children and infants: short-term outcome and long-term follow-up. Pediatr Transplant 2001;5(6): 457–62.
38. Baum D, Bernstein D, Starnes VA, et al. Pediatric heart transplantation at Stanford: results of a 15-year experience. Pediatrics 1991;88(2):203–14.
39. Baum M, Chinnock R, Ashwal S, et al. Growth and neurodevelopmental outcome of infants undergoing heart transplantation. J Heart Lung Transplant 1993;12(6 Pt 2):S211–7.
40. Chinnock R, Baum M. Somatic growth in infant heart transplant recipients. Pediatr Transplant 1998;2(1):30–4.
41. Ferrazzi P, Fiocchi R, Gamba A, et al. Pediatric heart transplantation without chronic maintenance steroids. J Heart Lung Transplant 1993;12(6 Pt 2): S241–5.

42. Peterson RE, Perens GS, Alejos JC, et al. Growth and weight gain of prepubertal children after cardiac transplantation. Pediatr Transplant 2008;12(4):436–41.
43. Cohen A, Addonizio LJ, Softness B, et al. Growth and skeletal maturation after pediatric cardiac transplantation. Pediatr Transplant 2004;8(2):126–35.
44. Mital S, Andron A, Lamour JM, et al. Effects of growth hormone therapy in children after cardiac transplantation. J Heart Lung Transplant 2006;25(7):772–7.
45. Elizur A, Faro A, Huddleston CB, et al. Lung transplantation in infants and toddlers from 1990 to 2004 at St. Louis Children's Hospital. Am J Transplant 2009;9(4):719–26.
46. Sweet SC, Spray TL, Huddleston CB, et al. Pediatric lung transplantation at St. Louis Children's Hospital, 1990–1995. Am J Respir Crit Care Med 1997;155(3):1027–35.
47. Nucci AM, Barksdale EM Jr, Beserock N, et al. Long-term nutritional outcome after pediatric intestinal transplantation. J Pediatr Surg 2002;37(3):460–3.
48. Sudan DL, Iverson A, Weseman RA, et al. Assessment of function, growth and development, and long-term quality of life after small bowel transplantation. Transplant Proc 2000;32(6):1211–2.
49. Qvist E, Pihko H, Fagerudd P, et al. Neurodevelopmental outcome in high-risk patients after renal transplantation in early childhood. Pediatr Transplant 2002;6(1):53–62.
50. Falger J, Latal B, Landolt MA, et al. Outcome after renal transplantation. Part I: intellectual and motor performance. Pediatr Nephrol 2008;23(8):1339–45.
51. Brouhard BH, Donaldson LA, Lawry KW, et al. Cognitive functioning in children on dialysis and post-transplantation. Pediatr Transplant 2000;4(4):261–7.
52. Warady BA. Neurodevelopment of infants with end-stage renal disease: is it improving? Pediatr Transplant 2002;6(1):5–7.
53. Warady BA, Belden B, Kohaut E. Neurodevelopmental outcome of children initiating peritoneal dialysis in early infancy. Pediatr Nephrol 1999;13(9):759–65.
54. Motoyama O, Kawamura T, Aikawa A, et al. Head circumference and development in young children after renal transplantation. Pediatr Int 2009;51(1):71–4.
55. Broyer M, Le Bihan C, Charbit M, et al. Long-term social outcome of children after kidney transplantation. Transplantation 2004;77(7):1033–7.
56. Groothoff JW, Cransberg K, Offringa M, et al. Long-term follow-up of renal transplantation in children: a Dutch cohort study. Transplantation 2004;78(3):453–60.
57. Karrfelt HM, Berg UB. Long-term psychosocial outcome after renal transplantation during childhood. Pediatr Transplant 2008;12(5):557–62.
58. Adeback P, Nemeth A, Fischler B. Cognitive and emotional outcome after pediatric liver transplantation. Pediatr Transplant 2003;7(5):385–9.
59. Kaller T, Schulz KH, Sander K, et al. Cognitive abilities in children after liver transplantation. Transplantation 2005;79(9):1252–6.
60. Krull K, Fuchs C, Yurk H, et al. Neurocognitive outcome in pediatric liver transplant recipients. Pediatr Transplant 2003;7(2):111–8.
61. Stewart SM, Campbell RA, McCallon D, et al. Cognitive patterns in school-age children with end-stage liver disease. J Dev Behav Pediatr 1992;13(5):331–8.
62. Stewart SM, Kennard BD, Waller DA, et al. Cognitive function in children who receive organ transplantation. Health Psychol 1994;13(1):3–13.
63. Wayman KI, Cox KL, Esquivel CO. Neurodevelopmental outcome of young children with extrahepatic biliary atresia 1 year after liver transplantation. J Pediatr 1997;131(6):894–8.
64. Kennard BD, Stewart SM, Phelan-McAuliffe D, et al. Academic outcome in long-term survivors of pediatric liver transplantation. J Dev Behav Pediatr 1999;20(1):17–23.

65. Gritti A, Di Sarno AM, Comito M, et al. Psychological impact of liver transplantation on children's inner worlds. Pediatr Transplant 2001;5(1):37–43.
66. Gilmour S, Adkins R, Liddell GA, et al. Assessment of psychoeducational outcomes after pediatric liver transplant. Am J Transplant 2009;9(2):294–300.
67. Grabhorn E, Schulz A, Helmke K, et al. Short- and long-term results of liver transplantation in infants aged less than 6 months. Transplantation 2004;78(2):235–41.
68. Newburger JW, Silbert AR, Buckley LP, et al. Cognitive function and age at repair of transposition of the great arteries in children. N Engl J Med 1984; 310(23):1495–9.
69. O'Dougherty M, Wright FS, Loewenson RB, et al. Cerebral dysfunction after chronic hypoxia in children. Neurology 1985;35(1):42–6.
70. Wright M, Nolan T. Impact of cyanotic heart disease on school performance. Arch Dis Child 1994;71(1):64–70.
71. Bellinger DC, Jonas RA, Rappaport LA, et al. Developmental and neurologic status of children after heart surgery with hypothermic circulatory arrest or low-flow cardiopulmonary bypass. N Engl J Med 1995;332(9):549–55.
72. Bellinger DC, Wypij D, Kuban KC, et al. Developmental and neurological status of children at 4 years of age after heart surgery with hypothermic circulatory arrest or low-flow cardiopulmonary bypass. Circulation 1999;100(5):526–32.
73. Miller G, Mamourian AC, Tesman JR, et al. Long-term MRI changes in brain after pediatric open heart surgery. J Child Neurol 1994;9(4):390–7.
74. Miller G, Tesman JR, Ramer JC, et al. Outcome after open-heart surgery in infants and children. J Child Neurol 1996;11(1):49–53.
75. Chinnock RE, Freier MC, Ashwal S, et al. Developmental outcomes after pediatric heart transplantation. J Heart Lung Transplant 2008;27(10):1079–84.
76. Freier MC, Babikian T, Pivonka J, et al. A longitudinal perspective on neurodevelopmental outcome after infant cardiac transplantation. J Heart Lung Transplant 2004;23(7):857–64.
77. Wray J, Radley-Smith R. Longitudinal assessment of psychological functioning in children after heart or heart-lung transplantation. J Heart Lung Transplant 2006;25(3):345–52.
78. Nixon PA, Morris KA. Quality of life in pediatric heart, heart-lung, and lung transplant recipients. Int J Sports Med 2000;21(Suppl 2):S109–11 [discussion: S112].
79. Ikle L, Hale K, Fashaw L, et al. Developmental outcome of patients with hypoplastic left heart syndrome treated with heart transplantation. J Pediatr 2003;142(1):20–5.
80. Thevenin DM, Baker A, Kato T, et al. Neurodevelopmental outcomes of infant multivisceral transplant recipients: a longitudinal study. Transplant Proc 2006; 38(6):1694–5.
81. Thevenin DM, Baker A, Kato T, et al. Neuodevelopmental outcomes for children transplanted under the age of 3 years. Transplant Proc 2006;38(6):1692–3.
82. Thevenin DM, Mittal N, Kato T, et al. Neurodevelopmental outcomes of infant intestinal transplant recipients. Transplant Proc 2004;36(2):319–20.
83. Riano-Galan I, Malaga S, Rajmil L, et al. Quality of life of adolescents with end-stage renal disease and kidney transplant. Pediatr Nephrol 2009;24(8): 1561–8.
84. Goldstein SL, Graham N, Burwinkle T, et al. Health-related quality of life in pediatric patients with ESRD. Pediatr Nephrol 2006;21(6):846–50.
85. Goldstein SL, Graham N, Warady BA, et al. Measuring health-related quality of life in children with ESRD: performance of the generic and ESRD-specific instrument of the Pediatric Quality of Life Inventory (PedsQL). Am J Kidney Dis 2008; 51(2):285–97.

86. Goldstein SL, Rosburg NM, Warady BA, et al. Pediatric end stage renal disease health-related quality of life differs by modality: a PedsQL ESRD analysis. Pediatr Nephrol 2009;24(8):1553–60.

87. Qvist E, Narhi V, Apajasalo M, et al. Psychosocial adjustment and quality of life after renal transplantation in early childhood. Pediatr Transplant 2004;8(2):120–5.

88. Sundaram SS, Landgraf JM, Neighbors K, et al. Adolescent health-related quality of life following liver and kidney transplantation. Am J Transplant 2007; 7(4):982–9.

89. Anthony SJ, Hebert D, Todd L, et al. Child and parental perspectives of multidimensional quality of life outcomes after kidney transplantation. Pediatr Transplant 2010;14(2):249–56.

90. Rosenkranz J, Reichwald-Klugger E, Oh J, et al. Psychosocial rehabilitation and satisfaction with life in adults with childhood-onset of end-stage renal disease. Pediatr Nephrol 2005;20(9):1288–94.

91. Rees L. Long-term outcome after renal transplantation in childhood. Pediatr Nephrol 2009;24(3):475–84.

92. Asonuma K, Inomata Y, Uemoto S, et al. Growth and quality of life after living-related liver transplantation in children. Pediatr Transplant 1998;2(1):64–9.

93. Burdelski M, Nolkemper D, Ganschow R, et al. Liver transplantation in children: long-term outcome and quality of life. Eur J Pediatr 1999;158(Suppl 2):S34–42.

94. Sokal EM. Quality of life after orthotopic liver transplantation in children. An overview of physical, psychological and social outcome. Eur J Pediatr 1995;154(3): 171–5.

95. Alonso EM, Neighbors K, Mattson C, et al. Functional outcomes of pediatric liver transplantation. J Pediatr Gastroenterol Nutr 2003;37(2):155–60.

96. Bucuvalas JC, Britto M, Krug S, et al. Health-related quality of life in pediatric liver transplant recipients: a single-center study. Liver Transpl 2003;9(1):62–71.

97. Bucuvalas JC, Britto M. Health-related quality of life after liver transplantation: it's not all about the liver. J Pediatr Gastroenterol Nutr 2003;37(2):106–8.

98. Cole CR, Bucuvalas JC, Hornung RW, et al. Impact of liver transplantation on HRQOL in children less than 5 years old. Pediatr Transplant 2004;8(3):222–7.

99. Alonso EM, Neighbors K, Barton FB, et al. Health-related quality of life and family function following pediatric liver transplantation. Liver Transpl 2008; 14(4):460–8.

100. Fredericks EM, Magee JC, Opipari-Arrigan L, et al. Adherence and health-related quality of life in adolescent liver transplant recipients. Pediatr Transplant 2008;12(3):289–99.

101. Petroski RA, Grady KL, Rodgers S, et al. Quality of life in adult survivors greater than 10 years after pediatric heart transplantation. J Heart Lung Transplant 2009;28(7):661–6.

102. Wray J, Radley-Smith R. Beyond the first year after pediatric heart or heart-lung transplantation: changes in cognitive function and behaviour. Pediatr Transplant 2005;9(2):170–7.

103. Rovera GM, DiMartini A, Schoen RE, et al. Quality of life of patients after intestinal transplantation. Transplantation 1998;66(9):1141–5.

104. Sudan D, Iyer K, Horslen S, et al. Assessment of quality of life after pediatric intestinal transplantation by parents and pediatric recipients using the child health questionnaire. Transplant Proc 2002;34(3):963–4.

Quality of Life After Pediatric Solid Organ Transplantation

Samantha J. Anthony, PhD(c), MSW[a], Stacey Pollock BarZiv, PhD[b],
Vicky Lee Ng, MD, FRCPC[c,d],*

KEYWORDS

- Quality of life • Pediatric transplantation
- Solid organ transplantation • Outcomes • Chronic diseases

Long-term survival after pediatric solid organ transplantation is now the rule rather than the exception for increasing numbers of children with end-stage kidney, heart, lung, liver, and small bowel diseases.[1] Although life-saving, solid organ transplantation is not curative; a fatal disease has been replaced by a chronic condition with its own associated morbidities, which may evolve or be present despite well-preserved allograft function.[2–4] While transplantation restores organ function, it does not necessarily return one to a normal life. Therefore, it is prudent to now focus on assessment of not only traditional biologic outcomes but also the quality of life of these children and their families. Health-related quality of life provides a more comprehensive evaluation than do disease parameters alone of the impact of an illness and its treatment on functioning and well-being. Improving long-term outcomes after solid organ transplantation must consider not only the quantity but also the quality of life years survived.[5–8] This article gives a brief overview of current definitions, conceptualizations, approaches to measurement, and unique considerations in the evaluation of quality of life in these children. Current understanding of quality of life in children who have undergone kidney, heart, lung, liver, or small bowel transplantation is reviewed,

[a] Department of Social Work, SickKids Transplant Center, The Hospital for Sick Children, Institute of Medical Science, University of Toronto, 555 University Avenue, Room 1109C, Toronto, ON M5G 1X8, Canada
[b] Department of Pediatrics, SickKids Transplant Center, The Hospital for Sick Children, University of Toronto, Toronto, ON, Canada
[c] Liver Transplant Program, SickKids Transplant Center, The Hospital for Sick Children, University of Toronto, Toronto, ON, Canada
[d] Division of Gastroenterology, Hepatology and Nutrition, SickKids Transplant Center, The Hospital for Sick Children, University of Toronto, 555 University Avenue, Black Wing Room 8262, Toronto, ON M5G 1X8, Canada
* Corresponding author. Division of Gastroenterology, Hepatology and Nutrition, SickKids Transplant Center, The Hospital for Sick Children, University of Toronto, 555 University Avenue, Black Wing Room 8262, Toronto, ON M5G 1X8, Canada.
E-mail address: vicky.ng@sickkids.ca

Pediatr Clin N Am 57 (2010) 559–574
doi:10.1016/j.pcl.2010.01.006
0031-3955/10/$ – see front matter © 2010 Elsevier Inc. All rights reserved.

followed by limitations of current knowledge. Clinical implications are discussed and future research directions suggested.

QUALITY OF LIFE: DEFINITIONS AND CONCEPTUALIZATION

In the World Health Organization's (WHO) 1948 landmark definition of health, the traditional considerations of physiologic factors and the absence of disease were expanded to encompass the broader multidimensional domains of "physical, mental, and social well-being."[9] While this commonly cited definition of health has remained the cornerstone of the quality of life construct, many varying definitions of quality of life have been proposed over the years. In excess of 100 definitions of the term 'quality of life' have been identified in the literature.[10] Although a precise and universally accepted definition of quality of life has yet to be framed, there is growing consensus around two fundamental concepts that are inherent in most definitions.[11,12] First, quality of life is primarily subjective, and should therefore be assessed from the patient's perspective whenever possible. Individuals have their own unique perspective on quality of life, which depends on present lifestyle, past experience, hopes for the future, dreams, and ambitions. Second, quality of life is generally conceptualized as a multidimensional construct encompassing several broad domains, with the most widely used domains reflecting those articulated by the WHO definition: physiologic, social, and psychological factors.[11,13,14]

Physiologic Factors

These factors include clinical indicators of health, energy level, and functional status (the ability to perform tasks of daily living).[15] Objective clinical indicators of health remain the cornerstone of medicine and provide standardization; however, individual factors such as tolerance of pain and individual perceptions can influence evaluations of well-being even in the face of normal physiologic parameters. Indeed, low levels of energy and limitations in functional health status can negatively influence ratings of global quality of life by creating, feelings of ineffectiveness, social restriction, and emotional distress.[11,16] Although there is a general reliance by clinicians on objective assessments, these frequently correlate poorly with subjective ratings of patients' well-being. Results from patient-driven tools may therefore better reflect functional status and quality of life.[11]

Social Factors

These factors include both social health and social support. Social health is the ability to perform normal social roles, how one gets along with others and how others react to them, and incorporates personality, social skills, and one's available social supports.[17,18] Social supports can directly influence physical health by easing the emotional or tangible burden of physical symptom, and can attenuate the effects of stressful life events and reduce severity of disease.[17] Measurement of social support typically includes self-administered rating scales, and interpreting results must reflect diverse social norms across individuals, cultures, and social strata.[15]

Psychological Factors

These factors include emotional status, self-esteem, body image, and cognitive variables. Evidence indicates that psychological factors affect health and physiologic responses to illness and treatments.[19,20] For example, anxiety and depression can affect adherence to treatments, hasten disease progression, and negatively affect one's quality of life.[16] These variables may be directly amenable to the development of interventions to alleviate suffering, improve treatment adherence, and in turn improve perceptions of quality of life and enhance long-term outcomes.[16] The relationship between physical health and psychological states is complex, with an impact that may be currently underappreciated due to a tendency toward a medicalized nature and focus of care.[19,20]

APPROACHES TO QUALITY OF LIFE MEASUREMENT

Meaningful assessment of patient quality of life mandates the ability to reliably and accurately assess well-being. Numerous generic and disease-specific indices and indicators have been developed that attempt to assess children's quality of life. Within the context of pediatric transplantation, there remains no gold standard instrument with the ability to measure concerns which may be specific to this particular patient population. As a result, it is very difficult to compare, generalize, or replicate findings. Important methodological considerations that require attention are discussed here.

Generic Versus Disease-specific Tools

Generic quality of life measures are multidimensional, consisting of, at minimum, the physical, psychological, and social health dimensions delineated by the WHO definition of health.[9] Generic measures are designed to be broadly applicable across many types of diseases, treatments, and groups of individuals, and permit comparisons across interventions and diagnostic conditions. In addition, data can be compared with general pediatric population norms to determine the impact of disease on quality of life.[11,12,21] Disease-specific measures, on the other hand, take into account aspects of disease and treatment relevant to a specific medical condition such as transplant-related issues (eg, medication side effects, worry about graft rejection, graft loss, and need for retransplant). Such measures may be more sensitive to changes in a child's condition, tend to be more effective at detecting treatment effects, and therefore may have greater salience for clinicians.[11,21] At present the use of both generic and disease-specific measures is likely to provide valuable and complementary information to further understand the quality of life in children who have undergone transplantation.[22]

Self-report Versus Proxy Report

Given the subjective nature of quality of life, there are strong arguments in favor of eliciting data directly from children wherever possible,[12,14,23] given data showing that information provided by proxy respondents is not equivalent to child self-report no matter how well-intentioned or informed the adult.[12] In a meta-analysis evaluating the agreement between child and proxy reports in chronically ill populations, researchers found greater agreement between children's and parents' reports for observable behaviors such as physical functioning than for nonobservable functioning such as emotional or social quality of life.[12]

Although the perspectives of children in evaluating quality of life are extremely important, direct assessment may be limited by age, medical condition, and developmental ability for comprehension, hence requiring a parent or caregiver to act as a proxy for the child. When it is not possible to elicit quality of life information from a child, the perspectives of parents are valuable in enabling the assessment of every child in population-based studies. Although there may be a degree of distortion in parental responses about their child's quality of life, parents nonetheless are usually a knowledgeable source of information about their child.[24]

Adult Versus Pediatric Measurement

Although published studies consistently report overall improvement in global quality of life for adults who have undergone transplantation, the focus on adult-specific issues such as employability, medical leave from work, marital relationships, and sexuality means these findings cannot be extrapolated onto the lives of children who have undergone transplantation. Issues that may be salient for children include school attendance, exercise capacity and sport participation, peer groups, bullying, growth retardation, and weight and body image. The challenge with measurement of pediatric quality of life relates to the wide developmental spectrum across the pediatric age group. Each developmental period is characterized by unique sets of issues, milestones, and developmental and psychosocial considerations. What might be important in the life of a young child may no longer apply once the individual reaches adolescence. Furthermore, adolescence is a particularly unique period, distinct from adulthood, and often described as emotionally turbulent and in transition. Issues unique to adolescents such as puberty, sexual development, search for autonomy and transition to adulthood have strong relevance for the study of quality of life and have been inadequately addressed in the literature.[25]

In summary, traditional posttransplantation outcomes such as number of biopsy-proven rejection episodes, graft function, hospitalization days or infections, or patient mortality rates do not adequately measure the impact of children's day-to-day life following transplant. Optimizing the future success of solid organ transplantation in children is defined by more than just excellent patient or graft survival rates. Further attention to strategies to achieve the goal of a health state that is desirable and a marked improvement from the pretransplant condition are needed. Assessment of quality of life will permit health care professionals to hear the voice and perspective of the patient, and has been found to predict, often better than physiologic measures, future health status, mortality, and resource use, which are critical issues in the care of children worldwide who have undergone, or will require, kidney, heart, lung, liver, or small bowel transplantation. The findings are now summarized.

Quality of life following pediatric kidney transplantation

Pediatric kidney transplantation is widely used, both with deceased and living donors. Among living donor recipients, 1- and 5-year patient survival rates exceed 98% and 96%, and deceased donor survival rates are 97% and 96% at 1 and 5 years, respectively.[1,26] Current literature conveys excellent long-term outcomes for children who have undergone kidney transplant.[1,7,27,28] However, these results are mostly limited to patient and graft survival, and freedom from rejection and morbidities. Quality of life research in pediatric kidney transplant patients remains scarce, with most existing studies relying on cross-sectional assessment or measurement of single dimensions of quality of life such as physical or social aspects.

Kidney transplant recipients experience better overall health and well-being after transplant as measured by a wide range of instruments of varying degrees of validity.[7,28–30] Variables used to assess psychosocial adjustment after transplantation include return to school and level of education attained, neurodevelopmental outcome, prevalence of psychological disorders, and later employment status, as well as more specific quality of life measurement tools including the Pediatric Quality of Life Inventory Generic Scale and End Stage Renal Disease Module, Child Health Questionnaire, and the Child Behavior Checklist, to name a few. These studies almost universally have reported good long-term psychosocial outcome after transplantation.[27,30–32] However, many physical and psychosocial issues remain salient after transplant. It has been shown that physical complaints such as headaches and fatigue are common in children after kidney transplant, as well as negative impacts of medications on growth (eg, short stature), weight gain, and general health.[7,33–36] Physical effects of medications can also influence behavioral adjustment. In particular, research has demonstrated a strong relationship between medication side-effects and nonadherence with medical regimens.[34,37] Medication adverse effects also have been shown to impact on social and psychological domains. It has been reported that somatic complaints and social problems are more common in boys after transplant,[30] and that children have increased emotional problems when there are overt signs of illness/treatment related to immunosuppressive medications (eg, short stature, weight gain, mouth sores).[38,39]

Issues pertaining to school function are of paramount importance. Difficulty with school re-entry and prolonged absence from school due to treatment-related issues impact on academic achievement, which then can lead to a detrimental effect on sustaining peer relationships, poor self-concept and self-esteem, all of which negatively influence quality of life.[27,30,40] Studies have shown that most children are enrolled in regular schools; however, research has demonstrated varying degrees of problems with learning and memory, inferior school performance on standardized achievement tests,[41] and attention problems that require intervention to maximize academic success in pediatric kidney transplant recipients.[30,40]

Children living with end-stage kidney disease are at risk for anxiety and depression.[42,43] In general, psychosocial factors such as depressive symptoms and anxiety, strained social relationships, and adjustment issues improve after organ transplantation, but they continue to warrant attention over the long term.[33,44] While several studies have assessed domains of psychological well-being, there is minimal research on actual rates of anxiety and depression in pediatric kidney transplant recipients; most available studies use screening tools rather than diagnostic criteria and therefore do not properly ascertain the true incidence and implications of these factors in children. Recent research compared 40 adolescent renal transplant patients with healthy peers and chronic kidney disease patients using psychiatric diagnostic interviews, and the Child Behavior Checklist self-rating scale.[43] The investigators demonstrated that 65% of transplant recipients met DSM-IV (*Diagnostic and Statistical Manual of Mental Disorders-IV*) criteria for a lifetime psychiatric disorder compared with 60% of chronic kidney disease and 37.5% of controls.

A recent exploratory study investigating multidimensional aspects of quality of life in 23 pediatric renal transplant recipients and their parents using the Pediatric Quality of Life Inventory Generic and End Stage Kidney Disease Modules[33] found that children reported good overall quality of life, yet results were lower than healthy children samples across all subscales. Parent ratings were lower across all domains especially on emotional, social, school, and physical summary scales. This study identified concerns in the following four areas: (1) physical symptoms (eg, fatigue and thirst); (2) body image and weight concern in adolescents; (3) school disruption due to medical follow-up; and (4) strained relationships with family and peers.[33]

Much of the research on quality of life in kidney transplant reflects long-term effects of an earlier era whereby higher levels of immunosuppression were used. Many kidney transplant programs now emphasize steroid minimization and steroid-free protocols, as well as more targeted immunosuppression. The impact of this on quality of life remains to be seen, but it can be speculated that kidney transplant recipients in the more recent era should expect better growth trajectories and less adverse drug effects, both of which are strongly linked to higher quality of life perceptions. Primary health care providers can actively screen for emotional distress, depression, and anxiety as well as the availability of social supports and adequate school function.

Assessing for the presence of physical effects of medications such as headaches and fatigue will provide opportunities for interventions and surveillance of adverse medication effects to improve the long-term quality of life of transplant recipients.

In summary, children who undergo kidney transplant can experience excellent survival and quality of life outcomes, yet there remain important issues regarding physical and psychosocial aspects after transplant that warrant further attention over the long term.

Quality of life following pediatric liver transplantation

Long-term survival after pediatric liver transplantation is now the rule rather than the exception. One-year and 5-year survival statistics are high, approximately 95% and 85%, respectively. More than 11,000 children in the United States (UNOS Web site, accessed October 2009) and Canada have received a liver transplant for the spectrum of indications, as discussed elsewhere in this issue. Advancing the understanding of health-related quality of life is an important issue to address to further improve the long-term well-being, health, and survival of this specific patient population.[5] Before 2000, most reports on quality of life in pediatric liver transplant recipients were cross-sectional investigations using several generic and some transplant-specific tools with varying degrees of validity. However, more recent single-center studies have used well-validated instruments, which have enabled the comparisons of quality of life in pediatric liver transplant recipients with other chronic disease groups. These validated generic tools have included the PedsQL 4.0 Generic Core Scales, Child Health Questionnaire Parent Report Form 50, Child Health Questionnaire Child Form 87, Health Utilities Index Mark 3, Infant Toddler Quality of Life Instrument, PedsQL Multidimensional Fatigue Scale, and PedsQL Cognitive Functioning Scale. Important findings from single-center studies as well as available published data from multicenter collaborations are highlighted here.

Quality of life in children and adolescents after liver transplantation has been evaluated in several single-center experiences and reviewed in a recent publication.[45] This critical systematic review of 11 of the most important published single-center studies, representing 395 children and adolescents who received liver transplants between 1981 and 2002, summarized that pediatric liver transplant recipients have (1) decreased quality of life compared with healthy children peers in the specific domains of physical, psychological, social, and family functioning; and (2) equal, or better, quality of life than comparison groups of children and adolescents with other chronic illnesses, such as pediatric juvenile arthritis, asthma, and epilepsy.[46–48] Decreased psychosocial function also identified concerns in the area of school function. One study assessing the academic outcome of a cohort of 50 children alive 3 to 9 years after pediatric liver transplantation revealed that almost 20% had an intelligence quotient score of less than 70.[49] It is as yet unknown whether an increased prevalence of developmental delays or learning disabilities exist in this population. Further, it is also possible that increased school absenteeism because of illness or doctor visits may be important contributors. School findings in a multicenter cohort of pediatric liver transplant recipients are discussed by Kamath and Olthiff elsewhere in this issue.

Subsequently, more recent single-center studies evaluating quality of life after pediatric liver transplantation have verified similar domain findings and raised additional relevant concepts.[50] Attention to the adolescent-age population have reiterated the previously noted discrepancy between self-report and proxy reports, with adolescents self-rating their physical, emotional, and social functioning as normal whereas their parent proxy did not.[51] A second single-center experience with adolescent survivors of liver and kidney transplantation demonstrated similar self-reported physical and psychological function to healthy controls, in contrast to parent-proxy reports viewing general health and physical function of these same patients to be poorer than the normative population.[7] This contrast in viewpoint supports the concept that ratings of both parents and patients should be considered to gain a fuller picture of quality of life outcomes. Finally, assessment of family functioning identified no difference between families with a pediatric liver transplant recipient compared with both a normative sample and families with a child with a chronic illness.

Understanding of the factors affecting quality of life for children after liver transplantation has been explored.[52] Pretransplant factors associated with improved quality of life include a primary diagnosis of biliary atresia, Caucasian race, and maternal education level,[47] whereas older age at time of liver transplant has been associated with decreased quality of life.[47,52] Posttransplant variables associated with better quality of life include fewer hospitalizations in the preceding year, improved height parameters, longer time since liver transplant, and higher self-esteem,[52] while not surprisingly, variables of medication side effects, headaches, the development of a second comorbid condition, and parental conflicts were associated with decreased quality of life.[47,52]

Realizing the limitations with even the most well-designed single-center experiences, the pediatric liver transplant community has capitalized on a research infrastructure called the Studies of Pediatric Liver Transplantation (SPLIT). Since its inception in 1996, SPLIT has worked to sustain a prospective collection of comprehensive pre- and posttransplant medical data on pediatric liver transplant candidates and recipients from pediatric liver transplant programs in the United States and Canada. Results from a large cross-sectional analysis of 873 pediatric liver transplant recipients from 20 pediatric liver transplant programs in the United States and Canada were reviewed by Alonso and colleagues[53] on behalf of the SPLIT Functional Outcomes Group (FOG). A subsequent preliminary subanalysis of 110 children with fulminant liver failure (from within the entire FOG study cohort) who underwent emergency liver transplant revealed that the patients themselves self-report similar quality of life to healthy children controls on the 23-item PedsQL Generic Core Scales self-report except in the domain of school functioning. This result is in contrast to their parents, who proxy reported impaired health-related quality of life across all domains compared with healthy controls, emphasizing the need to assess qualitative outcomes directly from the child's perspective whenever possible.[54]

Further to single-center experiences studying family function, Alonso and colleagues[55] conducted a 5-center cross-sectional analysis of quality of life and family function dynamics in a homogeneous population of 2-year survivors of pediatric liver transplantation, which showed that younger survivors (age <2 years) had lower scores in the domains of global health, general health perceptions, and change in health as compared with older transplant recipients (patient age >5 years at time of assessment) as reported by the completed parent-proxy reports of the Infant Toddler Quality of Life Instrument and the Child Health Questionnaire Parent Form 50, who had lower scores in the domains of physical health and general health. Median scores from the parent-proxy report suggest that younger survivors had fewer issues with discomfort and pain compared with the control group created for the study. Mean family assessment device scores indicated that families of a liver transplant recipient do not have increased levels of family dysfunction.

While physical function, mental health, cognitive development, and daily living skills are good examples of domains that can be assessed by all pediatric health care providers involved in the long-term follow-up for survivors of pediatric liver transplantation, it is also important to highlight dimensions that are uniquely relevant to pediatric liver transplant recipients.[5] Qualitative 1-to-1 interviews conducted with 63 children or adolescent liver transplant recipients and 84 parents from Canada and the United Kingdom identified a range of common and diverse childhood experiences and perceptions of quality of life following pediatric liver transplant.[56] These item generation interviews identified many generic items relevant to children with chronic medical conditions, and include physical health (restrictions), social (peer relationships, bullying, and teasing), emotional (fears and worries about future health, sadness due to knowledge of their parents worrying about them, and self-blame for imposing worry on family members), and school (attendance, ability to concentrate) domains. In addition, many disease-specific domains were identified as particularly relevant to a patient who has undergone liver transplantation as a child, which are not currently captured in available validated generic tools. Highlights of the top 9 disease-specific domains are: (1) vulnerability to specific posttransplant complications; (2) altered body image (living with a scar from the liver transplant surgery); (3) fear of infection; (4) thoughts about the future (rejection, retransplantation); (5) altered lifespan because of having a liver transplantation as a child; (6) living with a liver that is not the native one; (7) treatment-related challenges (side effects unique to immunosuppression medications, difficult procedures); (8) lifelong needs (medical team care, transition to adult-care teams), and (9) behavioral responses (compliance and nonadherence to surveillance and treatment regimens). To date, there is no published validated disease-specific health-related quality of life tool for use in pediatric liver transplantation patients, although work is ongoing toward this goal, so that in the near future such a tool is likely to become available.[54] Completion of psychometric testing is necessary to ensure broad cross-cultural applicability of an eventual health-related quality of life instrument for liver transplant recipients, thus ensuring that the assessment of quality of life in this population is culturally sensitive and will lead to a more nuanced understanding of the factors that influence transplant recipients' well-being.[57]

Quality of life following pediatric heart transplantation

In the last decade heart transplantation has proven to be an effective and accepted therapy in pediatric patients with lethal heart disease. One-, 5-, and 10-year survival statistics are high, approximately 95%, 75%, and 65%, respectively.[58] Since 1982 more than 7750 pediatric patients have received heart transplants, with an annual transplant rate of around 400.[58] In pediatric heart transplantation the investigative issues that have been most emphasized in past years pertain to mortality risk factors and morbidity, yet with improved medical outcomes, current research has shifted toward understanding and enhancing quality of life. Although data regarding survival have justified continued use of heart transplantation in children, there is a paucity of published data regarding the quality of life of these children. To date there is little literature available about the psychosocial effects on children who undergo heart transplantation, and their long-term psychological and social functioning remains unclear.

Early studies using functional status to evaluate the quality of life of pediatric heart transplant recipients indicated that quality of life after transplant improved and transplant recipients experienced a much improved physical status after recovery from the transplant process. The literature reported that postoperatively, children were active and could generally return to age-appropriate developmental, educational, social, and recreational activities.[59–62] In early retrospective clinical chart reviews, researchers reported that 89% to 100% of pediatric heart transplant recipients participated in or were capable of participation in normal activities for age and "lead an active and satisfying life."[63,64] In a multicenter study of 49 pediatric patients, it was revealed that most children experienced a dramatic improvement in functional status following heart transplant, with 93% attending school and participating in recreational activities including swimming, biking, skating, skiing, baseball, volleyball, and tennis.[61] Research examining the behavior and cognitive functioning of 65 and 81 children who had undergone heart or heart-lung transplantation found that most children had returned to activities appropriate for their age and had settled back into school, with academic performance attainments, evaluated by the British Ability Scales, as well as the Schonell graded spelling test, within normal limits.[65,66]

With a focus more on psychosocial outcomes as proxies for quality of life, a study examining the psychological functioning of 23 pediatric heart transplant recipients, which used clinician ratings on the Children's Global Assessment Scale, found that the majority of patients (78.3%) demonstrated improved psychological functioning after their transplant.[67] In a longitudinal follow-up study, improvement in psychological functioning was maintained over a decade, with 73% patients having improved emotional and psychological functioning.[68] Similarly, employing semistructured interviews as well as several standardized questionnaires including the Global Assessment of Functioning Scale, Children's Behavior Questionnaire Scale, and the Piers & Harris Self-Concept Scale, an assessment of psychosocial outcomes in 23 heart and 21 heart-lung transplant recipients found significant improvement in physical health and psychosocial functioning 12 months after transplant.[62] These results are consistent with 2 prospective evaluations of heart or heart-lung transplant recipients, which revealed that following transplantation overall physical and psychosocial functioning improved.[60,69] In 2003 Pollock-BarZiv and colleagues[70] examined the self-perceived quality of life of 8 heart transplant recipients, aged 10 to 18 years, and results demonstrated excellent overall quality of life and psychological well-being. A rare qualitative study found that most children described their lives in positive terms, such as "mostly good" or "fun," and valued the normal aspects of life.[71]

Despite significant improvements in functional status, quality of life, and psychosocial outcomes, results of some studies suggest that a significant minority of patients do experience psychological difficulties at some stage after transplantation. In a review of psychological outcomes of heart transplantation in children, Todaro and colleagues[72] reported that a proportion of recipients are at risk for psychological difficulties following heart transplantation.[70] Results indicated that pediatric heart transplant recipients are at increased risk of experiencing psychological distress, such as anxiety, depression, behavioral disorders, and poor self-concept, compared with normal, healthy peers.[61,62,73,74] There appears to be a higher prevalence of psychological difficulties and stress among pediatric heart transplant recipients, resulting in symptoms of negative affect, decreased social competence, and behavior problems.[61,67,72–75] These findings suggest that for some patients, there may be psychological difficulties coping with the demands or stressors of pediatric heart transplant.

It may be concluded that while problems do remain, the overall results of these studies support the adaptive potential of children and adolescents following heart transplantation, and indicate that the majority of pediatric recipients appear capable of healthy physical and psychological functioning after heart transplant.

Quality of life following pediatric lung transplantation

Since the first successful lung transplant was performed in the early 1980s, ongoing advances in surgical methods and improved medical management have led to 1- and 5- year patient survival rates of 83% and 50%, respectively.[8,76] The most recent report of the International Society for Heart and Lung Transplantation (ISHLT) registry reveals nearly 1000 pediatric lung transplants to date.[71] The most common reason for lung transplant in children is cystic fibrosis, but other etiologies include pulmonary hypertension, interstitial disease, congenital diseases, and other causes (http://www. unos.org).[8]

While lung transplantation is now widely used for advanced lung disease, research examining quality of life in lung transplant recipients has only begun to surface in the past decade.[77] Numerous clinical and registry studies demonstrate improved survival after lung transplant, yet studies focusing on quality of life remain scarce, particularly within pediatrics. In fact, due to the small numbers of pediatric lung transplants it is uncommon to find a study dedicated to quality of life in this cohort, and most published data to date in children are found embedded within adult studies, or along with research on heart transplant populations.

Issues specific to pediatric lung transplantation include a high need for mechanical ventilation before transplant, challenges in surveillance of rejection and chronic rejection using spirometry in younger children, and increased complications related to infection both before and after transplant.[8,66] Research thus far shows improved overall quality of life after lung transplantation.[77–79] A comprehensive literature review between 1980 and 1999 found only 13 published reports addressing quality of life after lung transplant, with most emanating from Canada, the United States, and the United Kingdom.[77] Additional studies have since emerged, yet limited published data exist that focuses on quality of life issues in pediatric lung transplant recipients. The recent ISHLT registry reported no activity limitations in 80% of children surviving 7 years following transplant[71]; as yet, the long-term psychosocial status remains unknown. A study by Durst and colleagues[80] used qualitative interviews to examine psychosocial issues after lung transplantation in adolescents with cystic fibrosis. The study reported that after transplant patients were able to develop long-term goals, and a wish to reclaim control over their lives as much as possible and adjust to a new lifestyle; yet common emotional responses included fear and anxiety over rejection, uncertainty over the future, and frustration with parent over protectiveness. These findings represent a cohort that has been chronically ill and has endured years of hospitalization and treatments, so results may not necessarily translate onto other pediatric lung diagnoses after transplant. Future studies are urgently required to decipher quality of life issues among short- and long-term survivors of pediatric lung transplantation.

Quality of life after pediatric small bowel transplant

Intestinal transplantation has become a standard treatment for intestinal failure in patients with life-threatening complications of parenteral nutrition. Over the last decade, 1- and 5- year patient survival rates are as high as 80% and 50%, respectively, with survival rates in high-volume centers in the United States and Europe even better, as reviewed in the article by Avitzur and colleagues elsewhere in this issue.

The quality of life after small bowel transplantation is probably equal to or better than quality of life on parenteral nutrition, and children report quality of life similar to normal school children, although these results require longer follow-up.[81] The achievement of oral tolerance in children who previously were dependent on parenteral nutrition is a disease-specific item unique to children with intestinal failure who survive intestinal transplantation. Indeed, a general assessment of quality of life by means of oral tolerance and the Karnofsky score, a general performance status tool, showed that the majority of surviving recipients tolerate enteral feeding and are capable of normal activities as recorded in the Intestine Registry (*Intestinal Registry Report*, Bologna, 2009).

LIMITATIONS AND FUTURE DIRECTIONS IN THE RESEARCH

With favorable long-term patient survival after pediatric solid organ transplantation, there has been an appropriate shift in focus toward understanding of quality of life issues in survivors. While it is encouraging to see a growing body of research attempting to address quality of life, it is prudent to review the current limitations of the available research. Studies vary with respect to the definition or operationalization of the term quality of life, the design of the study (prospective vs retrospective, cross-sectional vs longitudinal), the time of the assessment relative to transplant, and the age range of patients in the sample. Research samples have been composed of relatively small proportions of patients from single transplant centers. Much of the research relies heavily on the opinions or assessments of proxy informants (parents, teachers, or health care professionals); therefore there is little information available about the child's or adolescent's own perception of their psychological adaptation and quality of life following transplantation. To date the majority of studies are quantitative, and have used a variety of different assessment tools and measures, many of which do not address key aspects specific to being a pediatric recipient of a solid organ transplant. Quality of life studies using a qualitative approach have been sparse, thereby limiting researchers' and clinicians' comprehensive understanding of the personal, nuanced realities and quality of life of transplant recipients.

The current state of the pediatric transplant quality of life literature is awaiting further prospective and longitudinal studies, as well as larger samples potentially via multi-center collaborations, to enhance understanding of not only survival benefit but of quality of life benefit of solid organ transplantation. There is a need to combine research methodologies in future research, as using both quantitative and qualitative approaches will allow for a richer understanding of the quality of life in children after transplant. Finally, disease-specific instruments that would address important issues such as surgical concerns, the effects of immunosuppression medications, and recipient variables that impact quality of life in pediatric transplant recipients will be complementary additions to the clinician's armamentarium of instruments available for these patients.

OPPORTUNITIES FOR HEALTH CARE PROVIDERS

Primary healthy care providers, because of their longitudinal knowledge of, and unique relationship with, patients and their families, are in an advantageous position to regularly screen for many of the domains that constitute quality of life. These domains include knowledgeable inquiry for the presence of relevant adverse effects of medications including hirsutism, hair loss, headaches, and fatigue; screening for early signs of anxiety or emotional distress; monitoring neurocognitive development; integrating psychosocial care into an ongoing medical care program with early intervention services and prevention efforts before the development of more severe adjustment problems; and mobilizing community resources to aid the varying needs of siblings and extended family care providers. Prompt bidirectional communication between primary care providers and transplant centers about such important observations will facilitate involvement, set expectations, and provide guidance for both families and all health care professionals toward the goal of maximizing the success attainable by an ever-growing population of long-term survivors of pediatric solid organ transplantation.

SUMMARY

Life after transplantation in children is multifaceted, evolving, and requires the combined expertise of a dedicated multidisciplinary team to ensure optimal care.

Better understanding of the multiple domains comprising quality of life will add to the clinician's armamentarium so as to optimize future health status, mortality, and resource use of an ever-growing population of survivors of pediatric solid organ transplantation. Because of the limited research in this area and contradictory findings to date, there is a considerable amount that is not known about the impact of solid organ transplantation on the lives of children. Further study on the long-term physical, psychological, and social sequelae after transplantation will help elucidate important data and contribute to the development of strategies to optimize outcomes. Given the limited numbers of pediatric transplant patients in any one pediatric program, broad collaborative efforts are now required.

REFERENCES

1. Horslen S, Barr ML, Christensen LL, et al. Pediatric transplantation in the United States, 1996–2005. Am J Transplant 2007;7(5 Pt 2):1339–58.
2. Ng VL, Fecteau A, Shepherd R, et al. Outcomes of 5-year survivors of pediatric liver transplantation: report on 461 children from a North American multicenter registry. Pediatrics 2008;122(6):e1128–35.
3. McDonald SP, Craig JC. Long-term survival of children with end-stage renal disease. N Engl J Med 2004;350(26):2654–62.
4. Green A, Ray T. Attention to child development: a key piece of family-centered care for cardiac transplant recipients. J Spec Pediatr Nurs 2006;11(2):143–8.
5. Bucuvalas JC, Alonso E, Magee JC, et al. Improving long-term outcomes after liver transplantation in children. Am J Transplant 2008;8(12):2506–13.
6. McGuire BM, Rosenthal P, Brown CC, et al. Long-term management of the liver transplant patient: recommendations for the primary care doctor. Am J Transplant 2009;9(9):1988–2003.
7. Sundaram SS, Landgraf JM, Neighbors K, et al. Adolescent health-related quality of life following liver and kidney transplantation. Am J Transplant 2007;7(4):982–9.
8. Sweet SC. Pediatric lung transplantation. Proc Am Thorac Soc 2009;6(1):122–7.
9. WHO. World Health Organization Constitution. Geneva (Switzerland): World Health Organization; 1948.
10. Cummins RA. Assessing quality of life. In: Brown RI, editor. Quality of life for people with disabilities. 2nd edition. United Kingdom: Stanley Thornes Ltd; 1995. p. 116–50.
11. Matza LS, Swensen AR, Flood EM, et al. Assessment of health-related quality of life in children: a review of conceptual, methodological, and regulatory issues. Value Health 2004;7(1):79–92.
12. Eiser C, Morse R. Quality-of-life measures in chronic diseases of childhood. Health Technol Assess 2001;5(4):1–157.
13. Arnold R, Ranchor AV, Sanderman R, et al. The relative contribution of domains of quality of life to overall quality of life for different chronic diseases. Qual Life Res 2004;13(5):883–96.
14. Burra P, De Bona M. Quality of life following organ transplantation. Transpl Int 2007;20(5):397–409.
15. McDowell A, Newell C. Measuring health: a guide to rating scales and questionnaires. 2nd edition. New York: Oxford University Press; 1996.
16. Qvist E, Jalanko H, Homberg C. Psychosocial adaptation after solid organ transplantation in children. Pediatr Clin North Am 2003;50(6):1505–19.
17. Helgeson VS. Social support and quality of life. Qual Life Res 2003;12(1):25–31.
18. Cohen S. Social relationships and health. Am Psychol 2004;59(8):676–84.

19. Segerstrom SC, Miller GE. Psychological stress and the human immune system: a meta-analytic study of 30 years of inquiry. Psychol Bull 2004;130(4):601–30.
20. Testa MA, Simonson DC. Assessment of quality of life outcomes. N Engl J Med 1996;334(13):835–40.
21. Levi R, Drotar D. Critical issues and needs in health-related quality of life assessment of children and adolescents with chronic health conditions. In: Drotar D, editor. Measuring health-related quality of life in children and adolescents: implications for research and practice. Mahwah (NJ): Lawrence Erlbaum; 1998. p. 3–24.
22. Engstrom CP, Persson LO, Larsson S, et al. Health-related quality of life in COPD: why both disease-specific and generic measures should be used. Eur Respir J 2001;18(1):69–76.
23. Varni JW, Limbers CA, Burwinkle TM. Impaired health-related quality of life in children and adolescents with chronic conditions: a comparative analysis of 10 disease clusters and 33 disease categories/severities utilizing the PedsQL 4.0 Generic Core Scales. Health Qual Life Outcomes 2007;5:43.
24. Rosenbaum PL, Saigal S. Measuring health-related quality of life in pediatric populations: conceptual issues. In: Spilker B, editor. Quality of life and pharmacoeconomics in clinical trials. Philidelphia: Lippincott-Raven Publisher; 1996. p. 785–92.
25. Renwick R, Brown I, Nagler M. Quality of life in health promotion and rehabilitation. Thousand Oaks (CA): Sage Publications Inc; 1996.
26. Smith JM, Stablein DM, Munoz R, et al. Contributions of the transplant registry: the 2006 Annual Report of the North American Pediatric Renal Trials and Collaborative Studies (NAPRTCS). Pediatr Transplant 2007;11(4):366–73.
27. Goldstein SL, Graham N, Warady BA, et al. Measuring health-related quality of life in children with ESRD: performance of the generic and ESRD-specific instrument of the pediatric quality of life inventory (PedsQL). Am J Kidney Dis 2008; 51(2):285–97.
28. Bartosh SM, Leverson G, Robillard D, et al. Long-term outcomes in pediatric renal transplant recipients who survive into adulthood. Transplantation 2003;76(8): 1195–200.
29. Overbeck I, Bartels M, Decker O, et al. Changes in quality of life after renal transplantation. Transplant Proc 2005;37(3):1618–21.
30. Qvist E, Narhi V, Apajasalo M, et al. Psychosocial adjustment and quality of life after renal transplantation in early childhood. Pediatr Transplant 2004;8(2): 120–5.
31. Karrfelt UM, Berg UB. Long-term psychosocial outcome after renal transplantation during childhood. Pediatr Transplant 2008;12(5):557–62.
32. Broyer M, Le Bihan C, Charbit M, et al. Long-term social outcome of children after kidney transplantation. Transplantation 2004;77(7):1033–7.
33. Anthony SJ, Hebert D, Todd L, Korus M, et al. Child and parental perspectives of multidimensional quality of life outcomes after kidney transplantation. Pediatr Transplant 2009. [Epub ahead of print].
34. Neu AM. Special issues in pediatric kidney transplantation. Adv Chronic Kidney Dis 2006;13(1):62–9.
35. Simons LE, Anglin G, Warshaw BL, et al. Understanding the pathway between the transplant experience and health-related quality of life outcomes in adolescents. Pediatr Transplant 2008;12(2):187–93.
36. Uutela A, Qvist E, Holmberg C, et al. Headache in children and adolescents after organ transplantation. Pediatr Transplant 2009;13(5):565–70.

37. Noohi S, Khaghani-Zadeh M, Javadipour M, et al. Anxiety and depression are correlated with higher morbidity after kidney transplantation. Transplant Proc 2007;39(4):1074–8.
38. Dobbels F, Decorte A, Roskams A, et al. Health-related quality of life, treatment adherence, symptom experience and depression in adolescent renal transplant patients. Pediatr Transplant 2009. [Epub ahead of print].
39. Beck AL, Nethercut GE, Crittenden MR, et al. Visibility of handicap, self concept and social maturity among adult survivors of end stage renal disease. J Dev Behav Pediatr 1986;7(2):93–6.
40. Davis ID. Pediatric renal transplantation: back to school issues. Transplant Proc 1999;31(4A):61S–2S.
41. Brouhard BH, Donaldson LA, Lawry KW, et al. Cognitive functioning in children on dialysis and post-transplantation. Pediatr Transplant 2000;4(4):261–7.
42. Bakr A, Amr M, Sarhan A, et al. Psychiatric disorders in children with chronic renal failure. Pediatr Nephrol 2007;22(1):128–31.
43. Berney-Martinet S, Key F, Bell L, et al. Psychological profile of adolescents with a kidney transplant. Pediatr Transplant 2009;13(6):701–10.
44. Stuber ML. Psychiatric aspects of organ transplantation in children and adolescents. Psychosomatics 1993;4(5):379–87.
45. Taylor R, Franck LS, Gibson F, et al. A critical review of the health-related quality of life of children and adolescents after liver transplantation. Liver Transpl 2005; 11(1):51–60.
46. Alonso EM, Neighbors K, Mattson C, et al. Functional outcomes of pediatric liver transplantation. J Pediatr Gastroenterol Nutr 2003;37(2):106–8.
47. Bucuvalas JC, Britto M, Krug S, et al. Health-related quality of life in pediatric liver transplant recipients: a single-center study. Liver Transpl 2003;9(1):62–71.
48. Apajasalo M, Rautonen J, Sintonen H, et al. Health-related quality of life after organ transplantation in childhood. Pediatr Transplant 1997;1(2):130–7.
49. Kennard BD, Stewart SM, Phelan-McAuliffe D, et al. Academic outcome in long-term survivors of pediatric liver transplantation. J Dev Behav Pediatr 1999;20(1): 17–23.
50. Fredericks EM, Lopez MJ, Magee JC, et al. Psychological functioning, nonadherence and health outcomes after pediatric liver transplantation. Am J Kidney Dis 2007;7(8):1974–83.
51. Fredericks EM, Magee JC, Opipari-Arrigan L, et al. Adherence and health-related quality of life in adolescent liver transplant recipients. Pediatr Transplant 2008; 12(3):289–99.
52. Taylor RM, Franck LS, Gibson F, et al. Study of the factors affecting health-related quality of life in adolescents after liver transplantation. Am J Transplant 2009;9(5): 1179–88.
53. Alonso EM, Limbers CA, Neighbors K, et al. Cross-sectional analysis of health-related quality of life in pediatric liver transplant recipients. J Pediatr 2010;156(2):270–6, e1.
54. Ng VL, Martz K, Limbers C, et al. Health-related quality of life after pediatric liver transplantation for acute liver failure: results from the SPLIT functional outcomes group. Hepatology 2009;50(Suppl 4:237):417A.
55. Alonso EM, Neighbors K, Barton FB, et al. Health-related quality of life and family function following pediatric liver transplantation. Liver Transpl 2008;14(4):460–8.
56. Ng VL, Otley A, Gilmour S, et al. Development of PeLTQL: a disease specific health-related quality of life instrument for pediatric liver transplant recipients: item generation and item reduction. Hepatology 2009;50(Suppl 4:41):321A.

57. Jay CL, Butt Z, Ladner DP, et al. A review of quality of life instruments used in liver transplantation. J Hepatol 2009;51(5):949–59.
58. Kirk R, Edwards LB, Aurora P, et al. Registry of the International Society for Heart and Lung Transplantation: eleventh official pediatric heart transplantation report—2008. J Heart Lung Transplant 2008;27(9):970–7.
59. Lawrence KS, Fricker FJ. Pediatric heart transplantation: quality of life. J Heart Transplant 1987;6(6):329–33.
60. Wray J, Radley-Smith R. Effect of cardiac or heart-lung transplantation on the quality of life of the paediatric patient. Qual Life Res 1992;1(1):41–6.
61. Uzark KC, Sauer SN, Lawrence KS, et al. The psychosocial impact of pediatric heart transplantation. J Heart Lung Transplant 1992;11(6):1160–7.
62. Serrano-Ikkos E, Lask B, Whitehead B, et al. Heart or heart-lung transplantation: psychosocial outcome. Pediatr Transplant 1999;3(4):301–8.
63. Pennington DG, Sarafian J. Heart transplantation in children. J Heart Transplant 1985;9(4):441–5.
64. Sigfusson G, Fricker FJ, Bernstein D, et al. Long-term survivors of pediatric heart transplantation: a multicenter report of sixty-eight children who have survived longer than five years. J Pediatr 1997;130(6):862–71.
65. Wray J, Pot-Mees C, Zeitlin H, et al. Cognitive function and behavioural status in paediatric heart and heart-lung transplant recipients: the Harefield experience. BMJ 1994;309(6958):837–41.
66. Wray J, Long T, Radley-Smith R, et al. Returning to school after heart or heart-lung transplantation: how well do children adjust? Transplantation 2001;72(1):100–6.
67. DeMaso DR, Twente AW, Spratt EG, et al. Impact of psychologic functioning, medical severity, and family functioning in pediatric heart transplantation. J Heart Lung Transplant 1995;14(6 Pt 1):1102–8.
68. DeMaso DR, Douglas Kelley S, Bastardi H, et al. The longitudinal impact of psychological functioning, medical severity, and family functioning in pediatric heart transplantation. J Heart Lung Transplant 2004;23(4):473–80.
69. Spurkland I, Bjorbae T, Hagemo P. Psychosocial functioning in children after transplantation of the heart, and heart and lungs. Cardiol Young 2001;11(3):277–84.
70. Pollock-BarZiv S, Anthony S, Niedra R, et al. Quality of life and function following cardiac transplantation in adolescents. Transplant Proc 2003;35:2468–70.
71. Green A, McSweeney J. In my shoes: children's quality of life after heart transplantation. Prog Transplant 2007;17(3):199–208.
72. Todaro JF, Fennell EB, Sears SF, et al. Review: cognitive and psychological outcomes in pediatric heart transplantation. J Pediatr Psychol 2000;25(8):567–76.
73. Wray J, Radley-Smith R. Beyond the first year after pediatric heart or heart-lung transplantation: changes in cognitive function and behaviour. Pediatr Transplant 2005;9(2):170–7.
74. Wray J, Radley-Smith R. Longitudinal assessment of psychological functioning in children after heart or heart-lung transplantation. J Heart Lung Transplant 2006; 25(3):345–52.
75. Collier JA, Nathanson JW, Anderson CA. Personality functioning in adolescent heart transplant recipients. Clin Child Psychol Psychiatry 1999;4(3):367–77.
76. Aurora P, Boucek MM, Christie J, et al. Registry of the International Society for Heart and Lung Transplantation: tenth official pediatric lung and heart/lung transplantation report—2007. J Heart Lung Transplant 2007;26(12):1223–8.
77. Lanuza DM, Lefaiver CA, Farcas GA. Research on the quality of life of lung transplant candidates and recipients: an integrative review. Heart Lung 2000;29(3): 180–95.

78. Anyanwu AC, McGuire A, Rogers CA, et al. Assessment of quality of life in lung transplantation using a simple generic tool. Thorax 2001;56(3):218–22.
79. TenVergert EM, Essink-Bot ML, Geertsma A, et al. The effect of lung transplantation on health-related quality of life: a longitudinal study. Chest 1998;113(2): 358–64.
80. Durst CL, Horn MV, MacLaughlin EF, et al. Psychosocial responses of adolescent cystic fibrosis patients to lung transplantation. Pediatr Transplant 2001;5(1): 27–31.
81. Sudan D, Horslen S, Botha J, et al. Quality of life after pediatric intestinal transplantation: the perception of pediatric recipients and their parents. Am J Transplant 2004;4(3):407–13.

The Adolescent Transplant Recipient

Miriam Kaufman, MD[a,b,]*, Eyal Shemesh, MD[c,d],
Tami Benton, MD[e,f]

KEYWORDS

• Adolescent • Transplant • Adherence

Adolescents constitute a significant proportion of pediatric transplant patients, whether they have survived a transplant in early childhood (like most heart and liver recipients) or are transplanted in older childhood or adolescence, such as many renal transplant recipients. Their needs can be significantly different from either children or adults, as they are undergoing a major transformation that involves making educational and vocational decisions and commitments, establishing a new and more equal relationship with their parents, discovering their sexual identity, taking increasing responsibility for their health and creating the moral, philosophic, and ethical perspective that they will carry through their lives. Research addressing adolescence and transplantation should be an important focus in the future. Adolescent issues identified as research foci at a 2003 pediatric transplant consensus conference include adolescent graft survival, growth and the pubertal hormonal axis, quality of life, adherence, and alterations in drug metabolism.[1] This article discusses adolescent issues in transplantation.

THE ADOLESCENT INTERVIEW

Talking with adolescents does not have to be difficult nor particularly time consuming. To lay the groundwork, a discussion of confidentiality and its limits will make it clear what can be kept private and what cannot. This varies between jurisdictions, but

[a] The Transplant Centre, The Hospital for Sick Children, 555 University Avenue, Toronto, ON M5G 1X8, Canada
[b] Division of Adolescent Medicine, Department of Paediatrics, The University of Toronto, 555 University Avenue, Toronto, ON M5G 1X8, Canada
[c] Division of Behavioral Pediatrics, Department of Pediatrics, Mount Sinai Medical Center, Box 1198, 1 Gustave L Levy Place, New York, NY 10029, USA
[d] Mount Sinai School of Medicine, New York, NY, USA
[e] The Children's Hospital of Philadelphia, Behavioral Health Center, 3440 Market Street, Suite 200, Philadelphia, PA 19104, USA
[f] Department of Psychiatry, The Children's Hospital of Philadelphia, Behavioral Health Center, University of Pennsylvania School of Medicine, 3440 Market Street, Suite 200, Philadelphia, PA 19104, USA
* Corresponding author. Division of Adolescent Medicine, The Hospital for Sick Children, 555 University Avenue, Toronto, ON M5G 1X8, Canada.
E-mail address: miriam.kaufman@sickkids.ca

Pediatr Clin N Am 57 (2010) 575–592
doi:10.1016/j.pcl.2010.01.013
0031-3955/10/$ – see front matter © 2010 Elsevier Inc. All rights reserved.

pediatric.theclinics.com

confidentiality should not be promised for situations of suicide or homicide risk. Abuse must be reported (again, at varying ages) in most places. When discussing confidentiality, bring up any differences between what you will tell parents, what you will share with the team and what must be charted.

The HEADS acronym has been used to remind the clinician what to discuss. This originally stood for Home, Education, Activities, Drugs and Sex. Over the years other letters have been added: A for affect, D for depression, or S for suicidality; D for diet; S for safety.[2] The authors would also add A for adherence. Questions should be asked in a nonjudgmental fashion and some need to be fairly specific ("What were your grades on your last report card?" as opposed to "How is school?"). Questions about sexuality should use nongendered language ("Are you romantically interested in anyone?" as opposed to "Do you have a boyfriend?"). Younger adolescents tend to be concrete thinkers (see later discussion) and language should be nonambiguous.

ADOLESCENT DEVELOPMENT

Young people with solid organ transplants are young people first and foremost. Knowledge and expertise in addressing their developmental needs are important for all professionals involved in their care. There is a myth that teens see themselves as immortal and invulnerable but early adolescence is a time when many teens think about death and its permanency. As cognitive ability, knowledge of the world, physical prowess, and communication skills increase, adolescents desire and require increasing autonomy. Children learn what limits they should set for themselves by trying things out (and making mistakes) and by observing the limits that have been placed on them.

Cognitive Development

Although some adults with normal intelligence do not acquire significant abstract thinking skills, most teenagers move from concrete to sophisticated abstract thinking. Concrete thinkers do not see a spectrum of possibilities; things are black or white. As their reality shifts, they see today's truth as the only one, often surprising health care professionals as they espouse opposite views on sequential visits. This makes it difficult for providers to predict future behavior from current statements. Concrete thinkers have difficulty in deducing rules from their experiences, as each experience seems unique. They can be adherent as long as their situation remains constant, but when decisions have to be made, adherence is more challenging. For example, an adolescent may take his morning medication without reminder, but if he sleeps in, he might not take it as he has missed the appointed time. Difficulties can also arise when literal interpretations of health care advice are incorrect.[3]

Adolescent brain development is an active process, finishing in the third decade of life.[4] There is no literature on brain development in transplant recipients or in others with growth or pubertal delay. Executive functions, the last to fully develop, include organization, planning, self-regulation, selective attention, and inhibition. We expect young people to plan ahead for clinic appointments, arrange to be away from school to attend these appointments, focus on the dialog with their provider, and to restrain the impulse to miss medication. These are difficult tasks without significant executive function. This is not to say that we should have low expectations; rather we should develop strategies to aid them in developing these skills while their increasing brain maturity makes the tasks easier.

Cognitive function in pediatric transplant recipients has been examined in the pre- and posttransplant periods. Pretransplant, cognitive function was equally affected in young children awaiting heart or heart-lung transplants, those unlisted with congenital heart disease, and those awaiting bone marrow transplantation compared with healthy controls.[5] Almost half of tested heart transplant recipients showed significant delays in cognitive functioning, although most had scores in the average range for reading and spelling. Almost 25% of this sample had cognitive deficits pretransplant.[6]

Adolescent transplant recipients may have cognitive delays because of complications in the neonatal period, poor oxygenation before transplant, strokes, or other events surrounding transplantation, or as part of the syndrome that led to the need for transplant. It is key to remember that these young people are not equally delayed in all areas. Labeling them as being at a certain mental age can be a barrier to their development because of the provider's lower expectations.[7]

Puberty

Children and teens who are experiencing organ failure often have delayed puberty. Puberty and menarche have been showed to be delayed in girls who received liver or renal transplants prepubertally. (However, 1 study of 25 cardiac transplant patients showed normal onset and progression of puberty after transplant).[8] Adolescents may be reluctant to bring this up with the transplant team, because of embarrassment, worries that it is a sign of a major problem, confidentiality concerns, or because they doubt the expertise of the transplant team on pubertal issues. Sexual maturation rating (SMR, also known as Tanner Staging) should be offered every 6 months in younger teens and they should be kept up to date (without their parents) on where they are in their pubertal maturation. In a girl with no evidence of pubertal development who is at least 1 year posttransplant and who is more than 14 years old, investigations can include measurements of luteinizing hormone, follicle-stimulating hormone, estradiol, progesterone, and testosterone. Size of the ovaries on pelvic ultrasound can help determine if there is internal pubertal development.

Gynecomastia, common at SMR III in male adolescents, can also be caused by several drugs, including digoxin and isoniazid, as well as by marijuana. If gynecomastia is noted, the adolescent should be reassured that this is common, that it will get better, and that they are not changing gender. They should be counseled not to squeeze the breast tissue in an attempt to make it go away, as this will stimulate growth. Boys may also be concerned about the onset of nocturnal emission, or wet dreams. As they are unlikely to bring it up, it can be part of any discussion about puberty.

Boys and girls may have missed sexual health education at school, either because they are excused from gym or because they missed school on the day that it took place. Printed resources regarding puberty can be made available to address the questions of patients who are prepubertal or in the early stages of this development.

Emotional Development

Adolescence is a time when the experience, recognition and naming of emotions and emotional nuances is developing. As adolescents observe themselves experiencing their emotions, they learn how to behave in response to their emotions. Their expression of these observed feelings may seem dramatic or even histrionic. Adolescents need to believe that their feelings are being respected. If they are told what they are or are not (or should be) feeling, they may believe that their feelings are not valid. They will have difficulty expressing their needs to providers and might make decisions based on what they think the team wants them to say.

Adolescents develop their ability to interpret other people's emotions after they have developed their sense of their own feelings. It has been shown that they often misread facial expressions and body language, thinking that an adult is angry when he or she is actually sad.

Identity Development

Children learn to be like their parents and then spend their adolescence figuring out how they are different from them. Parental limit setting is an important part of this process. If limits are not clear, they may try many behaviors to learn when they have gone too far. If the limits are rigid and arbitrary, they may be punished for even minor infractions, which can interfere with learning about what their own personal limits are. Although experimentation with these boundaries is typically done in middle adolescence, transplant recipients may be delayed in this because of increased dependence on their parents or parental overprotection. Optimal identity formation must incorporate their health status and the transplant. If this is not part of their identity, they are unlikely to take care of their organ, but if it is the dominant part, they are unable to recognize all the other ways in which they are unique.[9]

The transplant team can have a positive influence on development. Adolescent recipients have access to more role models than most healthy teens and it is a testament to this that they often express the desire to become doctors, nurses, paramedics, social workers, or dieticians.

Adolescents who feel good about themselves are likely to incorporate this into their identity and will have increased self-confidence to move through the process of identity formation. When they acquire skills or use their abilities they tend to have a sense of themselves as globally more able.

Autonomy

In some cultures interdependence and communal values are tantamount; in the Western world, autonomy is the defining characteristic of adulthood. In either situation, some level of autonomy is expected, and parents give their children increasing levels of responsibility to foster this. Young people with chronic health conditions may see themselves as permanently dependent on parents, caregivers, medications, and technology, and may not recognize that they can achieve independence. Because they have always been cared for, these teenagers may assume that their care is the responsibility of others and that their role is to be helped rather than to be an active member of the health care team. Parents may be tempted to turn over all responsibility for medication or appointment making all at once, but a graduated approach works better, with the support of a transplant team that talks directly to the young person, sets specific stepwise goals around medical autonomy, and supports the young person as he or she inevitably makes mistakes.

PRETRANSPLANT ISSUES

Evaluation for transplant in the adolescent can be complicated by the young person's assumptions about the purpose of the psychosocial interview. Although the team uses this evaluation to assess motivation, capacity to consent, current adherence problems, and to delineate problems that might arise after transplant, the young person may think that the only reason for this interview is to see if they are psychologically suitable for transplant and do what they can to be seen as normal, mentally healthy, and optimistic. On the other hand, an ambivalent teen may present themselves as less stable, in an unconscious attempt to be rejected as a transplant candidate.

It has been shown that children and teens who have psychological problems before transplant have more hospitalizations after transplant,[10] therefore an assessment of the adolescent on their own is a crucial step in the transplant evaluation. Despite this, there is great variability between programs in terms of who does these assessments and how in-depth they are.

The assessment can be augmented with standardized psychiatric screening tools, such as the Beck Depression Inventory and the Minnesota Multiphasic Personality Inventory-Adolescent Version. One crucial thing to come out of this assessment is a determination of the teen's capacity to consent to treatment. Although laws regarding consent vary widely throughout the world, capacity to consent should still be determined in all adolescents. It would be a mistake to force a capable teen who does not want a transplant into having one, even though someone else is legally empowered to give consent.

A teen is capable of consenting if they understand their illness and understand the treatment, including having a reasonable idea of the negative and positive aspects of having or refusing the treatment. In general, the younger the child and the more complicated the disease and the treatment, the less likely they are to meet capacity criteria.

Adolescent and family expectations may become apparent during this assessment. As the teen describes the procedure and the positives and negatives of transplant, it may become clear that some or all family members have unreasonable expectations, or that they foresee a poor outcome but believe that they have no other choices.

The pretransplant assessment should also include questions about social supports. Extended family and friends are both important, but a young person may not want their healthy friends to know they are having a transplant. They may get more support from other teens they have met at the hospital or at functions held by disease-related foundations or agencies.

It is difficult to assess motivation and readiness for transplant as neither of these are fixed entities. Motivation fluctuates with mood, life events, and feelings of health or ill health. A young person's interest in transplant may be a statement of their relationship with their parents; if there is unresolved conflict, they may take the opposite point of view from the parents on everything. Enthusiasm or its absence for school, music, or work cannot be generalized to apply to their approach to transplant.

Asking a teen when the ideal time would be for a transplant can be illuminating. An otherwise enthusiastic adolescent may tell you that they will be ready in 6 months. A teen who says, "tomorrow," may be very ready or may see it as inevitable and just want to get it over with.

Adolescents and Waiting

The offer to list a teen for transplant may precipitate a realization of the seriousness of the situation. A previously cheerful, motivated adolescent may now be exhibiting anger (directed against parents or the transplant team), tearfulness, or silence. Those who are ambivalent or scared may show the most anger. Those with conduct disorders also react this way, having a narrow range of emotional options available to them. Concrete thinkers will focus on the practical details. If told average waiting times, they will interpret this as a promise that they will not have to wait any longer, so offering ranges (and adding a few months to your upper estimate) is a better approach. Almost everyone regresses in their cognitive abilities when stressed or overwhelmed, so a teen who has impressed the team with their abstract thinking skills may suddenly be reduced to asking very simple questions or making naive statements.

Waiting for transplant is particularly challenging for adolescents. A lack of ability to comprehend cause and effect, poor skills at seeing how a generalization might apply to a specific situation, poor impulse control, and less than optimal ability to pay attention can all have an effect. On the other hand, they might be better able to put the upcoming transplant out of their head and get on with life to their best ability.

Adolescents often appreciate practical advice about dealing with false alarms, what to have ready to take to the hospital, and asking a friend to text, twitter, or e-mail friends when the call comes.

The waiting period can be used to address underlying psychological issues. Adolescents who have had transplants have said they wanted more warning in the pretransplant period about postoperative pain, catheters, and the intensive care unit experience.[11]

Welcoming the adolescent's friends into the process of waiting will help them get the support they need and will set the stage for continued involvement after transplant. This can be as simple as bringing a friend to wait with them for appointments. The adolescent who wants the process kept secret should know that when they are suddenly out of school, many people will think they have gone to drug rehab or an eating disorder program.

IMMEDIATE POSTTRANSPLANT ISSUES

Many posttransplant issues are similar throughout the lifespan, such as pain, communicating while intubated, and medical issues. However, it is important for pediatric practitioners to remember that the older the adolescent, the more they will resemble an adult, and similarly for adult practitioners to keep in mind that their younger patients may seem like children in some ways.

In the absence of major complications, adolescents recover (and perceive themselves as recovering) more quickly than adults, but more slowly than younger children. Some adult sequelae (such as edema after cardiac transplant) are much more common in older adolescents than children. These young people can be much harder to mobilize than children. Adolescents may be apprehensive about leaving the protection of a critical care unit (small children are not), but are often more comfortable than their parents or an adult posttransplant.

Although the adolescent, like everyone else, is likely to regress in their thinking and behavior in the immediate postoperative period, they still have needs for control and independence. Any choices they can be given can help fill this need. Medication teaching, which should start early, must include the adolescent.

The reality of transplant is also starting to become clear. Despite what they are told before transplant, many expect to wake up feeling all better because of their new organ. In cases where the donor is a parent, they will be unable to fill their role as an important support to the adolescent during this time. When both are able to talk on the phone or communicate by computer, they should be given the opportunity to do so.

FAMILY ISSUES

Although many of the important tasks of adolescence involve differentiating oneself from one's family, the family is still the biggest influence on most teens. Teens with a chronic illness are dependent on their families for things that other teens do not even need, and many have intense relationships with their parents. Many teens who have transplants have family constellations that are nontraditional, with decisions being made by grandparents, siblings, or the partner of one of the parents.

Adolescents with chronic conditions often complain that their parents are overprotective.[12] Parents' concerns for their children's health may flow over into other aspects of life. The team may be able to help the family negotiate a contract that gradually gives more responsibility and autonomy to the teen.

When there is a living related donor, most often the donor is a parent. It seems to be a natural decision for parents, particularly mothers, and it can be difficult for parents when they cannot donate. However, adolescence is a time when there is often discord between parents and their offspring, and the donation of an organ can lead to increased strife, particularly when a parent expects ongoing gratitude for the gift of the organ.[9]

It has been shown in nontransplant populations that when the family can return to their usual parenting style, assume normal family routines, and otherwise have a normal family life, this mitigates the effect of an illness on the family.[13,14] This depends to some extent on what normal is. Parental nagging has been shown to correlate with poor adjustment in adolescents with cystic fibrosis.[14]

Some parenting patterns that are a result of long-standing illness are seen in transplant populations. The teens whose families have never set limits because their child is likely to die can be particularly frustrating for the transplant team which has to deal with an out of control youth and whose parents seem to have no authority. It is much easier to deal with the parentified young person, who for a variety of reasons (often including parental mental health issues) has been in charge of their care from a young age, ordering medications, discussing treatment changes with the team, and booking appointments. In the long run, these young people may feel stressed, present to the emergency department with big anxiety about small symptoms, and may not be capable of continually making all their health care decisions. Immigrant parents face multiple stressors including language barriers, employment, and insurance issues.[15]

Sibling concerns should not be ignored. The time surrounding a transplant is parent-intensive. The siblings may be in the care of different family members or left to their own devices for a significant time. Their daily routines often vanish. They often imagine that the parents and the recipient are having special bonding time while they are left out. Quality of life of siblings has been shown to be decreased in several conditions, including cancer and eating disorders.[16]

SCHOOL

School issues can be important before and after transplant. Some adolescents have to move to be closer to the transplant center. Starting a new school is challenging anyway, but frequent absences from school and low energy can make things worse. Schools are unlikely to make accommodations for undiagnosed cognitive problems.

After transplant, although some adolescents are anxious to get back to school and be with peers, others may be reluctant to restart their formal schooling. They may not want others to know they had a transplant, they may be fearful of having gotten behind academically, or they may not want people to see them looking cushingoid or otherwise different from the way they were before transplant. An early return to school should be encouraged, with supports in place to help the young person return if they are feeling hesitant.

Adolescents with transplants may have comorbidities that are known to negatively affect school performance, such as diabetes. Frequent absences from school for transplant clinic appointments and investigations are hard to avoid, especially in the first year after transplant. Many adolescent transplant recipients also have appointments with other subspecialists. Whenever possible, appointments should be grouped together on the same day.

PEERS

Friends are an important support and a mirror of what is normal to a young person in the transplant process. An assessment of the teen's peer network can be difficult, as a teen with few or no friends may not want to admit this. If they are attending school, asking who they eat lunch with, what they do after school and on the weekends will yield a better picture than asking directly about friends at first. Teens often feel deeply ashamed of being bullied and may deny it even when parents are presenting their concerns about bullying.

Most young people who have had heart transplants are concerned about the appearance of their scars and visible medication side effects such as weight gain, cushingoid features, gingival hypertrophy. These concerns can affect their willingness to see friends, and even more, acquaintances and classmates who do not know them well. Some adolescents find it helpful to address their classes (or have a health care provider do this), whereas others are embarrassed at being singled out in this way.

Peer support can come from within a school, neighborhood, religious institution, or disease- or organ-based support group, formal or informal. Adolescents who have a supportive friend who is aware of transplant issues seem to cope better than those who are isolated or whose condition is a secret.

SEXUALITY

Sexuality is a topic that many pediatric practitioners find difficult to discuss with their patients, but many transplant patients wonder if they are normal sexually. In a study of pediatric nephrologists, only about half interviewed patients alone, and about the same number took a sexual history.[17]

A good time to bring up the subject of sexuality is when young people are getting sexual health education at school. The message is that although there may be special concerns regarding fatigue, disclosure, sexually transmitted infections (STI) while immunosuppressed, and reproductive concerns, the adolescent will be able to have a normal sexual life. This may need to be tailored for adolescents who have genital abnormalities but sex encompasses more than just intercourse, so even if intercourse is not a possibility, the teen will still be able to have sex. Several large surveys have shown that youth with chronic conditions are more likely to be sexually active and start having sex at a slightly younger age than youth who identify themselves as healthy.[18,19]

Education should be focused on positive body image; assertiveness; information about anatomy, sexual functioning and the spectrum of sexual possibilities; communication skills; contraception and STI prevention. Gender roles should also be discussed, as girls who believe that it is their role to be passive and let men take care of the important decisions, and boys who believe that they should be in charge both have an increased risk of having unprotected intercourse, with the increased risk of pregnancy and STI that go along with this.[20] Beliefs, knowledge, and responsible behavior are integral to sexual health, which is strongly influenced by culture, class, cognitive ability, gender, sexual orientation, and general state of health.

Adolescents who are lesbian, gay, or bisexual may find it more difficult to reveal their sexual orientation to their parents than those without health issues, as they may believe they have already placed a significant burden on the family by needing a transplant.[21]

Effects of Transplantation on Sexual Functioning

Interviews with sexually active teens who have had transplants do not seem to reveal a higher incidence of sexual dysfunction than the general population but there is no published research on this topic. The literature does show a high rate of sexual dysfunction in adults who have had transplants.[22] In a study of adult women with pancreas/kidney transplant, one third reported that the transplant had a positive effect on their sexuality, another third reported no effect, and the remaining third reported negative effects, including fear of infection, decreased interest, and altered body image.[23]

Pretransplant, many teens are fatigued, which has a major effect on libido. Teens on dialysis may also be nauseated, something else that is not conducive to sexual behavior. Those with cardiac problems may worry that they will have an arrhythmia or heart attack if they have sex. Teens with breathing problems may also be concerned about the effect of having sex. Those with cystic fibrosis often have increased coughing with sex.

After transplant, the teen may have worries that sex will hurt their new organ, either from direct trauma or from over exertion. The teen can be advised to avoid anything that puts significant pressure on a transplanted kidney or on an incision. Adolescents with a small bowel transplant will have a stoma, at least for a while. Worries about leakage or the bag coming off during sex are common and realistic. Pressure on or just around the bag makes this more likely.

STI

Fear of infection is one of the factors that interferes with sexuality in adult transplant recipients. Research in this area in adolescents is lacking but it is known that fear is not a good motivator for adolescents.

Viral STI include human immunodeficiency virus (HIV), hepatitis B and C, herpes simplex (HSV), and human papilloma virus (HPV). HSV-2, commonly spread by sexual transmission, has not been shown to be increased in transplant recipients, although prevalence is high in women and men with HIV. HPV, on the other hand, has been shown to carry significant risk in the transplant population, with large treatment-resistant condylomata[24] and genital neoplasia.[25] Although HPV immunization is available and effective in immunocompetent girls and women[26] studies on transplant recipients have not been published. Based on other vaccine experience, it seems it would be sensible to immunize girls aged 10 years and higher pretransplant if possible. If this is not feasible, HPV immunization should be performed starting 1 year after transplant, when target immunosuppression levels are lower. Pap smears should be performed in sexually active adolescent girls on a schedule similar to that recommended for those who are HIV positive, yearly and indefinitely.[27]

Nonviral STI include chlamydia and gonorrhea. Local and systemic spread may be more likely and happen more quickly in immunosuppressed teens. Prevention of pelvic inflammatory disease, tubo-ovarian abscess, liver, and joint involvement are crucial. Genitourinary symptoms in sexually active teens should be empirically treated.[28]

Adolescent recipients having penetrative sex should be encouraged to use condoms every time they have sex. For those who are allergic to latex, there are condoms on the market made of polyurethane and, more recently, polyisoprene.

Contraception

Although adolescents should be told that women organ recipients have had successful pregnancies, they should also be informed of the risks and of current recommendations as to optimal timing of a pregnancy.[29] Adolescents of both genders should be counseled regarding contraceptive use. This should include a discussion of negotiating condom use with a sexual partner. If a teen seems to be considering a pregnancy, they should be referred to a high-risk obstetrician for a discussion of teratogenicity and other issues.

Barrier methods

The condoms that prevent STI also have a place in pregnancy prevention. Although not a very effective form of contraception, they are much better than no contraception, and their efficacy increases when used with a spermicidal agent. Spermicides come in a variety of forms including gel, foam, sponge, and film. Other barrier methods such as the diaphragm and the cervical cap have low acceptance rates in the adolescent population and do not protect against STI.

Hormonal contraception

Hormonal methods have been used in many transplant patients. Uncontrolled hypertension is an absolute contraindication to use, as are the other standard contraindications, such as a history of thrombophilia (unless anticoagulated). Hormonal methods that contain estrogen and progesterone include the birth control pill (daily), the patch (weekly) and the vaginal ring (monthly). There is a theoretic contraindication to use in heart transplant recipients, based on the high incidence of posttransplant coronary artery disease (CAD).[28] However, the mechanism and pathophysiology of CAD in this population is different from other CAD, and there is no evidence to indicate that estrogen-containing contraception will exacerbate posttransplant CAD. Cholestasis and, rarely, hepatocellular adenoma are known side effects of estrogen-containing contraceptives and many liver transplant programs recommend against their use, but they have been used with close follow-up. Hormonal contraception can affect immunosuppressant blood levels and doses made need to be adjusted because of this.[28]

Progestin-only contraception is often seen as a good alternative to contraceptives containing estrogen. However, the progestin-only pill is not as efficacious as a combined pill. The amount of progestin in these pills is low, so taking it at the same time every day is crucial, and patients complain of unpredictable bleeding. Injectable depo medroxy progesterone acetate has the advantage of only needing to be given every 3 months. Although heavy and irregular bleeding is common in the first few months, by 1 year almost all users are amenorrheic. However, these injections have been associated with decreased bone density, and as this is a population already at risk for osteoporosis, most clinicians avoid its use in transplant recipients. The progestin containing intrauterine device (IUCD) is effective, cost-effective if left in for 3 to 5 years, and is also associated with amenorrhea. It has not been reported to be associated with an increased rate of pelvic inflammatory disease, but no studies in transplant recipients have been published.

As the risks of pregnancy in this population are high, it seems reasonable to use an effective form of contraception, such as the combined pill or the progestin IUCD (in the absence of contraindications), and to monitor blood pressure and immunosuppressant levels.

Emergency contraception

Use of emergency contraception within 72 hours significantly reduces the risk of pregnancy, and there is some evidence that it can be used up to 120 hours after coitus.[30] The most used form contains only progestin (Plan B) taken as soon as possible after un- or under-protected intercourse. There are no contraindications to its use, and in some jurisdictions it is available over-the-counter. In places where it is not, clinicians should consider given patients a prescription to have on hand.

MENTAL HEALTH

Although most pediatric survivors of solid organ transplantation have good physical adjustment, healthy emotional functioning, and overall improvements in quality of life, more than 25% will have significant emotional difficulties, including psychiatric disorders.[31] Psychiatric symptoms or disorders may occur as a direct result of treatment including medications, response to the stress of an acute onset of illness or hospitalization, a new diagnosis, or the co-occurrence of a primary psychiatric condition that existed before transplantation. Given the risks for nonadherence associated with psychiatric comorbidities among transplant recipients, treatment is imperative.

Adolescence is a time of particular vulnerability for mental health conditions even in the absence of medical conditions or transplantation. Treatment of psychological conditions found during psychosocial and psychiatric assessments for adolescents pretransplant may prevent morbidity and mortality.

Depression and Anxiety

Symptoms of depression or anxiety are common in adolescents with chronic health conditions.[32] Although these symptoms may not meet threshold criteria for a psychiatric disorder, they can influence treatment adherence,[33] magnify physical symptom perceptions,[34] adversely affect medical outcomes,[35] and are associated with higher rates of adverse health behaviors,[36] increased risky sexual behaviors,[37] and substance abuse.[38]

Lifetime prevalence rates for depression among adolescents in community samples range from 5% to 14%.[39] Depression is highly comorbid with other disorders, with more than 60% of depressed adolescents meeting criteria for an anxiety disorder. Rates of depression increase during adolescence and begin to approach those found among adults.[40]

Anxiety disorders are the most prevalent psychiatric disorders among children and adolescents. Patients with chronic physical illnesses have higher adjusted lifetime prevalence rates for anxiety disorder.[41]

Studies of adults with solid organ transplants show high rates of psychological distress and psychiatric disorders, contributing to reduced quality of life[42] including a study showing that 25.5% of heart transplant recipients will experience a depressive episode in the first 3 years following transplantation. Pretransplantation factors correlated with risks for psychiatric disorders following transplantation included a prior psychiatric history, female gender, and low family supports.[43] Median lifetime rates for anxiety disorders of all types, excluding adjustment disorders, are approximately 5.9% following cardiac transplantation, with rates approaching 22% by 2 years after transplant.[44] Dew and colleagues[43] found posttraumatic stress disorder to be common in adults in the first year after cardiac transplantation.

Studies of mental health conditions among adolescents following solid organ transplantation reveal high rates of emotional problems.[31] A recent study in pediatric renal transplant recipients showed 65% meeting criteria for major depression and 20% having an anxiety disorder.[45]

Eating Disorders

The onset of eating disorders typically occurs during adolescence. These disorders are characterized by disturbances in eating behavior and over concern with body weight and shape and include anorexia nervosa (AN), bulimia nervosa (BN), and the more heterogeneous diagnosis of eating disorders not otherwise specified (EDNOS) These disorders are highly comorbid with other psychiatric disorders, are difficult to treat, are associated with significant medical morbidity and mortality, and frequently have a chronic and relapsing course. Risk factors include female gender, early feeding problems, childhood under-eating, and maternal weight. Identified protective factors are high self-esteem at 10 years of age and maternal well-being.[46] Few studies have examined the co-occurrence of these disorders among adolescents who undergo transplantation. Early feeding problems are common in those recipients who were ill or transplanted in the first few years of life. The use of high-dose steroids in some transplant groups can lead not only to weight gain but also a change in appearance. In addition, these adolescents are likely to share the same baseline risk factors for psychiatric disorder as those in the general population. Although most studies report an overall good quality of life for pediatric patients after transplantation, evidence regarding adolescent self-esteem following transplantation has been mixed with some studies showing that adolescents retain a positive body image and sense of self[47] and others showing significant dissatisfaction with body image following transplantation.[48]

Although there is no clear evidence of an increased rate of eating disorders after transplant, clinical experience would support discussing body image, following weight, and addressing diet with transplant recipients.

Substance Abuse

There are many theoretical risks for substance use and abuse in adolescent transplant patients: they may want to do things that they believe are normal for their age group; some may be short for their age and want to make it clear that they are not younger than their classmates or friends; or they may have learned that when one does not feel good, taking a medication helps. By far the most common substance used by North American adolescents is alcohol.

The 2007 Ontario Student Drug Use Survey (OSDUS) identified that approximately 16% of youth in grades 7 to 12 report hazardous drinking based on the Alcohol Use Disorders Identification Test (AUDIT) and 16% of students responded positively to 2 or more items on the 6 items CRAFFT scale, indicating a likelihood of problematic substance use and the need for further assessment and/or treatment. Only a few (1%) of those identified report receiving treatment.[49] Alcohol use is similar in other developed countries but Canadian youth use more marijuana and have less other drug use than in the United States.[50]

In adults, pretransplant substance abuse is associated with greater risk of post-transplant substance abuse, greater postoperative complications, increased frequency of hospitalizations and diminished quality of life.[51] As a result, most adult transplant programs require a period of abstinence before listing for transplantation. Similar data are not available in the adolescent transplant population.

Some pediatric transplant programs, particularly in the United States, have instituted zero tolerance for any substance use. This may make it unlikely that teens will disclose their use. Although there are medical concerns about some substances (such as alcohol in liver transplant recipients, tobacco effects on small blood vessels and the lungs, and cardiac and neurologic effects of ecstasy and cocaine) frank discussions of risks and how to mitigate them may be more helpful (and enforceable) than an outright ban on all substances. For example, although liver transplant recipients should not drink alcohol, a discussion with other organ recipients might include talking about the risks involved in getting drunk and forgetting to take medications, or the diuretic effect of alcohol and the importance of ensuring good fluid intake if they are going to drink alcohol.

Psychotherapies

Psychotherapeutic interventions have been effective for the treatment of psychiatric conditions among medically ill children and adolescents. Cognitive behavioral therapies (CBT) are problem-focused treatments that seek to identify maladaptive beliefs about one's environment, self, and others and to modify those beliefs, thus facilitating self-efficacy. This model takes into account developmental history, previous social learning, and important life experiences as the foundation for the unique set of assumptions that underlie how one perceives the world. Extreme, severe, or dysfunctional beliefs, and resistance to change are believed to underlie and maintain some psychiatric symptoms. This well-validated anxiety and depression treatment of non-medically ill pediatric populations,[52] also seems to be efficacious among those who are medically ill and those with eating disorders.[53,54]

Supportive therapy interventions can decrease distress by allowing the adolescent to identify and express feelings, accept and cope with the illness and demands of treatment, and provide the support needed to move beyond the psychological crisis generated by physical illness.

Family therapies attempt to alter interactions among family members for the purpose of improving functioning of the family unit. Medical family therapy emphasizes collaboration among the medical team, family, and family therapist, with the goals of involving the family in the medical treatment, recognizing the effect of illness on the family, using a biopsychosocial approach.[55] Group therapies have been helpful in adults after transplantation.[56]

Pharmacotherapy

Anecdotal evidence suggests that psychotropic medications may be helpful for the treatment of patients with severe depression and/or anxiety or those who have not responded to psychotherapy alone. It is important to remember that many immuno-suppressant agents may contribute to psychiatric symptoms, and that immunosuppressive and psychotropic medications may be metabolized by the cytochrome P450 (3A4) system, creating the potential for inhibited metabolism and toxicity.

Although no studies have demonstrated their efficacies for children and adolescents after transplantation, selective serotonin reuptake inhibitors have become the drugs of choice for depression and anxiety. Fluoxetine is the most commonly prescribed antidepressant for depression, despite its long half-life and potential for drug interactions. Citalopram and escitalopram tend to have more favorable side-effect profiles and fewer drug-drug interactions.

NONADHERENCE TO MEDICAL RECOMMENDATIONS

Patients' adherence to medical interventions becomes increasingly more important as interventions become more effective. Nonadherence is a major risk factor for poor outcomes in adolescent transplant recipients.[57] However, most adolescents are adherent and survive this period of growth, and conversely not all nonadherent patients are adolescents.

Specific tasks related to assuming responsibility over one's own care, becoming less dependent on parental advice, and other developmental achievements may complicate the task of maintaining adherence. A meta-analysis in adult transplant recipients concluded that slightly more than 20% of recipients are nonadherent to immunosuppressants in the course of 1 year.[58] The World Health Organization estimates a lifetime prevalence of 50% nonadherence in chronically ill patients in industrialized nations.[59] Using electronic monitoring devices and looking at adherence to medications in a small cohort (n = 14) of children with liver diseases,[60] we found that none of the patients took their medications as prescribed; more than 50% took them less than 70% of the time and in another study, we found that about 20% of the patients had unacceptable fluctuation of blood medication levels that put them at increased risk for poor medical outcomes.[61] Of course adherence to diet, exercise, spirometry, and physiotherapy recommendations are also important. In addition, immunosuppression is essential to survival in most transplant recipients, and the consequences of nonadherence can therefore be dire. Nonadherence, for example, is an important predictor of rejection episodes in long-term survivors.[61,62] And yet, methods to assess and treat nonadherence are rarely, if ever, incorporated into practice.[63]

Measuring Adherence

Nonadherence is dynamic[64]: a patient may present as nonadherent at one point in time and adherent at another. Therefore, any method used to measure adherence must be applied over time and continuously, rather than at only 1 time point. The importance of defining a method to assess adherence cannot be overstated. Without a valid standard method to measure adherence with a well-defined threshold, it is extremely difficult to proceed with clinical applications and evaluate interventions to improve adherence. The absence of a robust measure of adherence has been described as the Achilles Heel of much of such research.[65] The following methods have been used in the transplant setting.

Indirect measures

- Subjective measures: patient/caregiver self-report and clinicians' assessments are not reliable ways to assess adherence, especially in children and adolescents. Clinicians' assessments of adherence are unreliable.[61]
- Pill counts: a patient may engage in a variety of behaviors that would invalidate this method as a measure of adherence. Pills can be removed but not taken, or taken at an incorrect time.[64] The time spent counting pills is a barrier to a wide implementation of this method.
- Electronic event monitoring (EM) devices: pill boxes with electronic caps that register each opening of the device for dispensation of a pill. EMs are used in research settings, but are expensive, cannot be used for liquid preparations, and patients are reluctant to use them in pediatric transplant clinical settings.[65]
- Prescription refill rates: prescription refill data can be used to detect nonadherence.[66] Refilling a prescription is not synonymous with taking the prescribed dose, so this method provides only a crude estimate of adherence.

Direct measures

- Medication blood levels. Medication blood levels are routinely obtained for clinical care in transplant clinics. Blood levels are objective measures of adherence, and they are directly related to whether or not the patient took the medication. This method may mislabel a usually adherent patient who misses a dose the day before testing, and may miss the nonadherent patients who takes their medication for a few days before testing. A strategy of continuous surveillance, evaluating the degree of fluctuation over time, gives a clearer picture of medication use.[61] Calculating the degree of fluctuation of medication blood levels offers a unique opportunity to evaluate adherence in the transplant setting. However, medication levels may vary with personal pharmacokinetics and absorption.

Psychosocial Predictors and Risks

Psychosocial predictors for medication nonadherence are related to psychological symptoms of the patient or the caretaker, family interactions, the existence of barriers to adherent behavior, and health beliefs that may interfere with adherence, including responsibility shifts between caretaker and child. Other risks include factors associated with the disease process itself (ie, time because transplant), factors related to the provision of care (ie, prescription pattern), socioeconomic status, and others.

Interventions to Improve Adherence

There are currently no proven methods to improve adherence in pediatric and adolescent transplant recipients. However, many interventions have been suggested and are being tried. Educational interventions teach patients about adherence in general, or can be targeted at those who are at risk of nonadherence. Many young people use reminders, including electronic reminders or timing medications to a regular activity. Behavioral approaches target nonadherence as a dysfunctional behavior and include positive and negative reinforcements to modulate this behavior. In addition, specific risk factors can be targeted. Although this was not proved, it seems plausible that young people may be more likely to take medications if they believe that their health care provider likes them and explains the rationale for taking medications. Participating in decisions and having changes made that fit their lifestyle and schedule may also be helpful. If there are financial or structural (ie, clinic routine) barriers to adherence, interventions might attempt to target those issues as well.

SUMMARY

Adolescent transplant recipients are faced with many of the challenges that adults deal with: living with a chronic condition, being adherent, being different from one's peers. They must surmount these challenges while moving from childhood, with its dependence on parents, a black and white outlook often unfettered by a comprehension of cause and effect and lack of control, to an adult perspective that allows them to negotiate with parents, peers, partners, and employers; to know who they are; to accept the nuances and unpredictability of life and to become fully actualized adults. They can be helped in this journey by clinicians who respect and listen to them, who ask the right questions, pay attention to their mental health needs, and encourage them in their vocational aspirations. In addition to being good things to do, these interventions should improve adherence and long-term outcomes.

ACKNOWLEDGMENTS

The authors would like to thank Abigail Harrison, Karen Leslie, Ian Chen, and Melissa Keown for their help in preparing this manuscript.

REFERENCES

1. Bartosh SM, Ryckman FC, Shaddy R, et al. A national conference to determine research priorities in pediatric solid organ transplantation. Pediatr Transplant 2008;12:153–66.
2. Goldenring JM, Rosen DS. Getting into adolescent heads: an essential update. Contemp Pediatr 2004;21(1):64.
3. Kaufman M. Role of adolescent development in the transition process. Prog Transplant 2006;16:286–90.
4. Casey BJ, Giedd JN, Thomas KM. Structural and functional brain development and its relation to cognitive development. Biol Psychol 2000;54:241–57.
5. Wray J, Radley-Smith R. Developmental and behavioral status of infants and young children awaiting heart or heart-lung transplantation. Pediatrics 2004; 113:488–95.
6. Brosig C, Hintermeyer M, Zlotocha J, et al. An exploratory study of the cognitive, academic and behavioral functioning of pediatric cardiothoracic transplant recipients. Prog Transplant 2006;16:38–45.

7. Kaufman M. Transition of cognitively delayed adolescent organ transplant recipients to adult care. Pediatr Transplant 2006;10:413–7.
8. de Broux E, Huot CH, Chartrand S, et al. Growth and pubertal development following pediatric heart transplantation. Ann Chir 2001;126(9):881–7. English abstract accessed through Ovid Medline.
9. Franklin PM, Crombie AK. Live related renal transplantation: psychological, social and cultural issues. Transplantation 2003;76:1247–52.
10. DeMaso DR, Twente AW, Spratt EG, et al. Impact of psychological functioning, medical severity and family functioning in pediatric heart transplantation. J Heart Lung Transplant 1995;14(6):1102–8.
11. Anthony SJ, Kaufman M, Drabble A, et al. Perceptions of transitional care needs and experiences in pediatric heart transplant recipients. Am J Transplant 2009;9: 614–9.
12. Abrams A, Lewis D, Rahman A, et al. Young people have the last word. In: McDonagh JE, White PH, editors. Adolescent rheumatology. New York: Informa Healthcare; 2008. p. 404–12.
13. Vessey JA, Rumsey M. Chronic conditions and child development. In: Allen P, Vessey J, editors. Primary care of the child with a chronic condition. 4th edition. St. Louis (MO): Mosby; 2004. p. 23–43.
14. Graetz BW, Shute RH, Sawyer MG. An Australian study of adolescents with cystic fibrosis: perceived supportive and non-supportive behaviors from families and friends and psychological adjustment. J Adolesc Health 2000;26(1): 64–9.
15. Crockett M. New faces from faraway places: immigrant child health in Canada. Paediatr Child Health 2005;10(5):277–81.
16. Houtzager BA, Grootenhuis MA, Caron HN, et al. Quality of life and psychological adaptation in siblings of paediatric cancer patients, 2 years after diagnosis. Psychooncology 2004;13(8):499–511.
17. Hergenroeder AC, Brewer ED. A survey of pediatric nephrologists on adolescent sexual health. Pediatr Nephrol 2001;16:57–60.
18. Suris J-C, Parera N. Sex, drugs and chronic illness: health behaviours among chronically ill youth. Eur J Public Health 2005;15(5):484–8.
19. Tonkin R, Peters L, Murphy A, et al, & the McCreary Centre Society. Adolescent health survey: chronic illness and disability among youth in BC. Burnaby (BC): McCreary Centre Society; 1994.
20. Pleck J, Sonenstein L, Ku L. Masculine ideology: its impact on adolescent males' heterosexual relationships. J Soc Issues 1993;49(3):11–30.
21. Kaufman M, The Adolescent Health Committee. Adolescent sexual orientation. Paediatr Child Health 2008;13(7):619–23.
22. Raiz L, Davies E, Ferguson R. Sexual functioning following renal transplantation. Health Soc Work 2003;28:264–72.
23. Muehrer R, Keller M, Powwattana A, et al. Sexuality among women recipients of a pancreas and kidney transplant. West J Nurs Res 2006;28(2):137–50.
24. Gentile G, Formelli G, Selva S. Atypical picture of cervico-vaginal condylomatosis in a patient submitted to hepatic transplant. Clin Exp Obstet Gynecol 1990; 17(3–4):155–7.
25. Krebs HB, Schneider V, Hurt WG, et al. Genital condylomas in immunosuppressed women: a therapeutic challenge. Southampt Med J 1986;79(2): 183–7.
26. Koutsky LA, Ault KA, Wheeler CM, et al. A controlled trial of a human papillomavirus type 16 vaccine. N Engl J Med 2002;347:1645–51.

27. McLachlin CM, Mai V, Murphy J, et al. Ontario cervical cancer screening clinical practice guidelines. J Obstet Gynaecol Can 2007;29(4):344–53.
28. Sucato G, Murray P. Gynecologic health care for the adolescent solid organ transplant recipient. Pediatr Transplant 2005;9:346–56.
29. McKay DB, Josephson M, Armenti VT, et al. Reproduction and transplantation: report on the AST consensus conference on reproductive issues and transplantation. Am J Transplant 2005;5:1592–9.
30. Rodrigues I, Grou F, Joly J. Effectiveness of emergency contraceptive pills between 72 and 120 hours after unprotected sexual intercourse. Am J Obstet Gynecol 2001;184:531–7.
31. DeMaso DR, Kelley SD, Bastardi H, et al. The longitudinal impact of psychological functioning, medical severity, and family functioning in pediatric heart transplantation. J Heart Lung Transplant 2004;23:473–80.
32. Borowsky I, Mozayeny S, Ireland M. Brief psychosocial screening at health supervision and acute care visits. Pediatrics 2003;112:129–33.
33. DiMatteo MR, Lepper HS, Croghan TW. Depression is a risk factor for non-compliance with medical treatment: meta-analysis of the effects of anxiety and depression on patient adherence. Arch Intern Med 2000;160:2101–7.
34. Campo J, Comer D, Jansen-McWilliams L, et al. Recurrent pain, emotional distress, and health service use in childhood. J Pediatr 2002;141:76–83.
35. Katon W. Clinical and health services relationships between major depression, depressive symptoms, and general medical illness. Biol Psychiatry 2003;54:216–26.
36. Goodman E, Whitaker R. A prospective study of the role of depression in the development and persistence of adult obesity. Pediatrics 2002;110:497–504.
37. Lehrer JA, Shrier LA, Gortmaker S, et al. Depressive symptoms as a longitudinal predictor of sexual risk behaviors among US middle and high school students. Pediatrics 2006;118:189–200.
38. Bukstein OG, Brent DA, Kaminer Y. Comorbidity of substance abuse and other psychiatric disorders in adolescents. Am J Psychiatry 1989;146:1131–41.
39. Kessler RC, Walters EE. Epidemiology of DSM-III-R major depression and minor depression among adolescents and young adults in the National Comorbidity Survey. Depress Anxiety 1998;7:3–14.
40. Kessler RC, Aveneovoli S, Merikangas K, et al. Mood disorders in children and adolescents: an epidemiologic perspective. Biol Psychiatry 2001;49:1002–14.
41. Colon EA, Popkin MK. Anxiety and panic. In: Wise MG, Rundell JR, editors. The American psychiatric publishing textbook of consultation-liaison psychiatry. 2nd edition. Washington, DC: American Psychiatric Publishing; 2002. p. 394–415.
42. Dew MA, Switzer GE, DiMartini AF. Psychiatric morbidity and organ transplantation. Curr Opin Psychiatry 1998;29(11):621–6.
43. Dew MA, Kormos RL, DiMartini AF, et al. Prevalence and risk for depression and anxiety related disorders during the first three years after heart transplantation. Psychosomatics 2001;42:300–13.
44. Phipps L. Psychiatric aspects of heart transplantation. Can J Psychiatry 1991;36:563–8.
45. Berney-Martinet S, Key F, Bell L, et al. Psychological profile of adolescents with a kidney transplant. Pediatr Transplant 2009;13:701–10.
46. Nicholls DE, Viner RM. Childhood risk factors for lifetime anorexia nervosa by age 30 years in a national birth cohort. J Am Acad Child Adolesc Psychiatry 2003;48(8):791–9.
47. Durst CL, Horn MV, MacLaughin EF, et al. Psychosocial responses of adolescent cystic fibrosis patients to lung transplantation. Pediatr Transplant 2001;5:27–31.

48. Morel P, Almond P, Mata A, et al. Long term quality of life after kidney transplantation in childhood. Transplantation 1991;52:47–52.
49. Adlaf, EM, Paglia, A. Drug use among Ontario students, 1977–2005: detailed OSDUS findings CAMH research document series no. 16. Toronto: Centre for Addiction and Mental Health. 2005.
50. William A, Vega WA, Aguilar-Gaxiola S, et al. Prevalence and age of onset for drug use in seven international sites: results from the international consortium of psychiatric epidemiology. Drug Alcohol Depend 2002;68(3):285–97.
51. Shapiro PA, Williams DL, Foray AT, et al. Psychosocial evaluation and prediction of compliance problems and morbidity after heart transplantation. Transplantation 1995;60:1462–6.
52. Brent DA, Holder D, Kolko D, et al. A clinical psychotherapy trial for adolescent depression comparing cognitive, family and supportive treatments. Arch Gen Psychiatry 1997;54:877–85.
53. Szigethy E, Kenney BA, Carpenter J, et al. Cognitive–behavioral therapy for adolescents with inflammatory bowel disease and subsyndromal depression. J Am Acad Child Adolesc Psychiatry 2007;46:1290–8.
54. Schmidt U. Cognitive behavioral approaches in adolescent anorexia and bulimia nervosa. Child Adolesc Psychiatr Clin N Am 2009;18(1):147–58.
55. Sholevar P, Sahar C. Medical family therapy. In: Sholevar GP, Schwoeri LD, editors. Textbook of family and couples therapy: clinical applications. Washington, DC: American Psychiatric Publishing; 2003. p. 747–67.
56. Abbey S, Farrow S. Group therapy and organ transplantation. Int J Group Psychother 1998;48:163–85.
57. Shemesh E, Shneider BL, Savitzky JK, et al. Medication adherence in pediatric and adolescent liver transplant recipients. Pediatrics 2004;113(4):825–32.
58. Stuber ML, Shemesh E, Seacord D, et al. Evaluating nonadherence to immunosuppressant medications in pediatric liver transplant recipients. Pediatr Transplant 2008;12(3):284–8.
59. Shemesh E. Psychosocial adaptation and adherence. In: Fine RN, Webber S, Kelly D, et al, editors. Pediatric solid organ transplantation. 2nd edition. Oxford (UK): Blackwell Publishing; 2007. p. 418–24.
60. Dew MA, DiMartini AF, De Vito Dabbs A, et al. Rates and risk factors for nonadherence to the medical regimen after adult solid organ transplantation. Transplantation 2007;83(7):858–73.
61. World Health Organization. Adherence to long term therapies: evidence for action. Geneva (Switzerland): WHO Press; 2003.
62. Kerkar N, Annunziato RA, Foley L, et al. Prospective analysis of nonadherence in autoimmune hepatitis: a common problem. J Pediatr Gastroenterol Nutr 2006;43(5):629–34.
63. Johnson SB. Measuring adherence. Diabetes Care 1992;15(11):1658–67.
64. Shellmer DA, Zelikovsky N. The challenges of using medication event monitoring technology with pediatric transplant patients. Pediatr Transplant 2007;11(4):422–8.
65. Chisholm-Burns MA, Kwong WJ, Mulloy LL, et al. Nonmodifiable characteristics associated with nonadherence to immunosuppressant therapy in renal transplant recipients. Am J Health Syst Pharm 2008;65(13):1242–7.
66. Shemesh E, Annunziato R, Shneider BL, et al. Improving adherence to medications in pediatric liver transplant recipients. Pediatr Transplant 2008;12(3):316–23.

Transition of Care to Adult Services for Pediatric Solid-Organ Transplant Recipients

Lorraine E. Bell, MDCM, FRCPC[a,b],*,
Susan M. Sawyer, MBBS, MD, FRACP[c,d,e]

KEYWORDS

- Transition • Adolescent • Young adult
- Transplantation • Pediatric • Self-management

The path from childhood to adulthood is marked by a series of milestones. In the developed world, this ranges from the simple counting of years that are celebrated with birthday parties, to a series of educational milestones (such as commencement and completion of primary school, completion of secondary education, part-time work, and decision making about future work), to various social milestones (such as one's first boyfriend or girlfriend, leaving home), and to legal milestones (such as being able to vote and drive a car). For the growing number of young people with complex health conditions, transfer from pediatric to adult health care services is an event that equally deserves celebration by young people, parents, and health professionals alike, for the myriad achievements that are signified by this important event. As with increasing education and social participation, attainment of the milestone of transfer to adult services signals a beginning rather than an end point, with expectations of growing participation and competence. Thus the event of transfer to adult focused services is but part of the continuum of the process that constitutes transition to adult health care.

The importance of transition to adult health care for young people with chronic conditions is increasingly recognized by policy statements from various organizations.[1,2] These policy statements highlight that the goal of transitional care is to

[a] Department of Paediatrics, McGill University, Montréal, QC, Canada
[b] McGill University Health Centre - Montreal Children's Hospital, Division of Nephrology, 2300 rue Tupper, #E222, Montréal, QC H3H 1P3, Canada
[c] Department of Paediatrics, The University of Melbourne, Melbourne, Australia
[d] Centre for Adolescent Health, Royal Children's Hospital, Melbourne, Australia
[e] Murdoch Childrens Research Institute, Melbourne, Australia
* Corresponding author. McGill University Health Centre - Montreal Children's Hospital, Division of Nephrology, 2300 rue Tupper, #E222, Montréal, QC H3H 1P3, Canada.
E-mail address: lorraine.bell@mcgill.ca

Pediatr Clin N Am 57 (2010) 593–610
doi:10.1016/j.pcl.2010.01.007
0031-3955/10/$ – see front matter © 2010 Published by Elsevier Inc.

maximize lifelong functioning and potential through the provision of high-quality, developmentally appropriate health care services that continue uninterrupted as the individual moves from adolescence to adulthood.

Although successful transfer to adult focused health care is important for young people with a range of complex or severe chronic conditions, ensuring effective engagement with adult services for adolescents and young adult solid-organ transplant recipients is arguably as critical for immediate graft survival as it is for their future health and well-being.[3] Extrapolating from ANZDATA (Australia and New Zealand Dialysis and Transplant Registry)[4] and the Organ Procurement and Transplantation Network registry[5] reports, there are at least 7000 young people aged 15 to 24 years with functioning solid-organ transplants (kidney, liver, heart, and lung) in Australia, New Zealand, the United States, and Canada alone. Many of these patients would not have survived into adult life 2 decades ago. Now they are reaching adulthood in ever-increasing numbers. Some have underlying diseases or conditions that may be unfamiliar to adult physicians because patients with these conditions were previously far less likely to survive to adulthood. Some may have physical, social, or cognitive challenges, either directly related to their underlying disease or indirectly as a consequence of living with such a serious condition. Some may transfer to large well-resourced specialized adult transplant centers, whereas others may transfer to community-based specialists, with more variable support structures.

The Pediatric Committee of the American Society of Transplantation recognizes the importance of transition across the adolescent and young adult years and has called for greater focus by pediatric and adult teams on the tasks required to support successful transfer to and engagement with adult services.[3] Promoting acquisition of developmentally appropriate self-management skills and competencies by young people as they mature through adolescence into early adult life (as embodied in the term transition to adult health care) is equally critical.[6]

There is encouraging evidence from certain disease groups, such as cystic fibrosis, that the risk of major disruption to regular health care can be appropriately managed if it is carefully supported and resourced.[7] However, the situation is more concerning for other conditions. For example, studies of young people with type 1 diabetes report that 24% to 69% are lost to follow-up after transfer to adult health care.[8] In the United Kingdom, Kipps and colleagues[9] describe that 94% of young people were attending clinic at least 6 monthly in the 2 years before transfer, declining to 57% 2 years after transfer to adult health care. The attendance rate varied from 29% to 71%, which suggests the importance of local factors in influencing clinic attendance.

There have been few studies of young people with transplants to know how well they transfer to adult services and what effect this has on their health, well-being and transplant organ function. A report by Watson[10] was concerning, with 8 of 20 kidney allografts failing within 36 months of young people transferring to adult services. Particularly worrisome was that 7 of these failures were unexpected. A recent Australian study of all pediatric renal transplant recipients transferring to adult health care was more reassuring,[11] with 10 of 11 regularly receiving medical care within adult services 1 year after transfer, and none of the 11 having an unexpected clinical course. Clinic attendance reduced from 73% in the year before transfer to 57% during the year after transfer to adult focused care, raising questions about continuing engagement with adult focused care. This finding is consistent with an English study that followed up 16 of 28 kidney transplant recipients and showed a higher nonattendance rate at clinic in the year after transfer to adult services.[12] A small retrospective report of medication adherence in recently transitioned liver transplant recipients showed increased variability in tacrolimus trough level following transfer to adult care.[13] More disquieting are studies that suggest low levels of satisfaction with the process of transfer to adult health care. For example, Remorino and Taylor[12] recorded that 9 of 11 young people reported overall satisfaction with their transfer as being only "OK," and the remaining 2 described it as having gone "badly" and "really badly." Also concerning were statements by 9 of 10 young Australians that they did not feel involved in transition planning.[11] In a qualitative study about the process of transition for 17 organ transplant recipients (9 renal, 5 liver, 4 heart), McCurdy and colleagues[14] emphatically highlighted the greater need for investment in transition planning, with young people generally feeling poorly prepared to face the adult health care system, which they belatedly appreciated as being very different to pediatric services.

In light of these concerns this review explores the following broad areas: What do we want to achieve as adolescent transplant recipients move to adult health care? How do we reach that goal? Is the theory of emerging adulthood important in our concept of transition? What are the challenges during the process of transition? The bulk of the tasks required for young people to achieve successful transition to adult services occur during childhood and adolescence, and these are our primary focus. Thus this article (1) examines the definitions of adolescence and emerging adulthood and some of the challenges of these phases of life, including neurocognitive influences on decision making and behavior, (2) discusses elements that may influence motivation and engagement and enhance communication and adherence for adolescents and young adults, (3) highlights important areas in education, vocational planning, and quality of life (QOL) for transplant recipients, (4) reviews tasks and challenges during navigation of the transition journey, and (5) provides specific transition recommendations, for primary care providers practicing outside transplant centers and for transplant health care professionals.

WHAT DO WE WANT TO ACHIEVE AS ADOLESCENT SOLID-ORGAN TRANSPLANT RECIPIENTS MOVE TO ADULT HEALTH CARE?

Our health goals include maximizing young people's potential for longevity and an excellent quality of those lived years, with a minimum of health complications. Developmental goals include optimizing young people's potential to live as independently and self-sufficiently as they can, and to experience the same educational opportunities, employment possibilities, and social relationships as do their peers. These goals require a multifaceted comprehensive approach beginning early in care and a strong partnership between the health care team, the young person, and their parents or carers, and, increasingly, with schools. They ideally include attention to child and adolescent development, and focus on self-management skills, communication, and sustained attention to educational and social participation.

Adolescence and Emerging Adulthood

Adolescence is the period between childhood and adulthood encompassed by changes in physical, psychological, and social development. It is a time of significant change, associated with greater emotional reactivity and, for a range of reasons, a time of relative vulnerability.[15] In the early twentieth century adolescence was viewed as continuing into the mid-20s.[16–19] However, the World Health Organization[20] currently defines adolescence as the period between 10 and 19 years (starting from the onset of puberty); the teenage years are defined as spanning the age from 13 to 19 years. Although 18 years is the age of legal majority in most high-income countries,[21] this age does not denote any magical developmental imperative. Turning 18 years does not of itself signify achievement of adult functioning or mark that point when the perceived turbulence of adolescence disappears, rational decisions are consistently made, or risk taking is diminished. In defining youth as the period between 15 and 24 years, the World Health Organization has appreciated the growing capacity for more mature adult functioning beyond the age of legal majority. Similarly, Arnett[14] has used the term "emerging adulthood" to describe the period between 18 and 25 years, in recognition of ongoing maturation and social development. For most adolescents in the high-income world (defined by the World Bank as countries and regions in which the gross national income per capita [2008] is greater than 11,905 US dollars[21]), adolescence is a period of personal exploration and identity formation, which is still relatively free from major social and financial responsibilities.

The age at which patients typically transfer to adult health care coincides with the time of life when risk behaviors peak. This can be a challenging period for many young people, even in the absence of chronic disease. In the high-income world, the mortality of 15- to 19-year-olds is more than 3 times higher than that of 10- to 14-year-olds, whereas 19- to 24-year-olds have 4 times greater mortality than 10- to 14-year-olds.[22] Rates of substance use and abuse, mental disorders including suicide, and sexual health risks are all greater in young adults than in adolescents.[23] The burden of a serious health condition is an additional stressor, with higher rates of risk behaviors described in adolescents with chronic conditions than in healthy young people.[24] Challenges concerning treatment adherence become more evident in the adolescent and young adult years, as direct parental influence on behavior wanes and patient concerns about side effects of medication evolve. It is perhaps not surprising that young adult and adolescent renal transplant recipients have the highest rates of acute rejection, death-censored graft loss, and chronic rejection leading to graft loss than any other age group.[25,26] Outcome data for nonrenal organ transplant recipients during emerging adulthood are sparse; however, as with kidney recipients, long-term graft survival is worse for those transplanted during adolescence (age 12–17 years) than during childhood.[5]

Neurocognitive influences on adolescent and young adult decision making and behavior

Physical development antedates emotional maturity; most girls are physically mature by mid-adolescence, although boys are often not fully grown until the older teenage years. Cognitive abilities are also well established by the mid-teenage years.[27] However, the development of emotional regulation, reflective judgment, and thus social maturity lag behind achievement of physical maturity and cognitive skills. Contrary to common belief, young people do not have delusions of invulnerability.[28] Nonetheless, engagement in sensation-seeking activities peaks in adolescence and young adulthood and there is an exaggerated response to certain types of rewards.[15] Emotional and social factors may override more rational cognitive functions, leading to inconsistent choices and potentially dangerous risk taking.[29] These influences continue at least into the mid-20s.[28] On tests of risk perception, sensation seeking, impulsivity, resistance to peer influence, and future orientation, scores are similar at 10 and 15 years of age; differences begin to emerge at age 16 to 17 years, with a progressively increasing level of function up to at least the age of 30 years.[30] The complex interrelated skills of logical reasoning, reflective judgment, and emotional regulation evolve into adulthood.[31]

Advances in neuroimaging, particularly structural and functional magnetic resonance imaging, have led to a greater understanding of the neurobiological basis of these phenomena. Developmental changes in brain structure continue into the third decade of life.[28] The subcortical limbic regions, such as the amygdala and the nucleus accumbens in the basal ganglia, important for emotion and reward seeking, mature early. In contrast, the prefrontal cortex and associated areas, responsible for executive brain functions such as foresight, planning, evaluation of risk and reward, and the capacity to dissociate decision making and strong emotion, are among the last to reach adult levels; moreover, functional connectivity between these 2 regions is delayed.[15,32] When a young person makes a poor decision in a highly charged emotional or social context, he or she may well know better, and have different decision making in the absence of such influences.

The combination of heightened responsiveness to rewards and immaturity in brain areas for behavioral control may result in adolescents investing more in activities with immediate rather than long-term gains, and help explain their increase in risky decision making and emotional reactivity.[15] Thus there is some biologic basis for the emotional extremes and lack of mature executive planning that can be seen during adolescence and early adulthood.

Adolescent Motivation and Engagement

How adolescents view themselves in the present and into the future is important to their life goals, whether in relation to education, work and career, or intimate relationships. Young people do not commonly experience the notion of a future beyond the age of 30 years.[33,34] However, their goals are essential to their motivation and well-being and a key to understanding their behavior.[35] Although there are many theories of motivation, one with an important effect on health behavior, education, and child rearing is self-determination theory (SDT).[36–40] SDT emphasizes the importance of 3 basic psychological needs: autonomy, competence, and relatedness.[38,41] Autonomy involves experiencing a sense of choice and willingness rather than being controlled or pressured. Competence describes a feeling of self-confidence or self-efficacy, whereas relatedness is a sense of belonging, of having connection with others, of shared values and interests, and friendships. Aspects of SDT that are especially pertinent to working with adolescents and to parenting are (1) providing a rationale and explanation for behavioral requests; (2) recognizing the feelings and perspectives of the child or adolescent; (3) offering choices and encouraging initiative; and (4) minimizing the use of controlling techniques. Engagement of adolescents with their health care can be enhanced by clear and consistent goals, a perception of fairness, and participation and collaboration in decision making with the responsible adults in their lives (parents and health care staff).[42] Although peer groups have often been viewed as negative influences during adolescence, the provision of social support and acceptance from peers with chronic disease can also be harnessed positively.[43]

Education

Much success in later life depends on educational achievement.[44] Although many pediatric solid-organ transplant recipients do well academically and socially, a higher proportion have problems with school achievement, compared with the general population, and on reaching adulthood their unemployment rate is higher.[45–50] Contributing elements include neurocognitive factors as well as the extent of school absence. Children with chronic disease are at risk for experiencing more difficulty in academic areas that build on prerequisite skills and knowledge; this effect is present even after controlling for learning difficulties.[51] Frequent or prolonged school absence may lead children to miss out on key learning opportunities and mastery of core skills required to progress to a more advanced level. Equally critical are, long periods of absence that can make young people feel less confident about returning to school and re-establishing friendships or relationships that may be perceived to, or actually, have moved on. Organ transplant recipients in particular may miss a great deal of school before their transplant because of hospitalizations, frequent clinic visits, and fatigue or general malaise. Those with renal transplants may have additionally endured the burden of long hours of dialysis.

Areas that need to be explored to address these challenges are educational intervention programs (eg, tutoring, teaching of coping skills, peer-mediated supports) and school-reintegration programs for those who have missed prolonged periods of school.[51] A greater focus on coordination between hospital and school settings is also required.[51,52] At the very least, this should include dissemination of information to teachers about the effects of chronic illnesses and associated treatments which their pupils may be experiencing.[53] It is also important to balance the value of schools being informed with the patient's need for privacy and confidentiality. Thus, involving young people themselves in what information will be shared with whom is a critical aspect of communication with schools. Early recognition of learning problems or of educational deficits in children with chronic conditions, and ensuring timely remediation, are also likely to lead to greater success.[51,54] Other measures that may help augment school achievement include a stimulating home learning environment, positive parental role models, and favorable school experiences, such as individual attention to pupils' needs and giving them a voice in planning the content and evaluation of their learning.[54] Enhancing school engagement may help diminish high school dropout rates; research has shown that students who show a rapid decrease in engagement, or low levels of engagement, at the beginning of adolescence are more likely to drop out,[55] underlining the importance of well-timed intervention.

Health Related Quality of Life in Adolescent and Young Adult Transplant Recipients

Several small studies have investigated the QOL of adolescent transplant recipients and young adults transplanted in childhood, using instruments such as the 36-item Short-form Health Survey Version 2.0 (SF-36v2), the Child Health and Illness Profile, Adolescent Edition (CHIP-AE), and the Child Health Related Quality of Life Self Report Questionnaire (CHQ-CF87). Findings have been inconsistent, possibly because of small samples sizes, with mean scores ranging from similar to the general population to significantly lower in almost every domain.[46,56,57] However, questionnaires do not tell the whole story, and qualitative research, which seeks a deeper understanding of patients' experiences using careful analyses of in-depth interviews, can make important contributions. A recent systematic review of qualitative studies of more than 300 adolescent organ transplant recipients revealed the following information: adolescent patients' feelings and experiences included a sense of domination by their medical regimens, lowered self-esteem, resentment about feeling different, negative reaction by peers, loss of a sense of belonging, anxiety about rejection and how long their transplants would last, and uncertainty about life expectancy.[58] Some had suicidal thoughts. Some were thankful for the transplant having given them a second chance at life and for the new or restored vitality that it provided. Some desired more independence and felt overprotected by their parents. A wish to set long-term academic and vocational goals was prevalent. However, maintaining schoolwork was often a challenge; extensive school absenteeism caused some to fall behind in their studies, and many felt stressed and overwhelmed as they struggled to make progress and achieve satisfactory grades.[58] This work highlights the complexity and range of developmental issues experienced by young transplant recipients. It should reinforce to physicians, nurses, and other health care workers that our goals for medical stability during transition to adult health care need to be accompanied by support for our young patients' quests for fulfilling and productive lives.

Communicating with Adolescents

The quality of communication between clinicians and adolescents can affect their understanding of their medical condition, satisfaction with treatment, collaboration, and subsequent appointment keeping.[59–61] Positive influences on the health dialog include perceptions that the physician is trustworthy and completely honest with the adolescent patient, listens carefully and takes their concerns seriously, is patient-centered rather than condition-focused (eg, interested in the broader effect of their condition on their day-to-day life, particularly in discussing school difficulties or social and emotional problems), seeks permission before asking about personal issues, maintains confidentiality, provides understandable explanations, and involves the adolescent in decision making.[62] Physician willingness to discuss sensitive health topics is also associated with more positive perceptions of care by young people.[63] Adolescents are less likely to be engaged if their visit is brief or if they feel rushed, if they are seeing a health professional whom they have not previously met, or if there is a lack of privacy (including the presence of medical students in the room). Some young people with chronic disease have reported it takes at least 4 to 5 visits before they trust a physician.[64] Support of autonomy and competence is important; adolescents react poorly to the use of coercion, such as scare tactics, or techniques that make them feel badly about themselves. Sometimes parental presence at appointments is supportive and confidence building for adolescents; at other times it may hinder communication, particularly around personal or sensitive topics.[59,62] A study exploring specialists' perceptions of the health care preferences of chronically ill adolescents found physicians underestimated the importance of communicating as a friend, being trusted by the adolescent's parent or guardian, and showing a high level of proficiency in the medical or technical aspects of care (knowledge, experience, and careful clinical assessment) and a welcoming office.[62]

The knowledge, attitudes, and skills that underpin effective communication with young patients are increasingly recognized and taught at undergraduate and postgraduate levels. Skills-based training workshops incorporating interactive role play with simulated patients have led to significant improvement in the efficacy of screening and counseling practices for adolescents by medical students[65] and primary care physicians.[66] For health care teams treating adolescents and young adults with chronic conditions, a stronger focus on developing proficiency in core competencies that enhance engagement and communication with young people and their families may be one strategy to promote better transition to adult health care.

SPECIFIC RECOMMENDATIONS FOR TRANSITION OF PEDIATRIC TRANSPLANT RECIPIENTS
Tasks for the Pediatric Transplant Team

During the years before transfer, the development of a transition planning document may be a helpful resource to assist young people, families, and health care teams prioritize skill building that will support a successful transition to adult health care. Chronic organ failure (heart, kidney, intestine, liver, or lung), from an early age can be associated with delays in development, intellectual function, or attention deficit/hyperactivity disorders.[47,49,67–69] Emotionally and cognitively challenged children and adolescents need opportunities to develop aptitudes in problem solving, goal setting, and self-advocacy. Even those with significant impairment can usually make simple choices, such as which

Box 1
Critical milestones for patients to achieve before transfer to adult care

1. Understanding of and ability to describe the original cause of their organ failure and need for transplantation

   o Initial education may have been primarily provided to their parents; repetition is necessary to ensure they understand their condition

2. Ownership of their medical information in a concise portable accessible summary

3. Awareness of the long- and short-term implications of the transplant condition on their overall health and other aspects of their life (eg, infection prevention, cancer surveillance, academic and vocational aspirations)

4. Comprehension of the effect of their illness on their sexuality and reproductive health, including

   o The effect of pregnancy on their own well-being

   o The effect of their medications on fertility

   o Any potential teratogenicity of their medications

   o The role of genetic counseling, and genetic risk of their disease recurrence in future offspring, if pertinent to their condition

   o Their own increased susceptibility for sexually transmitted disease

5. Demonstration of a sense of responsibility for their own health care

   o Knowledge of the names (and shapes/colors), indications, and dosages of their transplant and ancillary medications (or carry that information in wallet/purse)

   o Call for their own prescription refills and renewals

   o Prepare their own medication dose boxes, if not done by their pharmacist

   o Independently communicate their health care needs to their providers

   o Know when and how to seek urgent medical attention, including health emergency telephone number(s)

   o Ability to make, keep a calendar of, and follow through with their own health care appointments

   o Understanding of their medical insurance coverage and eligibility requirements

6. Capacity to provide most self-care independently

7. An expressed readiness to move into adult care

Adapted from Bell LE, Bartosh SM, Davis CL, et al. Adolescent transition to adult care in solid organ transplantation: a consensus conference report. Am J Transplant 2008;8(11):2234; with permission.

pill to take first, and perform simple tasks.[70] **Box 1** illustrates some critical tasks and milestones that should ideally be achieved before transfer occurs.[3]

A designated transition coordinator can help facilitate the process of transfer to adult health care and ensure that all necessary preparations are made for this event. However as described earlier, assistance with many health care tasks is still commonly required at the time of transfer, for even the most highly functioning young people. At transfer, the patient and family should be provided with a portable concise, up-to-date summary of the patient's medical history, including medications.[2] The summary should be meaningful and may require special adaptation for those who are cognitively challenged. Thus, it may need to include pictures, tape recordings, and other nonwritten forms of communication.[70] In addition, a detailed health care professional summary, with all significant medical, surgical, and nursing history, relevant laboratory results, pathology reports, imaging results, operative reports, consultation letters, and pertinent psychosocial information should be sent directly to the adult treating team. Areas in need of specific attention should be respectfully communicated to adult providers. When necessary, resolution of guardianship issues should occur before the patient's 18th birthday.

Preparing the patient's parents

Parents of chronically ill children may be reluctant to set limits or push their child to do age-appropriate tasks. The pediatric team needs to encourage transplant recipients' parents to promote their independence and growing capacity for personal, family, and social responsibility. This encouragement might include discussion of participation in age and developmentally appropriate chores at home and after-school activities, including part-time jobs. Discussion also needs to focus on parents progressively involving their sons and daughters in their medical care, such as adherence with medication, appointment scheduling, medication preparation, and calling for prescription refills. Supporting young people to see clinicians by themselves for part of a consultation is another strategy that promotes growing responsibility with health care. These approaches are consistent with models of parenting that are embodied within SDT.[40] They can also be conceptualized as training in leadership in health care, in which parents gradually hand over more health care tasks to young people, who progressively take on greater responsibility. Thus parents can be viewed as transitioning from total caregivers or chief executive officers of care to managers, supervisors, and then consultants, as their children mature and become progressively more autonomous.[3,71] Parental modeling of healthy lifestyle behaviors can be considered equally fundamental to engagement of young people with health-promoting behaviors.[72]

Helping the pediatric team let go

It can sometimes be difficult for the pediatric team to break the bond of care that has developed over many years with the transplant recipient and his/her family. They may worry that neither the adolescent nor the adult transplant team is ready. Even if not explicitly stated, an attitude of mistrust may be transmitted to the patient and family that will inadvertently create barriers for the new adult providers.[3] These concerns may be diminished by working collaboratively with the adult team, sharing protocols to minimize treatment variation between centers, and assisting adolescent patients to access necessary adult system resources. The development of close affiliations between pediatric and adult transplant centers would clearly assist these processes.

Challenges for the Adult Transplant Team

The adult transplant team may assume the young person is an autonomous adult, who will come prepared with questions, be able to express any concerns, directly discuss treatment plans, and remember rapidly communicated instructions. But, no matter how well prepared, young people still need time to form trusting relationships with their new clinicians and adult health care team, as do their parents. Because adult transplant clinics frequently have a patient load at least 10-fold greater than those of pediatric centers, physician appointments are often shorter; this may delay the opportunity for relationship building. In the absence of a relationship, young people feel less comfortable sharing sensitive or personal issues, and mistakenly believe the adult physician neither understands nor cares.[59,62,64,73,74]

To minimize these concerns, the pediatric transplant team needs to prepare young people for the changes in practice style and culture between pediatric and adult services. Communication, coordination, and harmonization of approaches can be facilitated through bidirectional information sharing between pediatric and adult transplant colleagues. As with their pediatric confreres, adult site physicians and nurses may need to focus on competency development in communication skills that support engagement and relationship building with adolescents at various developmental levels and on understanding the effect of childhood chronic disease on development. They may also need to develop their skills in the management of childhood causes of end-stage organ failure and congenital diseases, infrequently seen in an adult practice.[2,3,75–77] Ideal adult site resources for transferring pediatric organ recipients would include a dedicated transfer coordinator, nurses and social workers with expertise in adolescent health, and access to reproductive specialists and urologists with proficiency in congenital urologic malformations.

A recent study of internists' perspectives on transition from pediatric to adult care revealed they had several major concerns, such as lack of training in congenital and childhood onset conditions, the need for superspecialists with expertise in adult manifestations of congenital and pediatric-onset disorders, lack of adolescent training, facing disability or end-of-life issues during youth and early in the relationship, insufficient family involvement, particularly when the patient was not ready for sole health care decision making, lack of resources to meet patients' psychosocial needs, financial pressures limiting time, and families' high expectations.[78]

Awareness that although 18- to 24-year-olds may look fully mature, their emotional regulation, risk behaviors, and adherence may differ from older adults, is the key to appreciating the importance of more focused engagement and communication. Specific questioning about the adolescent's feelings and concerns, and discussion of issues relevant to their lifestyle are important. These issues include sexuality, pregnancy, relationships, substance use, mental health, recreational activities, vocational and educational choices, and health care system expectations.[3,59,62,64,74] Age-appropriate peer support groups may also be valuable for young adults, whether face to face or electronically facilitated, such as through chat rooms or blogs.[39]

Primary and preventive health care

Partnerships with primary care providers should be established in advance of transfer to adult services, with discussion and clarification of the roles of primary and specialist health services.[2,3] There should be communication with patients and primary care providers about transplant-specific guidelines for issues such as immunization, dental health, reproductive health care, cancer screening, infection risks of everyday life, and the dangers of risky behaviors, including poor adherence with treatment. General guidelines for primary and preventive care for adolescents and young adults should equally be applied, recognizing that those who have undergone transplantation require more resources and services than others their age.

Enhancing Adherence

Organ transplant recipients need to adhere to lifelong immunosuppressive therapy, often in combination with other complex or demanding treatment regimens. Poor adherence jeopardizes health and QOL and may lead to graft loss, increased health care costs, and untimely death.[10,25,79,80] Nonrenal organ recipients, having no dialysis alternative, are at particular risk. Attention to adherence is a critical aspect of consultations with young people as the effects of poor adherence may not be immediately apparent to health care providers. Moreover, the consequences of poor adherence may sometimes be difficult for adolescents and young adults to appreciate.

For some young people, engaging in risky behaviors, such as binge drinking, casual sex, recreational drug use, or nonadherence with treatment, may be intentional. However, for many, these behaviors are not planned, deliberate, or even expected. Instead they are a reaction to situations, usually social, that were neither sought nor necessarily anticipated. A young person needs the opportunity to think in advance, with a cool head, about the risks and benefits of engaging in an activity, in order to be able to make a rational decision in the heat of the moment. Preparedness can decrease the likelihood of the adverse consequences of succumbing to a passionate moment of opportunity.[81] An interventional technique based on a dual-focus–dual-processing model of adolescent health risk behavior may be effective; it involves approaches that target the logical and emotional aspects of decision making, often using imagery.[81]

An example of this dual process intervention approach in transplant medication adherence involves 2 arms. One arm is presented to the parents and targets the reasoned path. The other arm is presented to the child or adolescent and targets an emotional or social reactive path. The aim of the first arm is to increase parenting skills such as communication with the child and to assist the parent in exploring potentially risky behaviors with their child ahead of time. The goal of the second arm is to help the child or adolescent learn about the consequences of poor adherence in ways that are relevant to their social/emotional decision making. The use of imagery is recommended to help the situation feel more real for the young person, for example through the use of photographs or video clips. Positive imagery might show a healthy transplant recipient doing an enjoyable activity that is feasible because of his or her health (eg, a sports or athletic event); negative imagery might be a graphic depiction of a transplanted organ lost to rejection compared with a healthy one, or a testimonial from a patient who has lost their graft, about the effect this has had on their life.

Adherence is influenced by aspects within individual patients, the range of resources around them that might support adherence behaviors (eg, family, friends, finances) as well as more interactive aspects of patients with the providers and the health care settings. A complementary approach that incorporates an understanding of adolescent development with SDT motivational techniques could help young people develop a sense of personal choice and autonomy in their behavior, rather than feeling controlled, pressured, or coerced. Other techniques include integrating more specific behavioral approaches (eg, use of wristwatch alarms, cell phone messaging), life coaching, and social support strategies (eg, peer support groups). Techniques that may help improve adherence for adolescents and young adults are summarized in **Box 2**.[3,79,80] Some other aspects of adolescent treatment adherence are discussed in another article elsewhere in this issue.

Systems Issues

Health and medication insurance

Patients and providers need to be alerted to insurance and health care service implications of transfer to adult health care. To prevent lapses in care or in provision of prescription medications, patients should apply early for insurance and special services requiring conversion.[3] Young adults have the lowest health insurance rate of any age group.[23] Promotion of public policy initiatives is needed to ensure problems with access to insurance and other services do not create disincentives for transfer to adult care.[3,82]

Transition clinics

There are many different understandings of what is meant by transition clinics. They range from the adult specialty physician or nurse having a single meeting with the adolescent and parent in the pediatric clinic before transfer, to a pediatric team

Box 2
Strategies to improve adherence among adolescents and young adults

1. A trusting, collaborative and open relationship that encourages dialog between the young person and the transplant health professional

2. Stepwise education regarding the treatment regimen, including purpose, names, dose, schedule, and side effects of prescribed medications

   • Enhance with booklets, pamphlets, videos, humor, and nonverbal materials (eg, medication labels and cartoon diagrams)

   • Assess comprehension

3. Behavioral strategies

   • Simplify the medication regimen

   • Tailor the medication schedule to individual patient's lifestyle

   • Prescribe more forgiving medications with longer half-lives

   • Recording of medication intake on calendars or pocket computers

   • Dose container aids

   • Wristwatch or mobile phone alarms

   • Linking of medication to daily routine cues such as meals, brushing teeth, shaving

4. Structured clinical and social network support

   • More frequent clinic/nursing visits

   • System for open communication with transplant clinic staff, such as Internet, e-mail, and phone

   • Health care provider continuity

   • Peer group support and mentoring

5. A clinic environment that is welcoming to young adults and adolescents

   • Relevant educational and age-appropriate reading material and diversional activities (eg, computer, Internet)

   • Youth-friendly decor

Adapted from Bell LE, Bartosh SM, Davis CL, et al. Adolescent transition to adult care in solid organ transplantation: a consensus conference report. Am J Transplant 2008;8(11):2237; with permission.

member accompanying the patient to their first adult site visit, to overlapping or alternating visits between the pediatric and adult sites, to fully shared adolescent and young adult clinics.[52,75,77,83]

An attractive model is a joint adolescent and young adult transplant clinic staffed with pediatric and adult transplant physicians and nurses, a social worker, and other health professionals as needed. Such clinics would ideally be staffed with clinicians more experienced in working with young people, and it is hoped would be more engaging for young people because of the presence of others similar in age (rather than a larger number of older and often sicker people), provision of youth-focused reading material, and availability of other diversionary activities in waiting spaces (eg, computers, Internet access). This model creates opportunities for interaction, role modeling, and mentoring, and provides additional support to transplant recipients in their early 20s, who are often relatively invisible within a demographic twilight zone that is no longer pediatric but not fully integrated into the adult realm.[3,83]

If a transition clinic is not feasible, having a single individual designated as the key contact person with whom to communicate can be helpful. Other options include having an adult site transplant transition coordinator, who, depending on numbers, might be shared with other specialty services. At the very least, efforts to schedule age-related transplant recipients together is a strategy to help young people understand that they are not the only ones experiencing such complex health issues at their age.

Transition policy and health care systems

Although national, local, hospital, and payer policies may influence the timing of transfer of care, the decision should ideally be collaborative, involving the patient, family, and pediatric and adult health care providers.[3] Availability of services, continuity of care, and patient safety all need to be taken into consideration, with an appreciation that transfer to adult health care services is a time of risk for young people and their transplanted organs, in terms of dropping out of care. Institutional policies need to be sufficiently flexible to accommodate individual patient and family circumstances. Ideally, patients should be medically stable at the time they transfer.[76,77] Young people who are terminally ill should not be acutely transferred. However, for a range of reasons, young people may sometimes have access to more community-based palliative care services within the adult setting, which, for example, might prompt the development of a shared care arrangement.

SUMMARY

The notion of transition to adult health care has gradually emerged as the survival of young people with previously fatal conditions has improved, bringing with it high expectations from families and young people alike of an appropriate quality of care continuing beyond the realm of pediatric services. Health care providers and services are encouraged to appreciate the wider challenges faced by young people with chronic illness and disability, and by their families, as they negotiate a change in place as well as a change in orientation from family-centered to individually focused care.[84]

Pediatric providers may believe that the increasing numbers of young people transferring to adult services constitute a tsunami that will inevitably lead to changes in adult practice. However, the significantly larger numbers of older adults with organ transplants means that the transfer of pediatric transplant recipients will only ever be felt as a ripple.[84] Rather than arguments based on size or numbers, it is more likely that clinical service developments will be driven by a quality agenda based on equity of health outcomes. This approach helped propel the creation of specialist adolescent and young adult cancer services in the United Kingdom, where research showed that the survival gains achieved in other age groups had not been similarly experienced by this cohort.[85]

The data are clear: registry reports for all solid-organ transplant recipients show reduced long-term graft survival for those transplanted during the teenage years[5]; more detailed analysis shows adolescent and young adult renal transplant recipients have the highest rates of acute rejection, death-censored graft loss, and chronic rejection leading to graft loss than any other age group.[25,26] The challenge is how clinical services should respond. At this stage, there is little evidence supporting one specific model of health care transition. However, there are clear indications that young people risk dropping out of health care at around the age they transfer to adult services, and that continued close engagement with developmentally appropriate health care matters. A major challenge is to ensure that this developmentally appropriate care is provided in pediatric and adult services; current evidence suggests there is significant room for improvement within both settings. Prospective studies are needed on factors influencing health care engagement during emerging adulthood, the life stage when most transplant recipients move to the adult milieu. As great a challenge relates to how best to harness consumer input; arguably it is ultimately this perspective that will be more influential in obtaining funding for evidence-based clinical initiatives.

REFERENCES

1. American Academy of Pediatrics, American Academy of Family Physicians, American College of Physicians-American Society of Internal Medicine. A consensus statement on health care transitions for young adults with special health care needs. Pediatrics 2002;110(6):1304–6.
2. Rosen DS, Blum RW, Britto M, et al. Transition to adult health care for adolescents and young adults with chronic conditions: position paper of the Society for Adolescent Medicine. J Adolesc Health 2003;33(4):309–11.
3. Bell LE, Bartosh SM, Davis CL, et al. Adolescent transition to adult care in solid organ transplantation: a consensus conference report. Am J Transplant 2008; 8(11):2230–42.
4. Australia and New Zealand Dialysis and Transplant Registry. ANZDATA - The 31st annual report–2008, 2009. Available at: http://www.anzdata.org.au/v1/report_2008.html. Accessed December 10, 2010.
5. 2008 Annual Report of the US Organ Procurement and Transplantation Network and the Scientific Registry of Transplant Recipients: Transplant Data 1998–2007. Rockville (MD): US Department of Health and Human Services, Health Resources and Services Administration, Healthcare Systems Bureau, Division of Transplantation; 2009. Available at: http://optn.transplant.hrsa.gov/data/. Accessed February 10, 2010.
6. Kennedy A, Sawyer S. Transition from pediatric to adult services: are we getting it right? Curr Opin Pediatr 2008;20(4):403–9.
7. Dugueperoux I, Tamalet A, Sermet-Gaudelus I, et al. Clinical changes of patients with cystic fibrosis during transition from pediatric to adult care. J Adolesc Health 2008;43(5):459–65.
8. Pacaud D, Crawford S, Stephure DK, et al. Effect of type 1 diabetes on psychosocial maturation in young adults. J Adolesc Health 2007;40(1):29–35.
9. Kipps S, Bahu T, Ong K, et al. Current methods of transfer of young people with type 1 diabetes to adult services. Diabet Med 2002;19(8):649–54.
10. Watson AR. Non-compliance and transfer from paediatric to adult transplant unit. Pediatr Nephrol 2000;14(6):469–72.
11. Chaturvedi S, Jones C, Walker R, et al. The transition of kidney transplant recipients: a work in progress. Pediatr Nephrol 2009;24:1055–60.
12. Remorino R, Taylor J. Smoothing things over: the transition from paediatric to adult care for kidney transplant recipients. Prog Transplant 2006;16:303–8.
13. Annunziato RA, Emre S, Schneider B, et al. Adherence and medical outcomes in pediatric liver transplant recipients who transition to adult services. Pediatr Transplant 2007;11(6):608–14.
14. McCurdy C, DiCenso A, Ludwin D, et al. There to here: young adult patients' perceptions of the process of transition from pediatric to adult transplant care. Prog Transplant 2006;16:309–16.
15. Casey BJ, Jones RM, Hare TA. The adolescent brain. Ann N Y Acad Sci 2008; 1124(1):111–26.
16. Arnett JJ, Taber S. Adolescence terminable and interminable: when does adolescence end? J Youth Adolesc 1994;23(5):517–37.

17. Arnett JJ. Adolescent storm and stress, reconsidered. Am Psychol 1999;54(5): 317–26.
18. Bynner J. Rethinking the youth phase of the life-course: the case for emerging adulthood? J Youth Stud 2005;8(4):367–84.
19. Hall SGIn: Adolescence: its psychology and its relations to physiology, anthropology, sociology, sex, crime, religion, and education, vols. I & II. New York: D. Appleton & Co; 1904.
20. McIntyre P. Adolescent friendly health services. World Health Organization, Geneva Switzerland 2002 WHO reference number: WHO/FCH/CAH/02.14 2002. Available at: http://www.who.int/child_adolescent_health/documents/fch_cah_02_14/en/index.html. Accessed December 13, 2009.
21. The World Bank country classification. The World Bank data & statistics, 2009. Available at: http://go.worldbank.org/K2CKM78CC0. Accessed January 3, 2010.
22. Patton GC, Coffey C, Sawyer SM, et al. Global patterns of mortality in young people: a systematic analysis of population health data. Lancet 2009; 374(9693):881–92.
23. Park MJ, Paul Mulye T, Adams SH, et al. The health status of young adults in the United States. J Adolesc Health 2006;39(3):305–17.
24. Suris JC, Michaud PA, Akre C, et al. Health risk behaviors in adolescents with chronic conditions. Pediatrics 2008;122(5):e1113–8.
25. Keith DS, Cantarovich M, Paraskevas S, et al. Recipient age and risk of chronic allograft nephropathy in primary deceased donor kidney transplant. Transpl Int 2006;19(8):649–56.
26. Ekstrand LE. End-stage renal disease: characteristics of kidney transplant recipients, frequency of transplant failures, and cost to Medicare, 2007. Available at: http://www.gao.gov/new.items/d071117.pdf. Accessed December 13, 2009.
27. Weithorn LA, Campbell SB. The competency of children and adolescents to make informed treatment decisions. Child Dev 1982;53(6):1589–98.
28. Steinberg L. A social neuroscience perspective on adolescent risk-taking. Dev Rev 2008;28(1):78–106.
29. Luna B, Padmanabhan A, O'Hearn K. What has fMRI told us about the development of cognitive control through adolescence? Brain Cogn 2010;72(1): 101–13.
30. Steinberg L, Cauffman E, Woolard J, et al. Are adolescents less mature than adults? Minors' access to abortion, the juvenile death penalty, and the alleged APA "flip-flop". Am Psychol 2009;64(7):583–94.
31. Fischer KW, Stein Z, Heikkinen K. Narrow assessments misrepresent development and misguide policy: comment on Steinberg, Cauffman, Woolard, Graham, and Banich (2009). Am Psychol 2009;64(7):595–600.
32. Giedd JN. The teen brain: insights from neuroimaging. J Adolesc Health 2008; 42(4):335–43.
33. Nurmi JE. Development of orientation to the future during early adolescence: a four-year longitudinal study and two cross-sectional comparisons. Int J Psychol 1989;24(2):195.
34. Nurmi JE. How do adolescents see their future? A review of the development of future orientation and planning. Dev Rev 1991;11(1):1–59.
35. Massey EK, Gebhardt WA, Garnefski N. Adolescent goal content and pursuit: a review of the literature from the past 16 years. Dev Rev 2008;28(4):421–60.
36. Williams GC, Cox EM, Kouides R, et al. Presenting the facts about smoking to adolescents: effects of an autonomy-supportive style. Arch Pediatr Adolesc Med 1999;153(9):959–64.

37. Williams GC, McGregor H, Sharp D, et al. A self-determination multiple risk intervention trial to improve smokers' health. J Gen Intern Med 2006;21(12):1288–94.
38. Deci EL, Ryan RM. Facilitating optimal motivation and psychological well-being across life's domains. Can Psychol 2008;49(1):14–23.
39. Williams GC, Cox EM, Hedberg V, et al. Extrinsic life goals and health risk behaviors in adolescents. J Appl Soc Psychol 2000;30:1756–71.
40. Joussemet M, Landry Re, Koestner R. A self-determination theory perspective on parenting. Can Psychol 2008;49(3):194–200.
41. Ryan RM, Deci EL. Self-determination theory and the facilitation of intrinsic motivation, social development, and well-being. Am Psychol 2000;55:68–78.
42. Fredricks JA, Blumenfeld PC, Paris AH. School engagement: potential of the concept, state of the evidence. Rev Educ Res 2004;74(1):59–109.
43. Olsson CA, Boyce M, Toumbourou JW, et al. Chronic illness in adolescents: the role of peer support groups. Clinical child psychology and psychiatry 2005;1078–87.
44. Bynner J. Childhood risks and protective factors in social exclusion. Child Soc 2001;15(5):285–301.
45. Alonso EM, Limbers CA, Neighbors K, et al. Cross-sectional analysis of health-related quality of life in pediatric liver transplant recipients. J Pediatr 2010; 156(2):270–6.
46. Petroski RA, Grady KL, Rodgers S, et al. Quality of life in adult survivors greater than 10 years after pediatric heart transplantation. J Heart Lung Transplant 2009; 28(7):661–6.
47. Qvist E, Jalanko H, Holmberg C. Psychosocial adaptation after solid organ transplantation in children. Pediatr Clin North Am 2003;50(6):1505–19.
48. Ross M, Kouretas P, Gamberg P, et al. Ten- and 20-year survivors of pediatric orthotopic heart transplantation. J Heart Lung Transplant 2006;25(3):261–70.
49. Slickers J, Duquette P, Hooper S, et al. Clinical predictors of neurocognitive deficits in children with chronic kidney disease. Pediatr Nephrol 2007;22(4):565–72.
50. Uzark K, Spicer R, Beebe DW. Neurodevelopmental outcomes in pediatric heart transplant recipients. J Heart Lung Transplant 2009;28(12):1306–11.
51. Martinez YJ, Ercikan K. Chronic illnesses in Canadian children: what is the effect of illness on academic achievement, and anxiety and emotional disorders? Child Care Health Dev 2009;35(3):391–401.
52. White PH. Transition: a future promise for children and adolescents with special health care needs and disabilities. Rheum Dis Clin North Am 2002;28(3): 687–703.
53. Brook U, Galili A. Knowledge and attitudes of high school teachers towards pupils suffering from chronic diseases. Patient Educ Couns 2001;43:37–42.
54. Cassen R, Feinstein L, Graham P. Educational outcomes: adversity and resilience. Soc Pol Soc 2009;8(01):73–85.
55. Janosz M, Archambault I, Morizot J, et al. School engagement trajectories and their differential predictive relations to dropout. J Soc Issues 2008;64(1):21–40.
56. Riano-Galan I, Malaga S, Rajmil L, et al. Quality of life of adolescents with end-stage renal disease and kidney transplant. Pediatr Nephrol 2009;24(8):1561–8.
57. Taylor RM, Franck LS, Gibson F, et al. A. study of the factors affecting health-related quality of life in adolescents after liver transplantation. Am J Transplant 2009;9(5):1179–88.
58. Tong A, Morton R, Howard K, et al. Adolescent experiences following organ transplantation: a systematic review of qualitative studies. J Pediatr 2009;155(4): 542–9.

59. Beresford BA, Sloper P. Chronically ill adolescents' experiences of communicating with doctors: a qualitative study. J Adolesc Health 2003;33(3):172–9.
60. Litt IF, Cuskey WR. Satisfaction with health care: a predictor of adolescents' appointment keeping. J Adolesc Health Care 1984;5(3):196–200.
61. Freed LH, Ellen JM, Irwin CE, et al. Determinants of adolescents' satisfaction with health care providers and intentions to keep follow-up appointments. J Adolesc Health 1998;22(6):475–9.
62. Britto MT, Slap GB, DeVellis RF, et al. Specialists understanding of the health care preferences of chronically ill adolescents. J Adolesc Health 2007;40(4):334–41.
63. Brown JD, Wissow LS. Discussion of sensitive health topics with youth during primary care visits: relationship to youth perceptions of care. J Adolesc Health 2009;44(1):48–54.
64. McDonagh JE, Kaufman M. The challenging adolescent. Rheumatology 2009; 48(8):872–5.
65. Feddock CA, Hoellein AR, Griffith CH, et al. Enhancing knowledge and clinical skills through an adolescent medicine workshop. Arch Pediatr Adolesc Med 2009;163(3):256–60.
66. Lustig JL, Ozer EM, Adams SH, et al. Improving the delivery of adolescent clinical preventive services through skills-based training. Pediatrics 2001; 107(5):1100–7.
67. Baum M, Freier MC, Chinnock RE. Neurodevelopmental outcome of solid organ transplantation in children. Pediatr Clin North Am 2003;50(6):1493–503.
68. Falger J, Latal B, Landolt M, et al. Outcome after renal transplantation. Part I: intellectual and motor performance. Pediatr Nephrol 2008;23(8):1339–45.
69. Gipson DS, Hooper SR, Duquette PJ, et al. Memory and executive functions in pediatric chronic kidney disease. Child Neuropsychol 2006;12(6): 391–405.
70. Kaufman M. Transition of cognitively delayed adolescent organ transplant recipients to adult care. Pediatr Transplant 2006;10(4):413–7.
71. Kieckhefer GM, Trahms CM. Supporting development of children with chronic conditions: from compliance toward shared management. Pediatr Nurs 2000; 26(4):354–63.
72. Gutgesell ME, Payne N. Issues of adolescent psychological development in the 21st century. Pediatr Rev 2004;25(3):79–85.
73. Dovey-Pearce G, Hurrell R, May C, et al. Young adults' (16–25 years) suggestions for providing developmentally appropriate diabetes services: a qualitative study. Health Soc Care Community 2005;13(5):409–19.
74. Grant C, Elliott A, Dimeglio GD, et al. What teenagers want: tips on working with today's youth. Paediatr Child Health 2008;13(1):15–8.
75. McDonagh JE, McDonagh JE. Growing up and moving on: transition from pediatric to adult care. Pediatr Transplant 2005;9(3):364–72.
76. Knauth A, Verstappen A, Reiss J, et al. Transition and transfer from pediatric to adult care of the young adult with complex congenital heart disease. Cardiol Clin 2006;24(4):619–29.
77. Rosen DS. Transition of young people with respiratory diseases to adult health care. Paediatr Respir Rev 2004;5(2):124–31.
78. Peter NG, Forke CM, Ginsburg KR, et al. Transition from pediatric to adult care: internists' perspectives. Pediatrics 2009;123(2):417–23.
79. Dobbels F, Van Damme-Lombaert R, Vanhaecke J, et al. Growing pains: non-adherence with the immunosuppressive regimen in adolescent transplant recipients. Pediatr Transplant 2005;9(3):381–90.

80. Rianthavorn P, Ettenger RB, Malekzadeh M, et al. Noncompliance with immuno-suppressive medications in pediatric and adolescent patients receiving solid-organ transplants. Transplantation 2004;77(5):778–82.

81. Gibbons FX, Houlihan AE, Gerrard M. Reason and reaction: the utility of a dual-focus, dual-processing perspective on promotion and prevention of adolescent health risk behaviour. Brit J Health Psychol 2009;14(2):231–48.

82. White PH. Access to health care: health insurance considerations for young adults with special health care needs/disabilities. Pediatrics 2002;110(6 Pt 2): 1328–35.

83. Jordan A, McDonagh JE. Recognition of emerging adulthood in UK rheuma-tology: the case for young adult rheumatology service developments. Rheuma-tology 2007;46(2):188–91.

84. Sawyer SM. In search of quality care for young people with chronic conditions. J Paediatr Child Health 2008;44(9):475–7.

85. National Institute for Health and Clinical Excellence Guidance on Cancer Services. Improving outcomes in children and young people with cancer. National Institute for Health and Clinical Excellence, London, 2005. United Kingdom, Available at: http://www.nice.org.uk/nicemedia/pdf/C&YPManual.pdf. Accessed December 13, 2009.

Most Commonly Asked Questions from Parents of Pediatric Transplant Recipients

Maria DeAngelis, MScN, NP(Paediatrics)[a],*,
Kathy Martin, MN, NP(Paediatrics)[b],
Angela Williams, MS, NP(PHNCP)[c],
Beverly Kosmach-Park, MSN, CRNP[d]

KEYWORDS

- Pediatric solid-organ transplant • Immunosuppression
- Growth and development • Quality of life

This article provides brief responses to many of the questions commonly asked by children and their parents after organ transplantation. This is by no means a complete list of commonly asked questions but an attempt to address those that have implications specifically related to transplantation. Individual transplant center guidelines may vary and consultation with the patients' transplant team is important. From a list of more than 40 questions generated by the authors' clinical experience more than 25 are included here. As with other chronic illnesses, children and parents may have difficulty attributing certain behaviors to normal growth and development versus the transplant. Counseling regarding issues such as discipline and sleep disturbance, for example, should be guided by general principles of parenting a child with a chronic illness.

[a] Liver and Intestinal Transplant Program, Transplant Centre, The Hospital for Sick Children, 555 University Avenue, Toronto M5G 1X8, Canada
[b] Heart Transplant Program, Transplant Centre, The Hospital for Sick Children, 555 University Avenue, Toronto M5G 1X8, Canada
[c] Renal Transplant Program, Transplant Centre, The Hospital for Sick Children, 555 University Avenue, Toronto M5G 1X8, Canada
[d] Department of Transplant Surgery, Starzl Transplantation Institute, Children's Hospital of Pittsburgh of UPMC, Faculty Pavillion, 6B 45th street and Penn Avenue 15524 Pittsburgh, PA, USA
* Corresponding author.
E-mail address: maria.deangelis@sickkids.ca

Pediatr Clin N Am 57 (2010) 611–622
doi:10.1016/j.pcl.2010.01.010
0031-3955/10/$ – see front matter © 2010 Published by Elsevier Inc.
pediatric.theclinics.com

RECOVERING FROM TRANSPLANT
When Can My Child Return to School After Transplant?

Transplant center recommendations regarding the return to school after transplant varies from a few weeks to up to 3 months. The intent of this recommendation is that the child is healthy and on baseline or near baseline levels of immunosuppression by the time they return to school so that they are not at undue risk of infection.[1] Many children are ready to return to school within a few weeks of their transplant. It is important for children to resume normal activities and be with peers.[2,3]

Transplant recipients typically tolerate common community-acquired infections, however, exposure to certain viruses such as varicella or measles necessitates prophylactic treatment of the transplant recipient.[4] Parents should alert school staff to this and any other special needs their child may have.

Can My Child Attend Daycare After Their Transplant?

Recommendations regarding daycare will vary between transplant centers but the guiding principles are similar to returning to school. The child should feel well enough to cope with the daycare setting and immunosuppression should be near baseline levels so that the child is not at undue risk of infection.[1] Daycare staff should be aware of reporting exposure to communicable disease (eg, varicella) to parents.

Can My Child Exercise After Transplantation?

Returning to normal activities and participation in exercise is recommended for children after solid-organ transplantation (SOT). Regular exercise helps to maintain a healthy body weight, improves endurance and flexibility, and can contribute to an improved quality of life.[5] After the early transplant period when wound healing is complete, there are few restrictions related to exercise. Some renal transplant centers recommend avoidance of activity that could result in a direct hit to the transplanted kidney.[5,6] Use of protective equipment may mitigate some of this risk for children who intend to play contact sports, however the literature in this area is sparse. Heart transplant recipients experience slower heart rate increases with exercise and slower return to baseline heart rate after exercise as a result of autonomic denervation of the transplanted heart.[7] Pediatric heart transplant recipients participating in competitive sports will benefit from warm-up and cool-down routines to assist in modulation of their heart rate.

Poor bone mineral density can place children at risk for bone fractures.[8] Children with markedly reduced bone density or a history of fractures may be cautioned against participating in contact sports until bone density is improved. Moderate weight-bearing exercise should be encouraged to improve bone density. Appropriate activities should be encouraged and tailored to the child with physical disabilities.

Many pediatric transplant recipients participate in competitive sports. The World Transplant Games is an international biannual competition that profiles transplant athletes, the success of transplant surgery, and the need for organ donation.[9] Participation in these events can be a positive experience for transplant recipients and their families.[10]

IMMUNOSUPPRESSION AND OTHER MEDICATIONS
What Happens When My Child Has Organ Rejection?

Organ rejection is the result of the body's attempt to attack tissue that is recognized as foreign. Transplant recipients take immunosuppression medications to suppress or fool the body into accepting the transplanted organ. Most transplant recipients will have some organ rejection. This is most common early after the transplant but can happen at any time. Patients and parents can do their part to help prevent rejection by ensuring that immunosuppression medications are taken precisely as prescribed.

The transplant team often detects signs of rejection through laboratory tests and routine biopsies long before physical symptoms are noticed. Detection of rejection means that immunosuppression medications need adjustment. In most cases, this is successful in treating the rejection. Please refer to organ-specific articles in this issue for further discussion of organ rejection.

What Happens if My Child Vomits up His/Her Medications?

The decision to re-administer a vomited immunosuppressant dose involves several factors including but not limited to time from transplant, previous levels, concurrent infection, and rejection status.

For this reason, patients/families are asked to call their transplant center if the patient has vomited an immunosuppressant dose. The following general guidelines have been created based on review of population pharmacokinetic characteristics of the immunosuppressants. Doses vomited more than an hour from the time of administration do not need to be repeated (**Table 1**).

If My Child Has a Fever Can They Take Acetaminophen and/or Ibuprofen?

In general, transplant recipients may take acetaminophen for fever or pain according to the manufacturer's dose guidelines. Patients with liver dysfunction may require a decreased dose of acetaminophen and these patients should consult their transplant team. Ibuprofen and nonsteroidal antiinflammatory drugs are discouraged and require consultation from the transplant center because of potential renal impairment. After consultation with the transplant center, some patients without renal impairment may be permitted occasional doses of ibuprofen. Prolonged fever and/or a sick child with a fever will need to be investigated further.

Are There Medications That My Child Should Avoid?

Many drugs can interact with immunosuppression medication. For example, macrolide antibiotics such as erythromycin are inhibitors of tacrolimus, cyclosporine, and sirolimus metabolism and can cause toxic levels within a few concurrent doses.[11] Health care professionals and transplant recipients should check with the transplant center before starting a new medication to ensure no adverse interactions are known. The same precautions should be taken with over-the-counter and prescription medications as well as herbal remedies.

Table 1 Repeat dosing guidelines		
Immunosuppressant	Vomited Dose <0.5 Hour After Dose Time	Vomited Dose Within 0.5 to 1 Hour of Dose Time
Tacrolimus or cyclosporine	Give dose again	Give half dose (or as close to half as possible)
Sirolimus (rapamycin)	Give dose again	
Mycophenolate mofetil	Give dose again	Do not repeat dose
Azathioprine	Give dose again	
Prednisone or prednisolone	Give dose again	

When Should My Child Start Looking After Their Own Medications?

Developing skills to care for their transplanted organ(s) is a long-term process. Learning about medications, their purposes, and self-administration are all important steps. In early adolescence, the young teen should begin preparing and self-administrating medications with supervision. More complex tasks such as re-ordering medications should be mastered by the time transition to adult health care setting takes place.[12]

GENERAL MEDICAL CARE AND VACCINES
What Is the Role of My Child's Pediatrician and Family Doctor?

The pediatrician or family doctor will collaborate with the transplant team. Your child should be seen by their pediatrician or family doctor for routine immunizations, monitoring of growth and development, and initial assessment of illnesses. The pediatrician or family doctor is key in the initial examination and medical plan for a transplant recipient with acute illness and other long-standing health issues. There are many common childhood illnesses that will also affect the transplant patient and the pediatrician can examine and determine the appropriate steps for treatment. Fevers, coughs, sore throat, ear aches, obesity, and difficulty paying attention in school are some examples of health issues that the pediatrician or family doctor can assess initially and treat. If the acute issue does not resolve or worsens, the pediatrician or family doctor may contact the transplant center for further discussion.

When Should I Call My Transplant Center?

The transplant center is always there as a resource and can be called for direction if uncertain about who to call. If there are questions about immunosuppression the transplant center is a first contact. Acute issues that may necessitate a call to the transplant will vary for each organ group. Some examples include jaundice in the liver transplant patient, decreased spirometry readings in the lung transplant patient, and blood in the urine for the renal transplant recipient. One is always encouraged to call if uncertain and advice can be offered by phone.

Should My Child Receive Vaccinations Before Transplant?

The pediatric transplant candidate should receive a full complement of routine vaccines before transplant according to national immunization guidelines. The use of live vaccines should be discussed with the transplant team before transplant as deferral of transplantation for a few weeks after immunization may be necessary. Accelerated vaccine schedules are warranted in many children before transplant.[4,13]

How Will My Child Be Immunized After Organ Transplantation?

There are several important points regarding the immunization of children after organ transplantation. Posttransplantation immunosuppression interferes with the immune responses that are needed for successful immunization. There are limited data regarding the exact timing of vaccination after transplant, however the general consensus is that vaccination can resume approximately 6 months following transplantation, when baseline immunosuppression levels are attained.[14,15]

Live-attenuated vaccines such as MMR (measles, mumps, rubella) and varicella are contraindicated in SOT recipients as immunosuppression increases the risk of acquiring disease from a live vaccine.[4,15] Siblings and household contacts can receive live virus vaccines without risk to the transplant recipient, however oral polio vaccine should be avoided because of possible viral shedding after administration. There may be dose or schedule alterations for some immunizations such as hepatitis B vaccine. Check with the transplant center regarding their immunization protocol.

What Happens if My Child Is Exposed to or Develops Chicken Pox?

Chicken pox (varicella) is a common childhood infection. Most transplant patients have minimal complications from the disease, however, there is a risk of disseminated infection. Prophylaxis with varicella zoster immunoglobulin is recommended within 96 hours of exposure to varicella to prevent or ameliorate the disease.[4]

Some transplant recipients on minimal immunosuppression with a mild varicella may recover without intervention.[16] However, treatment with acyclovir is the most common standard of care. Acyclovir is typically given intravenously until lesions are crusted and no new lesions have developed. The remainder of the treatment course can be given orally.[4]

What Happens if My Child Gets Fifth Disease?

Fifth disease is a common childhood illness caused by human parvovirus (PV B19). Most transplant recipients handle PV B19 like their immunocompetent peers. However, a small number of patients may develop hematologic complications such as aplastic anemia, leucopenia, and thrombocytopenia.[17] Screening for PV B19 is therefore important in an immunocompromised SOT recipient who presents with severe, unexplained, or prolonged anemia.[18]

There is no treatment required for uncomplicated PV B19 in the transplant recipient. Intravenous immunoglobulin has been shown to neutralize the virus, thus reducing the viral load and is the treatment of choice in PV B19 disease with associated severe persistent anemia.[17]

Are There Any Important Differences in Dental Care for Children Who are Transplant Recipients?

Oral hygiene and preventative dental care routines for children following organ transplantation should follow the same guidelines as for the general population. Gingival hyperplasia is seen in patients who are on cyclosporine-based immunosuppression and is more common in children.[19] A soft toothbrush can be used to avoid bleeding gums and routine dental examinations should be scheduled to assess gum overgrowth and complications. In some cases, surgery may be required for tissue reduction to decrease infection and for an improved appearance.

Oral candidiasis is another potential complication after transplant and may develop during periods of higher immunosuppression. Candidiasis is usually treated with nystatin oral suspension. Resistant candidasis may require oral fluconazole, although this treatment usually increases serum levels of tacrolimus and cyclosporine and requires close monitoring of trough levels of these medications.[20,21]

Oral ulceration induced by medication (eg, sirolimus) or infection (eg, herpes simplex) should be addressed based on the likely cause. Antibiotic prophylaxis before invasive dental work is controversial and there are few guidelines and no clinical trials that address appropriate care for transplant recipients. The American Heart Association's standard regimen for endocarditis prophylaxis can be used as a guideline (http://www.americanheart.org).[22]

GENERAL QUALITY OF LIFE
Does My Child Have Dietary Restrictions After Transplant?

Most transplant recipients have no dietary restrictions and a healthy diet based on national guidelines is recommended.[23,24] Some children may have restrictions related to their individual circumstances (eg, low potassium diet for children with hyperkalemia related to renal dysfunction). Transplant recipients should avoid grapefruit and grapefruit juice as it is an inhibitor of calcineurin metabolism (eg, tacrolimus, cyclosporine) and can contribute to high serum levels of these medications.[25] Other citrus fruits do not have this effect and are safe to eat.

Some transplant centers may recommend avoiding foods perceived to have increased risk for food-borne bacteria such as unpasteurized cheese. There is little evidence for the benefit of this practice and food guidelines are variable from one institution to another.[26] Safe food storage, handling, and cooking practices are important in preventing food-borne illness for SOT recipients.[5]

Will Transplantation Affect My Child's Sleep Patterns?

Some pretransplant conditions such as pruritus in liver failure or breathing problems in chronic lung disease may hinder sleep; sleep disturbance after transplant is more likely to be related to anxiety or behavioral problems.[1] Having a transplant is not specifically associated with sleep problems but hospitalizations, anxiety about diagnostic tests, or other parts of the health care regimen can contribute to disruption in sleep patterns. Parents and children should be encouraged to practice regular sleep routines including a consistent bedtime routine (eg, regular bedtime, bath, stories, quiet talking, or music) and a quiet sleep environment. Daily exercise and avoidance of caffeine can also improve sleep.

Can My Child Have a Pet After Transplant?

Most pets do not seem to present a major health risk to a child who is immunosuppressed.[27] With good hygiene practices, health maintenance, proper handling, and common sense practices, the transplant recipient should be able to experience the benefits of having a pet. Transplant recipients should be encouraged to wash their hands well after petting and playing with pets or other animals, particularly before eating and handling food. Pet's health maintenance is equally important. Pets should have routine examinations and immunizations as recommended by the veterinarian. If the pet is ill, it should be seen by a veterinarian as soon as possible.

Some transplant centers may recommend avoiding reptiles, which are at higher risk of carrying salmonellosis. Some transplant centers also recommend that amphibians (frogs), hamsters, guinea pigs, and caged birds are not kept as pets in the home. Additional information on caring for common pets after transplant can be found at the Centers for Disease Control Web site at http://www.cdc.gov/HEALTHYPETS/bonemarrow_transplant.htm.

Our Family Wants to Go on Vacation. Can My Child Travel After Their Transplant?

Transplant recipients can travel with a few common sense precautions.

- Purchase adequate travel insurance to ensure coverage of expenses if the transplant recipient or other family member becomes ill when traveling.
- Bring all medications needed during travel plus a few extra doses in case medication is spilled or vomited. Keep medications with you at all times; do not put them in checked luggage.
- Determine if additional vaccinations are needed for travel to a particular area. Assessment through an Infectious Disease Travel Clinic should be considered. Vaccination recommendations should be reviewed by the transplant center as not all vaccinations (eg, live virus vaccines) are indicated after transplant.[4]

Transplant recipients and their families should follow other common precautions during travel with respect to food safety and hygiene. Family travel or travel for business or school is part of achieving optimal quality of life after transplant and should be encouraged and facilitated.

Will My Child Get Cancer After Transplant?

Immunosuppression promotes acceptance of the allograft by the SOT recipients, but it also increases the risk of malignancy.[28] Malignancy after pediatric SOT transplantation is most commonly related to Epstein-Barr virus (EBV) infection through either a primary infection or reactivation of latent EBV. EBV infection can cause proliferation, and in some cases malignant transformation, of lymphoid tissue resulting in posttransplant lymphoproliferative disease (PTLD).[28]

PTLD can range from mild EBV disease to lymphoma. Treatment may involve antiviral agents for simple EBV disease or chemotherapy for lymphoma.[29] The incidence of PTLD varies based on the EBV status of the organ donor and recipient, degree of immunosuppression, type of organ transplantation, and elapsed time after transplant. The frequency ranges between 4% and 20%.[30] PTLD has many possible manifestations. Nonspecific signs and symptoms such as malaise, recurrent fever without cause, nausea, vomiting, diarrhea, weight loss, and adenopathy are cues that often lead to further investigation for PTLD.[30]

Although actual malignancy is not typically seen until adulthood, the risk of skin cancer is increased for SOT recipients.[31] Use of sun screen and avoidance of prolonged unnecessary sun exposure are common measures recommended to reduce the risk of skin cancer.

GROWTH AND DEVELOPMENT
My Child has been Through So Much. What is the Best Way to Discipline My Child After Transplantation?

Discipline is an important part of the ongoing development of a child after transplantation. As with many parents of children who have faced a life-threatening illness, parents of transplant recipients may be over protective of their child or over lenient in their behavioral expectations.[1,32] Both of these approaches will hinder the development of positive behavior and coping skills in the pediatric transplant recipient. For example, a child who is not expected to follow family rules may have more difficulty adjusting to school routines. By the same token, a child who is kept home from peer-social events misses the opportunity to build independence and social skills. Parents should be encouraged to provide fair consistent discipline for their child.

Will My Child Grow Like Their Friends?

Normal growth patterns are the goal after transplantation. However, there are multiple factors involved in the individual's ability to attain age-matched linear growth. Before transplant, end-stage organ failure often leads to malnutrition because of increased energy needs, malabsorption, and anorexia. Posttransplant growth is affected by organ function, age at transplant, steroid use, and transplant complications.[33] Height and weight generally increase after transplant. Catch up growth can occur but height remains reduced in a percentage of transplant patients compared with their peers.[34–36]

There is increasing awareness of the importance of bone health in the child after transplant. Many children experience poor bone mineral density related to pretransplant chronic illness and immunosuppressive medications. Ensuring adequate dietary calcium and vitamin D intake as well as weight-bearing exercise will help to optimize bone health.[8]

Will My Child Experience Developmental Delay/Normal Cognitive Development?

Most transplant patients without prior neurologic injury will continue to develop appropriately. Individual differences in illness trajectory and transplant complications may affect neurologic development. Most pediatric transplant recipients attend school and participate in all aspects of the curriculum. In the limited research available, most pediatric transplant recipients fall into the normal or low-normal range for cognitive ability.[37–42] Some children will benefit from neurodevelopmental assessment and an education plan tailored to their needs and strengths.

ENTERING ADOLESCENCE
What Is the Best Approach to the Treatment of Acne After Transplantation?

Acne is a difficult outward sign of pubertal growth for many teenagers. For some teenagers with transplants, steroids and sirolimus may accentuate this normal process. Treatment options are the same as those recommended by the Expert Committee for Acne Management.[43] Topical antibiotics, retinoids, and benzyl peroxide can all be used. Oral antibiotics can be used with the exception of oral macrolides as they interact with immunosuppressant medications (see section on medication). Hormonal therapy should be reviewed based on patient risk factors such as hypertension, and coronary artery disease may preclude their use.

Can My Child Become Pregnant or Father a Child?

Female transplant recipients can become pregnant and male transplant recipients can father children. Prepregnancy planning is essential to ensure appropriate immunosuppression, stable graft function, and good general health.[44,45] Immunosuppression may need to be altered before pregnancy as the safety of mycophenolate mofetil and sirolimus in pregnancy is not established. However, pregnancies fathered by male transplant recipients taking these medications have outcomes similar to the general population.[45] Although pregnancy in the SOT recipient is considered high risk, in a well-planned stable situation, many common risks of pregnancy are similar to the general population.[44,46]

Unplanned pregnancy in the transplant recipient poses risks for mother and baby. Adolescent transplant recipients should receive information and the opportunity to discuss birth control measures. Barrier methods and low-dose oral contraceptives can be considered[44] but should be selected in the context of the adolescents' clinical status and individual preferences. Regardless of birth control method, condom use to prevent sexually transmitted infection should be advocated.

What if My Child Experiments with Smoking, Alcohol, or Nonprescription Drugs?

Risk-taking behaviors are a common feature of adolescence. Data are limited but information regarding the dangers of smoking, alcohol, and illicit drugs for the transplant patient should be provided. The risks of cigarette smoking are well known. Alcohol is a diuretic that can lead to difficulty in maintaining hydration. Marijuana smoking can lead to lung infections with *Aspergillus* (mold). Parents and health care providers can provide information, support, counseling, and intervention if needed (see the article by Kaufman and colleagues elsewhere in this issue for further explanation of this topic).

I'm Worried That My Child Will Want to Get a Tattoo or Have Body Piercing

Many transplant centers indicate that tattooing and piercing should be discouraged in transplant recipients. Immunosuppression increases the risk of infectious complications with these procedures. However, because some transplant recipients may pursue these procedures, information about tattooing and piercing should be provided during routine visits and reinforced as needed. If the patient intends on obtaining a tattoo or piercing, licensed facilities with ideal safety procedures should be advocated and adherence to follow-up appointments and care for any complications should be stressed.[47,48]

How Will my Child's Care Change During Adolescence? Will They Always Be a Pediatric Patient?

Transition from pediatric to adult care is an important process for adolescent SOT recipients. An international consensus statement emphasizes the importance of early preparation for transitioning the child and family to adult care.[49] Although, 10 to 14 years of age is recommended as a starting point for a transition program, the timing should be individualized based on the adolescent's developmental level and family characteristics. Adolescents can become increasingly involved with their care with activities including scheduling of follow-up appointments, calling the pharmacy for repeat prescriptions, discussing laboratory results with their transplant team, or attending clinic independently.

Insurance coverage and special health care issues should be explored before transition to highlight of the implications of transition to an adult setting, particularly in the United States. It is important that this is done early to avoid lapses in insurance coverage.[50]

SUMMARY

Pediatric SOT recipients and their parents are often challenged to cope with new transplant regimens as well as common situations in the context of organ transplantation. Health care professionals will receive questions from parents and children regarding clinical transplant care as well as general pediatric concerns that seem unfamiliar to families now that their child has a transplant. The literature is limited in some areas of pediatric care after SOT, and there is little guidance for the health care practitioner. To help address gaps in the literature and provide guidance for health care professionals, this article reviews some of the most commonly asked questions regarding general care after SOT, parenting the child with a chronic illness, and growth and development. The answers provided stem from the literature in part but also the combined clinical experiences of transplant centers that over time have moved toward decreased limitations and full social integration.

REFERENCES

1. Klein MS, Martin K. Organ transplantation. In: Allen PJackson, Vessey JA, Shapiro NA, editors. Primary care of the child with a chronic condition. 5th edition. St Louis (MO): Mosby Elsevier; 2010. p. 715–38.
2. Well CM, Rodgers S, Rubovits S. School re-entry of the pediatric heart transplant recipient. Pediatr Transplant 2006;10(8):928–33.
3. Selekman J, Vessey JA. School and the child with a chronic illness. In: Allen P-Jackson, Vessey JA, Shapiro NA, editors. Primary care of the child with a chronic condition. 5th edition. St Louis (MO): Mosby Elsevier; 2010. p. 42–59.

4. American Academy of Pediatrics Committee on Infectious Diseases. Red book: 2009 report of the Committee on Infectious Diseases. In: Pickering LK, editor. 28th edition. Elk Grove Village (IL): American Academy of Pediatrics; 2009.

5. International Transplant Nurses' Society. What you should know: diet and exercise after transplant. Available at: http://www.itns.org/ITNS_transplant_educational_materials.php. Accessed October 30, 2009.

6. Addenbrooke's Hospital NHA. Physical activity after renal transplant. Available at: http://www.cambridge-transplant.org.uk/program/renal/physical.htm. Accessed October 30, 2009.

7. Singh TP, Gauvreau K, Rhodes J, et al. Longitudinal changes in heart rate recovery after maximal exercise in pediatric heart transplant recipients: evidence of autonomic re-innervation? J Heart Lung Transplant 2007;26(12):1306–12.

8. Chan JC. Post-transplant metabolic bone complications and optimization of treatment. Pediatr Transplant 2007;11(4):349–53.

9. World Transplant Games Federation. Available at: http://www.wtgf.org/. Accessed November 1, 2009.

10. Wray J, Lunnon-Wood T. Psychological benefits for children and adolescents who have undergone transplantation of the heart from participation in the British Transplant Games. Cardiol Young 2008;18(12):185–8.

11. Taketomo CK, Hodding JH, Kraus DM, editors. Pediatric dosage handbook. 14th edition. Hudson (OH): Lexicomp; 2007.

12. Good 2 go transition program. Help them grow so they're good 2 go. Available at: www.sickkids.ca/good2go. Accessed November 12, 2009.

13. National Advisory Committee on Immunization. Canadian immunization guide. 7th edition. Ottawa (Canada): Public Health Agency of Canada; 2006.

14. Verma A, Wade J. Immunization issues before and after solid organ transplantation in children. Pediatr Transplant 2006;10:536–48.

15. American Society of Transplantation. Guidelines for vaccination of solid organ transplant candidates and recipients. Available at: http://www.a-s-t.org/files/pdf/mobile/Vaccinations.pdf. Accessed November 15, 2009.

16. Dodd D, Burger J, Edwards K, et al. Varicella in a pedatric heart transplant population on nonsteroid maintenance immunosuppression. Pediatrics 2001;108(5):80–4.

17. Broliden K. Parvovirus B19 infection in pediatric solid-organ and bone marrow transplantation. Pediatr Transplant 2001;5:320–30.

18. Chisaka H, Morita E, Yaegashi N, et al. Parvovirus B19 and the pathogenesis of anemia. Rev Med Virol 2003;13:347–59.

19. National Institute of Dental and Craniofacilar Research. Dental management of the organ transplant patient. Available at: www.nidcr.nih.gov. Accessed November 2, 2009.

20. Hurst P. Dental issues before and after organ transplantation. In: Stuart FP, Abecassis MM, Kaufman DB, editors. Organ transplantation. Georgetown (TX): Landes Bioscience; 2000. p. 517–22.

21. Guggenheimer J, Eghtesad B, Stock DJ. Dental management of the solid organ transplant patient. Oral Surg Oral Med Oral Pathol Oral Radiol Endod 2003;95:383–9.

22. Wilson W, Taubert K, Gerwitz M, et al. Prevention of infective endocarditis: guidelines from the American Heart Association: a guideline from the American Heart Association Rheumatic Fever, Endocarditis, and Kawasaki Disease Committee, Council on Cardiovascular Disease in the Young, and the Council on Clinical

Cardiology, Council on Cardiovascular Surgery and Anesthesia, and the Quality of Care and Outcomes Research Interdisciplinary Working Group. Circulation 2007;116:1736–54.

23. Health Canada. Canada's food guide. Available at: http://www.hc-sc.gc.ca/fn-an/food-guide-aliment/index-eng.php; 2007. Accessed October 30, 2009.

24. Department of Health and Human Services and Department of Agriculture. Dietary guidelines for Americans 2005. Available at: http://www.healthierus.gov/dietaryguidelines/; 2006. Accessed October 30, 2009.

25. Mertens-Talcott SU, Zadezensky I, De Castro WV, et al. Grapefruit-drug interactions: can interactions with drugs be avoided? J Clin Pharmacol 2006;46(12): 1390–416.

26. Mank MP, Davies M. Examining low bacterial dietary practice: a survey on low bacterial food. Eur J Oncol Nurs 2008;12(4):342–8.

27. Hemsworth S, Pizer B. Pet ownership in immunocompromised children. A review of the literature and survey of existing guidelines. Eur J Oncol Nurs 2006;10(2): 117–27.

28. Colins MH, Montone KT, Leahey A, et al. Post-transplant lymphoproliferative disease in children. Pediatr Transplant 2001;5:250–7.

29. Toyoda M, Moudgil A, Bradley A, et al. Clinical significance of peripheral blood Epstein-Barr viral load monitoring using polymerase chain reaction in renal transplant recipients. Pediatr Transplant 2008;12:778–84.

30. Webber S, Green M. Post-transplant lymphoproliferative disorders and malignancy. In: Fine R, Webber S, Olthoff K, et al, editors. Pediatric solid organ transplantation. 2nd edition. Philadelphia: Blackwell Publishing; 2007. p. 114–23.

31. Stitt N, Barone M, Castellese M, et al. Transplant complications: noninfectious diseases. In: Ohler L, Cupples S, editors. Core curriculum for transplant nurses. St Louis (MO): Mosby Elsevier; 2008. p. 201–63.

32. Vessey JA, Sullivan BJ. Chronic conditions and child development. In: Allen PJackson, Vessey JA, Shapiro NA, editors. Primary care of the child with a chronic condition. 5th edition. St Louis (MO): Mosby Elsevier; 2010. p. 22–41.

33. Fuqua JS. Growth after organ transplantation. Semin Pediatr Surg 2006;15: 162–9.

34. Alonso EM, Sheperd R, Martz KL, et al. Linear growth patterns in prepubertal children following liver transplantation. Am J Transplant 2009;9:1389–97.

35. Vasudevan A, Phadke K. Growth in pediatric renal transplant recipients. Pediatr Transplant 2007;39:753–5.

36. Peterson RE, Perens GS, Alejos JC, et al. Growth and weight gain of prepubertal children after cardiac transplantation. Pediatr Transplant 2008;12:436–41.

37. Alonso EM, Sorensen LG. Cognitive development following pediatric solid organ transplantation. Curr Opin Organ Transplant 2009;4(5):522–5.

38. DeMaso D, Kelley SD, Bastardi H, et al. The longitudinal impact of psychological functioning, medical severity, and family functioning in pediatric heart transplantation. J Heart Lung Transplant 2004;23:473–80.

39. Chinnock RE, Freier C, Ashwal S, et al. Developmental outcomes after pediatric heart transplantation. J Heart Lung Transplant 2008;27:1079–84.

40. Wray J, Radley-Smith R. Beyond the first year after pediatric heart or heart-lung transplantation: changes in cognitive function and behavior. Pediatr Transplant 2005;9:170–7.

41. Ng LV, Fecteau A, Sheperd R, et al. Outcomes of 5 year survivors of pediatric liver transplantation: report on 461 children from a North American multicenter registry. Pediatrics 2008;122:e1128–35.

42. Ferraresso M, Ghio L, Raiteri M, et al. Pediatric kidney transplantation: a snapshot 10 years later. Transplant Proc 2008;40:1852–3.
43. Zaenglem AL, Thiboutot DM. Expert recommendations for acne management. Pediatrics 2006;118:1188–99.
44. International Transplant Nurses' Society. What you should know: pregnancy and parenthood after transplant: things you should know. Available at: http://www.itns.org/ITNS_transplant_educational_materials.php. Accessed November 1, 2009.
45. Armenti VT, et al. Report from the National Transplantation Pregnancy Registry (NTPR): outcomes of pregnancy after transplantation. Clin Transplant 2005;69–83.
46. Wielgos M, Pietrzak B, Bobrowska K, et al. Pregnancy after organ transplantation. Neuroendocrinol Lett 2009;30(1):6–10.
47. Betz C. To tattoo or not: that is the question. Pediatr Nurs 2009;24(4):241–3.
48. Centers for Disease Control and Prevention. Body art. Retrieved November 12, 2009. Available at: http://www.cdc.gov/niosh/topics/bbp/bodyart/; 2008. Accessed November 2, 2009.
49. Bell LE, Bartosh SM, Davis CL, et al. Adolescent transition to adult are in solid organ transplantation: a consensus conference report. Am J Transplant 2008;8:2230–42.
50. Little JW, Lawrence RL, Zwanfer L, editors. Extending medicare coverage of the medically compromised patient. 6th edition. St Louis (MO): Mosby, Inc; 2002. p. 501–25.

Index

Note: Page numbers of article titles are in **boldface** type.

Moving?

Make sure your subscription moves with you!

To notify us of your new address, find your **Clinics Account Number** (located on your mailing label above your name), and contact customer service at:

Email: journalscustomerservice-usa@elsevier.com

800-654-2452 (subscribers in the U.S. & Canada)
314-447-8871 (subscribers outside of the U.S. & Canada)

Fax number: 314-447-8029

Elsevier Health Sciences Division
Subscription Customer Service
3251 Riverport Lane
Maryland Heights, MO 63043

*To ensure uninterrupted delivery of your subscription, please notify us at least 4 weeks in advance of move.

ELSEVIER

Printed and bound by CPI Group (UK) Ltd, Croydon, CR0 4YY

08/06/2025

01896875-0004